TAKING SIDES

Clashing Views on

Bioethical Issues

FIFTEENTH EDITION

Selected, Edited, and with Introductions by

Gregory E. Kaebnick
The Hastings Center

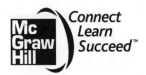

Mc Graw Hill

Connect
Learn
Succeed™

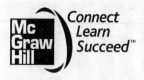

Connect
Learn
Succeed™

TAKING SIDES: CLASHING VIEWS ON BIOETHICAL ISSUES, FIFTEENTH EDITION

1 2 3 4 5 6 7 8 9 0 DOC/DOC 1 0 9 8 7 6 5 4 3

MHID: 0-07-813949-X
ISBN: 978-0-07-813949-9
ISSN: 1091-8809

Acquisitions Editor: *Joan L. McNamara*
Marketing Director: *Adam Kloza*
Marketing Manager: *Nathan Edwards*
Developmental Editor: *Dave Welsh*
Lead Project Manager: *Jane Mohr*
Buyer: *Jennifer Pickel*
Cover Designer: *Studio Montage, St. Louis, MO.*
Cover Image: *CDC/Greg Knobloch*
Content License Specialist: *DeAnna Dausener*
Media Project Manager: *Sridevi Palani*

Compositor: MPS Limited

www.mhhe.com

Editors/Academic Advisory Board

Members of the Academic Advisory Board are instrumental in the final selection of articles for each edition of TAKING SIDES. Their review of articles for content, level, and appropriateness provides critical direction to the editors and staff. We think that you will find their careful consideration well reflected in this volume.

TAKING SIDES: Clashing Views on BIOETHICAL ISSUES
Fifteenth Edition

EDITOR
Gregory E. Kaebnick
The Hastings Center

ACADEMIC ADVISORY BOARD MEMBERS

Editors/Academic Advisory Board continued

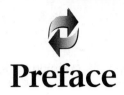

Preface

T his is a book about choices—hard and tragic choices. The choices are hard not only because they often involve life and death but also because there are convincing arguments on both sides of the issues. An ethical dilemma, by definition, is one that poses a conflict not between good and evil but between one good principle and another that is equally good. The choices are hard because the decisions that are made—by individuals, groups, and public policymakers—will influence the kind of society we have today and the one we will have in the future.

Although many of the views expressed in the selections in this volume are strong—even passionate—they are also subtle, concerned with the nuances of the particular debate. How one argues matters in bioethics; you will see and have to weigh the significance of varying rhetorical styles and appeals throughout this volume.

Although there are no easy answers to any of the issues in the book, the questions will be answered in some fashion—partly by individual choices and partly by decisions that are made by professionals and government. We must make them the best answers possible, and that can only be done by informed and thoughtful consideration. This book, then, can serve as a beginning for what ideally will become an ongoing process of examination and reflection.

In approaching each new edition, the editor also must make some hard choices. In trying to keep the selections up to date, sometimes older ones must be replaced. In other instances, newer articles are just that—newer, but not necessarily better. Striking a balance between timeliness and timelessness is challenging. For each issue, additional points of view are noted in the follow-up section titled "Exploring the Issue," and readers are encouraged to pursue these references.

Changes to this edition   Many popular issues and the basic structure of the book remain from the previous edition. There are now six units: Medical Decision Making; End-of-Life Dilemmas; Choices in Reproduction; Professional Integrity; The Development and Use of Biotechnology; and Access to Health Care. The issues have been reorganized to fit this structure. There are three completely new issues: "May Surrogate Decision Makers Terminate Care for a Person in a Persistent Vegetative State?" (issue 2); "Should Fertility Doctors Be Allowed to Transfer Multiple Embryos into a Woman Who Wants to Be Pregnant?" (issue 8); and "Should Physicians Be Allowed to Participate in Executions?" (issue 10). Also, issue 17 ("Is There an Ethical Duty to Provide Health Care for All Immigrants to the United States?") appeared only in the expanded version of edition 14, and both selections for issue 16 ("Is an Individual Mandate to Purchase Health Insurance Fair?") are new. There are new YES selections in issue 9 ("Should a Pregnant Woman Be Punished for Exposing Her Fetus to Risk?"), issue 12 ("Is the Use of Medical Tools to Enhance Human Beings Morally Troubling?"), issue 15 ("Should Scientists Create

Artificial Organisms?"), and issue 19 ("Should Vaccination for HPV Be Mandated for Teenage Girls?"). In all there are 14 new selections. Unit introductions, issue introductions, and postscripts have been updated as necessary.

A word to the instructor   An *Instructor's Resource Guide with Test Questions* (multiple choice and essay) is available through the publisher, and a general guide book, *Using Taking Sides in the Classroom*, which discusses methods and techniques for using the pro–con approach in any classroom setting, is also available. An online version of *Using Taking Sides in the Classroom* and a correspondence service for *Taking Sides* adopters can be found at www.mhhe.com/cls/usingts/.

   Taking Sides: Clashing Views on Bioethical Issues is only one title in the *Taking Sides* series. If you are interested in seeing the table of contents for any of the other titles, please visit the *Taking Sides* website at http://www.mhhe.com/cls/takingsides/.

   The current edition owes very much to the work of Carol Levine, who was editor of this title up through the 14th edition. I am indebted to Carol both for her excellent work and for encouraging me to take over the project. I am also indebted to Thomas H. Murray, Daniel Callahan, and Nancy Berlinger, as well as to several members of the Academic Advisory Board, for their comments and suggestions on various portions of the book.

Gregory E. Kaebnick
The Hastings Center

For Hannah, Rebecca, and Gwen

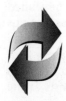

The Educational Experience of Disciplinary Controversy*

BRENT D. SLIFE
Brigham Young University

As a long-time user of the *Taking Sides* books, I have seen first-hand their educational impact on students. A student we will call "Brittany" is a prime example. Until her role in a *Taking Sides* panel discussion, she had not participated once in class discussions. It is probably fair to say that she was sleepwalking through the course. However, once she was assigned to a "side" of the panel discussion, she vigorously pitched in "to do battle," as she put it, with the opposing team. She described a "kind of energy" as she and the rest of her team prepared for the upcoming debate. In fact, she found herself and her teammates "talking trash" good-naturedly with the opposing team before the actual discussion, despite her usual reserve. Because she wanted to win, she "drilled down" and even did extra research.

The panel discussion itself, she reported, was exhilarating, but what I noticed afterward was probably the most intriguing. Not only did she participate in class more frequently, taking more risks in class discussions because she knew her teammates would support her, she also found herself having a position from which to see other positions in the discipline. Somehow, as she explained, her advocating a particular position on the panel, even though she knew I had arbitrarily assigned it, gave her a stake in other discussions and a perspective from which to contribute to them. Brittany's experience nicely illustrates the unique educational impact of the *Taking Sides* series.

Taking Sides is designed quite intentionally to shore up some of the weaknesses of many contemporary educational settings. The unique energy that Brittany experienced is a result of *Taking Sides'* specific focus on the controversial side of academic disciplines. For several good reasons, instructors and textbooks have traditionally focused almost exclusively on the more factual or settled aspects of their disciplines. This focus has led, in turn, to educational strategies that can rob the subject matter of its vitality.

Taking Sides, on the other hand, is uniquely structured to highlight the more issue-oriented aspects of a discipline, allowing students to care about and even invest in the subject matter as did Brittany. Involvement can spur a deeper understanding of the topic and help students to appreciate how knowledge advancement is sometimes driven by passionate positions.

---

*The full text of this essay and references are available online at: http://highered
.mcgraw-hill.com/sites/0076667771/information_center_view0/

Including the Controversial

A case could be made that a complete understanding of any discipline includes its controversies. Controversies may not be considered "knowledge" per se, depending on the discipline, but there is surely no doubt that they are part of the process of advancing knowledge. The conflicts generated among disciplinary leaders often produce problem-solving energy, if not disciplinary passions. In fact, they can drive entire disciplinary conferences and whole programs of investigation. In this sense, disciplinary controversies are not just "error" or an indication of the absence of knowledge; they can be viewed as a positive part of the discipline, a generator of disciplinary vigor if not purpose.

If this is true, then de-emphasizing the controversial elements of a discipline is de-emphasizing a vital part of the discipline itself. Students may learn accepted aspects of the discipline, but they may not learn, at least directly, the disputed aspects. This de-emphasis may not only produce an incomplete or inaccurate sense of the discipline, but it may also mislead the student to understand the field as more sterile, less emotional, and less "messy" than it truly is. The more rational, factual side is clearly important, perhaps even more important. The question, however, is: Do these more settled and perhaps rational aspects of the discipline have to monopolize courses for beginning students?

Another way to put the question might be: Couldn't some portion of the course be devoted to the more controversial, thus allowing the student to engage the field in a more emotional manner? In some sense, the more settled and accepted the information is, the less students can feel they are truly participating in the disciplinary enterprise. After all, this information is already decided; there is no room for involvement in developing and "owning" the information. Students may even assume they will be punished for challenging the disciplinary status quo.

Specific Educational Benefits

Engaging the Discipline. When controversy is placed in the foreground of an educational experience, it gives disciplinary novices (students) permission to participate in and perhaps even form their own positions on some of the issues in the field. After all, some issues have not been addressed; some problems have not been solved. As Brittany put it, she was ready to "do battle" with the alternative position, even though she was quite aware of the arbitrariness of her own positional assignment. She was aware that something was at stake; something was to be decided.

In other words, it is the very *lack* of resolution in a controversy that invites students to make sense of the issues themselves and perhaps even venture their own thoughts. Obviously, students should be encouraged to be humble about these positions, understanding that their perspective is fledgling, but even novice positions can facilitate greater engagement with the materials. In a sense, the controversy, and thus a vital part of the discipline, becomes their own, as the example of Brittany illustrates. She not only "owned" a disciplinary position, she used it as a conceptual bridge to engage other settled and unsettled aspects of the discipline.

Appreciating the Messy. Students can also experience the messiness of disciplines using *Taking Sides.* I use the term "messiness" because conventional texts are notorious for representing the field too neatly and too logically, as if there were no human involvement. If disciplines are more than their settled aspects, there are also unsettled elements, including poorly defined terms and inadequately understood concepts, which also need to be appreciated. This messiness is what led Brittany to "drill down" and do "extra research" in her preparation for her panel discussion. She knew that some of the basic terms and understandings were at play.

Good conventional texts may attempt to include these unsettled aspects, but they typically do so in a deceptively logical fashion, as though the controversy is solely rational. This presentation may not only distort these aspects of the discipline but also deliver merely a secondhand report. By contrast, *Taking Sides* books—in pitting two authors against one another—facilitate an *experience* with actual published authorities, who are struggling with the issues from completely different perspectives. In reading both articles, students cannot help but struggle *with* the authors. They do not need to be *told* that the terms of the debate are problematic; the students *experience* these terms as problematic when they attempt to understand what is at stake in the authors' positions.

Preventing Premature Closure. The *Taking Sides* structure also serves to prevent students from prematurely closing controversies. Premature closure can occur by underestimating the controversy's depth or deciding it without a proper appreciation for the issues involved. *Taking Sides* prevents this prematurity by helping the student to experience how two reasonable and highly educated people can so thoroughly disagree. In other words, premature closure is discouraged because real experts are countering each other, sometimes point by point.

A student would almost have to ignore one side of the controversy, one of the experts, to prematurely close the issue. Brittany, for example, reported that she became "absolutely convinced" of the validity of the first authors' position, only to have the second reading put this position into question! Obviously, if the issue could be closed or settled so easily, presumably the experts or leaders of the discipline would have done so already. Controversies are controversies because they are *deeply* problematic, so it is important for the student to appreciate this, and thus have a more profound understanding of the disciplinary meanings involved.

Rehabilitating the Dialectic. One of the truly unique benefits of the *Taking Sides* experience is its rehabilitation of the age-old educational tradition of the dialectic. Since at least the time of Socrates, educators have understood that a *full* understanding of any disciplinary meaning, explanation, or bit of information requires not only knowing what this meaning or information is but also knowing what it isn't. The dialectic, in this sense, is the educational relation of a concept to its alternative (see Rychlak, 2003). As dialectician Joseph Rychlak (1991) explains, all meanings "reach beyond themselves" and are thus clarified and have implications beyond their synonyms. It may be trivial to note, for example, that one cannot fully comprehend what "up" means without understanding what "down" means. However, this dialectic is not trivial when the meanings are disciplinary, such as when the political science student realizes that justice is incomprehensible without some apprehension of the meaning of injustice.

One of the more fascinating educational moments, when using *Taking Sides* books, occurs when students recognize that they cannot properly understand even one side of the controversy without taking into account another side. Brittany described learning very quickly that she clarified and even became aware of important aspects of her own position only *after* she understood the alternative to her position. This dialectical awareness is also pivotal to truly critical thinking.

Facilitating Critical Thinking. I say "truly" critical thinking because critical thinking has sometimes been confused with rigorous thinking (see Slife et al., 2005). Rigorous thinking is the application of rigorous reasoning or analytical thinking to a particular problem, which is surely an important skill in most any field. Still, it is not truly *critical* thinking until one has an alternative perspective from which to criticize a perspective. Recall that Brittany did not participate in class until she developed a perspective to view other perspectives. In other words, one must have a (critical) perspective "outside of" or alternative to the perspective being critiqued. Otherwise, one is "inside" the perspective being critiqued and cannot "see" it as a whole.

As many recent educational formulations of critical thinking attest, this approach means that critical thinkers should develop at least a dialectic of perspectives (one plus an alternative). That is to say, they should have an awareness of their own perspective as *facilitated* by an understanding of at least one alternative perspective. Without an alternative, students assume either they have no position or their position is the *only* one possible. A point of comparison, on the other hand, prevents the reification of one's perspective and allows students to have a perspective on their perspectives. A clear strength of the *Taking Sides'* juxtaposition of alternative perspectives is that it facilitates this kind of critical thinking.

These five benefits—engaging the discipline, appreciating the messy, preventing premature closure, rehabilitating the dialectic, and facilitating critical thinking—are probably not exclusive to controversy. However, they are, I would contend, a relatively unique *package* of educational advantages that students can gain with the inclusion of a *Taking Sides* approach in the classroom. Controversy, of course, is rarely helpful on its own; settled information and sound reasoning must buttress and perhaps even ground controversy. Otherwise, it is more heat than light. Even so, an *exclusive* focus on the settled and more cognitive aspects can deprive students of the vitality of a discipline and prevent the ownership of information that is so important to real learning.

Contents In Brief

xi

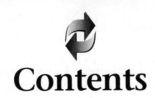

Contents

UNIT 1   MEDICAL DECISION MAKING   1

Issue 1.   Is Autonomy Still Central to Medical Ethics?   2

YES: Robert M. Arnold and Charles W. Lidz, from "Informed Consent: Clinical Aspects of Consent in Health Care," in Stephen G. Post, ed., *Encyclopedia of Bioethics,* vol. 3, 3rd ed. (Macmillan, 2003)   *5*

NO: Onora O'Neill, from *Autonomy and Trust in Bioethics?* (Cambridge University Press, 2002)   *16*

Physician Robert M. Arnold and professor of psychiatry and sociology Charles W. Lidz assert that informed consent in clinical care is an essential process that promotes good communication and patient autonomy despite the obstacles of implementation. Philosopher Onora O'Neill argues that the most evident change in medical practice in recent decades may be a loss of trust in physicians rather than any growth of patient autonomy. Informed consent in practice, she says, often amounts simply to a right to choose or refuse treatments, not a deeper and more meaningful expression of self-mastery.

Issue 2.   May Surrogate Decision Makers Terminate Care for a Person in a Persistent Vegetative State?   24

YES: Jay Wolfson, from *A Report to Governor Jeb Bush and the 6th Judicial Circuit in the Matter of Theresa Marie Schiavo* (December 2003)   *27*

NO: Tom Koch, from "The Challenge of Terri Schiavo: Lessons for Bioethics," *Journal of Medical Ethics* (2005)   *36*

Jay Wolfson, a lawyer and the special guardian ad litem appointed for Theresa Marie Schiavo, explains the clinical and legal considerations that justified removal of Ms. Schiavo's feeding tube, causing her to die. Tom Koch, an independent writer and researcher, holds that helping a person die cannot be said to benefit the person and that questions of personhood and sanctity of life gave reason to help her live.

Issue 3.   Should Adolescents Be Allowed to Make Their Own Life-and-Death Decisions?   43

YES: Robert F. Weir and Charles Peters, from "Affirming the Decisions Adolescents Make About Life and Death," *Hastings Center Report* (November–December 1997)   *45*

Ethicist Robert F. Weir and pediatrician Charles Peters assert that
adolescents with normal cognitive and developmental skills have the
capacity to make decisions about their own health care. Advance
directives, if used appropriately, can give older pediatric patients a voice
in their care. Pediatrician Lainie Friedman Ross counters that parents
should be responsible for making their child's health care decisions. Children need to develop virtues, such as self-control, that will enhance their
long-term, not just immediate, autonomy.

UNIT 2   END-OF-LIFE DILEMMAS   61

Psychologist Angela Fagerlin and law professor Carl E. Schneider believe
not only that living wills have failed to live up to their advocates' expectations
but also that these expectations were unrealistic from the start. Susan E.
Hickman, Bernard J. Hammes, Alvin H. Moss, and Susan W. Tolle,
multidisciplinary specialists in end-of-life care, recognize the limitations of
traditional advance directives but argue that newer processes of
introducing advance directives can achieve their original aims.

The American Medical Association affirms that in cases of extreme
suffering the physician's duty to relieve pain and suffering includes
palliative sedation—using drugs that result in unconsciousness and may
hasten death. Philosopher Margaret P. Battin believes that palliative or
terminal sedation is an unsatisfying compromise that offers no greater
protection against abuse than do institutional safeguards established for
direct physician aid in dying.

Physician Marcia Angell asserts that a physician's main duties are to respect patient autonomy and to relieve suffering, even if that sometimes means assisting in a patient's death. Physician Kathleen M. Foley counters that if physician-assisted suicide becomes legal, it will begin to substitute for interventions that otherwise might enhance the quality of life for dying patients.

UNIT 3   CHOICES IN REPRODUCTION   135

Philosopher Patrick Lee and professor of jurisprudence Robert P. George assert that human embryos and fetuses are complete (though immature) human beings and that intentional abortion is unjust and objectively immoral. Philosopher Margaret Olivia Little believes that the moral status of the fetus is only one aspect of the morality of abortion. She points to gestation as an intimacy, motherhood as a relationship, and creation as a process to advance a more nuanced approach.

Professor of medicine David Orentlicher argues that the practice of transferring multiple embryos to a woman's uterus, which came to public attention with the case of Nadya Suleman in 2009, is dangerous for both children and mothers and should be discouraged by federal policy. Lawyer John A. Robertson holds that professional guidelines on embryo transfer are enough, and that hard and fast legal limits on embryo transfer would be seen as violating parents' rights.

Liles Burke sets out the majority opinion of the Alabama Court of Criminal Appeals in a case involving a pregnant woman who was found to have used cocaine while pregnant. Burke argues that Alabama law that forbids adults from exposing children to controlled substances applies in cases involving pregnant women and their fetuses. Attorney Lynn M. Paltrow argues that treating drug-using pregnant women as criminals targets poor, African American women while ignoring other drug usage and fails to provide the resources to assist them in recovery.

UNIT 4   PROFESSIONAL INTEGRITY   193

Issue 10.   Should Physicians Be Allowed to Participate in Executions?   194

David Waisel, a professor of medicine, argues that if the state is to administer capital punishment, then physicians may honorably seek to help the condemned die as painlessly as possible. Physician and journalist Atul Gawande supports capital punishment but believes physicians, as healers, should play no role in it.

Issue 11.   Should Pharmacists Be Allowed to Deny Prescriptions on Grounds of Conscience?   225

Law student Donald W. Herbe asserts that pharmacists' moral beliefs concerning abortion and emergency contraception are genuinely fundamental and deserve respect. He proposes that professional pharmaceutical organizations lead the way to recognizing a true right of conscience, which would eventually result in universal legislation protecting against all potential ramifications of choosing conscience. Julie Cantor, a lawyer, and Ken Baum, a physician and lawyer, reject an absolute right to object, as well as no right to object, to these prescriptions but assert that pharmacists who cannot or will not dispense a drug have a professional obligation to meet the needs of their customers by referring them elsewhere.

UNIT 5   THE DEVELOPMENT AND USE OF BIOTECHNOLOGY   247

The President's Council on Bioethics, a presidential body formed by President Bush, argues that biotechnological interventions for making people better than normal raise profound concerns about the relationship between humans and nature, human identity, and human happiness. Physician Howard Trachtman says that the medical community should embrace enhancement as a never-ending quest for health that recognizes that perfection can never be achieved.

Social psychologist Thomas H. Murray contends that the ban on performance-enhancing drugs should continue because it furthers the true meaning of sports—which is to compare athletes on their natural talent and abilities. Philosopher Julian Savulescu and research colleagues Bennett Foddy and Megan Clayton argue that legalizing drugs in sport may be fairer and safer than banning them.

Nurse Sarah E. Shannon believes that ethically and legally parents have the right and duty to make decisions and to care for their family members who are unable to do so themselves and that we should not abandon parents of severely developmentally disabled children to the harsh social and economic realities that are barriers to good care. Nurse Teresa A. Savage believes that children like Ashley should have independent advocates, preferably persons with disabilities, to weigh the risks and benefits of proposed interventions.

Philosopher Mark A. Bedau argues that the effort to "create life"—the goal
of the field known as synthetic biology—would be both socially useful and
a huge step forward in the quest to understand what life is. Christopher J.
Preston, an environmental ethicist, warns that synthetic biology is a threat
to the concept of "natural" that has guided moral thinking about the
environment in North America.

UNIT 6   ACCESS TO HEALTH CARE   311

Karen Davenport, a health policy analyst, argues that an individual
mandate to purchase health insurance emphasizes conservative ideals of
personal responsibility and is necessary to ensure that health care is
available and affordable for all citizens. Michael F. Cannon, also a health
policy analyst, argues that it will promote irresponsibility, restrict personal
freedom, increase the cost of health care, and lead ultimately to
government rationing.

Rajeev Raghavan and Ricardo Nuila, physicians who work with end-
stage renal disease patients, argue that standardized coverage for dialysis
treatments would alleviate the burden on taxpayers where the most
undocumented residents live and would improve these patients' health,
allowing them to return to work. James Dwyer, a philosopher and
bioethicist, looks at another response to treatments for immigrants—
deporting them. While he opposes deportation, he asserts that placing
the financial responsibility on individual hospitals or regions is unfair.

Physician Emil J. Freireich believes that patients with advanced cancer and limited life expectancy should have the same privilege as all individuals in a free society. Law professor George J. Annas argues that there is no constitutional right to demand experimental interventions, and that fully open access would undermine the FDA's ability to protect the public from unsafe drugs.

Law professor R. Alta Charo argues that vaccination against the human papillomavirus, which causes most cases of cervical cancer, should be mandatory except in cases of medical, religious, or philosophical objection. Law professors Gail Javitt and Lawrence O. Gostin and physician Deena Berkowitz believe that, given the limited data and experience, and the fact that HPV does not pose imminent and significant risk to others, mandating HPV vaccine is premature.

Psychiatrist Sally Satel contends that a regulated and legal system of rewarding organ donors will not only save lives but also stop the illegal trafficking that offers no protections for poor people around the world. The Institute of Medicine Committee on Increasing Rates of Organ Donation argues that a free market in organs is problematic because in live organ donation, both buyers and sellers may not have complete or accurate information, and selling organs of dead people raises concerns about commodification of human bodies.

Correlation Guide

The *Taking Sides* series presents current issues in a debate-style format designed to stimulate student interest and develop critical thinking skills: Each issue is thoughtfully framed with an issue summary, an issue introduction, and a post-script. The pro and con essays—selected for their liveliness and substance—represent the arguments of leading scholars and commentators in their fields.

Taking Sides: Clashing Views on Bioethical Issues, 15/e is an easy-to-use reader that presents issues on important topics such as *Advance Directives, Palliative Sedation,* and *Synthetic Biology*: For more information on *Taking Sides* and other *McGraw-Hill Contemporary Learning Series* titles, visit www:mhhe:com/cls.

This convenient guide matches the issues in **Taking Sides: Clashing Views on Bioethical Issues, 15/e,** with the corresponding chapters in two of our best-selling McGraw-Hill Ethics textbooks by DeGrazia et al. and Steinbock et al.

Taking Sides: Bioethical Issues, 15/e	Biomedical Ethics, 7/e by DeGrazia et al.	Ethical Issues in Modern Medicine: Contemporary Readings in Bioethics, 8/e by Steinbock et al.
Issue 1: Is Autonomy Still Central to Medical Ethics?	**Chapter 1:** General Introduction	**Part One, Section 2:** Informed Consent and Truth Telling
Issue 2: May Surrogate Decision Makers Terminate Care for a Person in a Persistent Vegetative State?	**Chapter 2:** The Professional-Patient Relationship	**Part One, Section 2:** Informed Consent and Truth Telling
Issue 3: Should Adolescents Be Allowed to Make Their Own Life-and-Death Decisions?	**Chapter 5:** Death and Decisions Regarding Life-Sustaining Treatment	**Part One, Section 2:** Informed Consent and Truth Telling
Issue 4: Have Advance Directives Failed?	**Chapter 5:** Death and Decisions Regarding Life-Sustaining Treatment	**Part Three, Section 1:** Decisional Capacity and the Right to Refuse Treatment **Part Three, Section 2:** Advance Directives **Part Three, Section 3:** Choosing for Once-Competent Patients **Part Three, Section 4:** Choosing for Never-Competent Patients
Issue 5: Is "Palliative Sedation" Ethically Different from Active Euthanasia?	**Chapter 6:** Suicide, Physician-Assisted Suicide, and Active Euthanasia	**Part Four, Section 5:** Physician-Assisted Death
Issue 6: Should Physicians Be Allowed to Assist in Patient Suicide?	**Chapter 2:** The Professional-Patient Relationship **Chapter 6:** Suicide, Physician-Assisted Suicide, and Active Euthanasia	**Part Four, Section 5:** Physician-Assisted Death

Taking Sides: Bioethical Issues, 15/e	Biomedical Ethics, 7/e by DeGrazia et al.	Ethical Issues in Modern Medicine: Contemporary Readings in Bioethics, 8/e by Steinbock et al.
Issue 7: Is Abortion Immoral?	**Chapter 7:** Abortion and Embryonic Stem-Cell Research	**Part Four, Section 2:** The Morality of Abortion
Issue 8: Should There Be Legal Limits on How Many Embryos Can Be Transferred into a Woman Who Wants to Be Pregnant?	**Chapter 8:** Genetics and Human Reproduction **Chapter 9:** Social Justice and Health-Care Policy	**Part Five, Section 1:** Procreative Responsibility
Issue 9: Should a Pregnant Woman Be Punished for Exposing Her Fetus to Risk?	**Chapter 2:** The Professional-Patient Relationship	
Issue 10: Should Physicians Be Allowed to Participate in Executions?	**Chapter 2:** The Professional-Patient Relationship	
Issue 11: Should Pharmacists Be Allowed to Deny Prescriptions on Grounds of Conscience?	**Chapter 3:** Contested Therapies and Biomedical Enhancement	**Part Seven, Section 2:** Enhancing Humans and Remaking Nature
Issue 12: Is the Use of Medical Tools to Enhance Human Beings Morally Troubling?	**Chapter 1:** General Introduction	
Issue 13: Should Performance-Enhancing Drugs Be Banned from Sports?	**Chapter 3:** Contested Therapies and Biomedical Enhancement	**Part Seven, Section 2:** Enhancing Humans and Remaking Nature
Issue 14: May Doctors Offer Medical Drugs and Surgery to Stop a Disabled Child from Maturing?	**Chapter 1:** General Introduction	**Part Six, Section 2:** The Ethics of Randomized Clinical Trials
Issue 15: Should Scientists Create Artificial Organisms?	**Chapter 13:** Contested Therapies and Biomedical Enhancement	**Part Seven, Section 2:** Enhancing Humans and Remaking Nature
Issue 16: Is an Individual Mandate to Purchase Health Insurance Fair?	**Chapter 9:** Social Justice and Health-Care Policy	**Part Two, Section 1:** Justice, Health, and Health Care
Issue 17: Is There an Ethical Duty to Provide Health Care for All Immigrants to the United States?	**Chapter 9:** Social Justice and Health-Care Policy	**Part Two, Section 1:** Justice, Health, and Health Care
Issue 18: Should New Drugs Be Given to Patients Outside Clinical Trials?	**Chapter 1:** General Introduction **Chapter 13:** Contested Therapies and Biomedical Enhancement	**Part One, Section 2:** Informed Consent and Truth Telling
Issue 19: Should Vaccination for HPV Be Mandated for Teenage Girls?	**Chapter 1:** General Introduction **Chapter 9:** Social Justice and Health-Care Policy	
Issue 20: Should There Be a Market in Human Organs?	**Chapter 9:** Social Justice and Health-Care Policy	**Part Two, Section 3:** Organ Transplantation: Gifts Versus Markets

Topic Guide

T his Topic Guide suggests how the selections in this book relate to the subjects covered in your course. You may want to use the topics listed on these pages to search the web more easily. On the following pages, a number of websites have been gathered specifically for this book. They are arranged to reflect the units of this *Taking Sides* reader. You can link to these sites by going to www.mhhe.com/cls.

All the articles that relate to each topic are listed below the bold-faced term.

Abortion

7. Is Abortion Immoral?

Advance Directives

4. Have Advance Directives Failed?

Alzheimer's Disease

14. May Doctors Offer Medical Drugs and Surgery to Stop a Disabled Child from Maturing?

Autonomy

1. Is Autonomy Still Central to Medical Ethics?
3. Should Adolescents Be Allowed to Make Their Own Life-and-Death Decisions?
4. Have Advance Directives Failed?
16. Is an Individual Mandate to Purchase Health Insurance Fair?

Capital Punishment

9. Should a Pregnant Woman Be Punished for Exposing Her Fetus to Risk?

Children and Adolescents

3. Should Adolescents Be Allowed to Make Their Own Life-and-Death Decisions?

Conscience

10. Should Physicians Be Allowed to Participate in Executions?

Dementia

14. May Doctors Offer Medical Drugs and Surgery to Stop a Disabled Child from Maturing?

Disability

13. Should Performance-Enhancing Drugs Be Banned from Sports?
14. May Doctors Offer Medical Drugs and Surgery to Stop a Disabled Child from Maturing?

Enhancement

11. Should Pharmacists Be Allowed to Deny Prescriptions on Grounds of Conscience?
12. Is the Use of Medical Tools to Enhance Human Beings Morally Troubling?

Health Insurance

16. Is an Individual Mandate to Purchase Health Insurance Fair?
17. Is There an Ethical Duty to Provide Health Care for All Immigrants to the United States?

Informed Consent

1. Is Autonomy Still Central to Medical Ethics?

Medical Research

18. Should New Drugs Be Given to Patients Outside Clinical Trials?

Organ Transplantation

20. Should There Be a Market in Human Organs?

Palliative Care

5. Is "Palliative Sedation" Ethically Different from Active Euthanasia?

Persistent Vegetative State

2. May Surrogate Decision Makers Terminate Care for a Person in a Persistent Vegetative State?

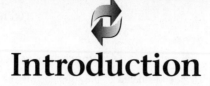

Introduction

Biology, Medicine, and Ethics

Gregory E. Kaebnick

The term "bioethics" is usually attributed to the biologist Van Rensselaer Potter, who proposed it in a book in 1971 as a way of creating a bridge between the "two cultures" that had been identified a dozen years earlier by the British novelist C.P. Snow. The "two cultures" are the sciences and the humanities, which Snow lamented were growing increasingly far apart from each other, to the point that they seemed no longer to share a language. Bioethics, then, was supposed to provide that language. Potter's idea was that the broad set of scientific disciplines that go under the heading of "the biological sciences" or "the life sciences" was the scientific outcrop on which the bridge could be built.

Too, they were particularly in need of input from the humanities. The period in which Potter was developing these thoughts was a fertile period for biology, with scientific insights and biotechnologies that suggested a change in the human relationship with the natural world and certainly began to change medical practice. One of the most dramatic of these developments was the avail-ability of kidney dialysis, which turned what had been a fatal diagnosis (kidney failure) into a potentially chronic condition. Because dialysis was exceedingly expensive and very scarce, not everybody who needed it could get it. In Seattle, as a 1962 story in *Life Magazine* explained to an amazed nation, a committee was formed to decide which patients would. The committee was making life-and-death decisions, of course, and it came to be known as the "God committee." In 1972, the national unease with these decisions led to a decision to provide coverage under Medicare for nearly any patient who needed it. Dialysis was not the only major new biomedical development in the 1960s and early 1970s, however. Organ transplantation became feasible thanks to the development of drugs to prevent the body's immune system from destroying a transplanted organ, the contraceptive pill was approved, and artificial respirators came into widespread use. Incrementally, doctors acquired tools that allowed them to actually help patients get well. Before antibiotics, of course, doctors mostly just presided over the sick.

Meanwhile, another revolution was also occurring on the other side of the bridge that bioethics was meant to be. The 1960s and 1970s were a period, famously, of intense cultural ferment, in which entrenched values were questioned and overturned. Authority and social inequality were widely challenged, and individual rights and social justice became prominent concerns both in popular culture and in academia, as illustrated in the civil rights movement, the protests against the Vietnam War, and Lyndon Johnson's Great Society. In medicine, the civil right movements generated a spin-off patients' rights movement, and the authority that had been granted physicians and the expectation of passivity from patients came under withering criticism. In health policy, a renewed effort was made to extend access to medical care, culminating in the creation of Medicaid in 1965.

In the late 1960s and early 1970s, bioethics emerged not just as a label but as the beginnings of a special area of scholarly research and writing. The Hastings Center, an independent research center known initially as the Institute for Society, Ethics, and the Life Sciences (later renamed after the town of Hastings-on-Hudson, New York, where it was originally located), and the Kennedy Institute of Ethics at Georgetown University launched this process. There is no one master discipline for bioethics: Instead, people come to it from many other disciplines—often from philosophy and from medicine, but also from other professions in the health sciences, from the law, from the social sciences, and from religion and literature among other disciplines in the humanities. Bioethics is seen as rigorously interdisciplinary— in this way, too, it is a kind of bridge. Today, it is possible to specialize in bioethics: A number of universities offer advanced degrees in bioethics, and some larger hospitals have "clinical ethicists" on staff, but even clinical ethicists usuallyhave primary training in some other field. The scholarly work conducted in bioethics— on human subjects research, public health, health care policy, and the development and use of biotechnologies, in addition to clinical care issues that range from child-bearing to end-of-life decisions—reflects many professional, political, and disciplinary viewpoints.

Bioethics and Moral Philosophy

Because bioethics incorporates many fields, there are many ways of approaching bioethical problems. The challenge of how to increase the number of organs available for transplantation not only involves moral problems but also lends itself to sociological and economic analysis, for example. One possible way of increasing the number of organs would be to create a market for them, so that patients or their families would have some perhaps modest financial incentive to make organs available. But then sociological and economic questions arise: What would be the effect on society? Would the market work? Similarly, the question of whether to offer patients experimental drugs only in the context of clinical trials involves, in addition to a debate about individual rights versus public safety, some legal and regulatory concerns.

Often, in bioethical debates, discussion focuses on the relevant facts. How many people are infected with HPV and with what consequences, and which interventions are likely to have what consequences for this public health problem? Underneath all bioethical debates, however, are questions about the relative significance and implications of various moral values or principles. Particularly important are debates about individual freedom and responsibility versus the public good, equity, and responsibility for others. Given these foundational concerns, bioethics is often said to be a subset of ethics generally—the application to an interesting set of cases, all of which have to do with the life sciences, of moral philosophy.

A common account of how bioethics fits into academia is therefore that it is one kind of "applied ethics" or "professional ethics" (alongside, e.g., environmental ethics, business ethics, and journalism ethics), which itself fits under the broader heading of "moral philosophy." The other branches of moral philosophy are "normative ethics," which examines and clarifies the basic standards that govern action and character, and "metaethics," which examines the ultimate justifications and meaning of morality—asking, for example, where the basic standards come from and whether an answer to a moral question can be described as "true" or "false." (These branches are not always distinct from each other, however, and a single discussion in moral philosophy may delve into all of them. A defense of a fundamental moral standard may have metaethical implications and may lead to a discussion of applications.)

Moral Theories

Because bioethics draws heavily on moral philosophy, and is indeed sometimes seen as a kind of subfield of moral philosophy, books that explore a range of bioethical debates often include an outline of the most widely discussed theories of morality in the Western philosophical canon. Just how moral theories can be legitimately used in moral deliberation is itself an interesting question, both for bioethics and for moral philosophy. It is a little odd, to say the least, to imagine a hospital ethicist who has been brought in to discuss a life-or-death decision launching into an explanation of what his chosen moral theory leads him to say. But even if moral theories are not invoked to reach specific judgments, they might still be useful in other ways. One might rely on general theories, for example, to reach mid-level moral rules—that lying is wrong, or that touching a person's body without that person's permission is wrong—that then lead to judgments in specific cases.

The oldest of the theoretic approaches that still has currency today is virtue theory, which has its roots in the writings of Aristotle. Virtue theory holds that the fundamental standards of morality are not standards of conduct, but standards of character. These standards, the virtues, are dispositions to behave in certain ways—to be honest, to be brave, and to be temperate. There is no one agreed-upon list of the virtues, nor can the virtues be articulated in such a way that one can develop an account of the virtues and straightforwardly deduce good judgments from that account. One must instead internalize these standards, through a process of long training. If one has gone through this process and acquired the virtues, then one will respond to new circumstances appropriately.

In bioethics, virtue theory has been used primarily to try to give an account of how doctors should treat patients. Virtue theory lends itself less well to discussions of public policy, although virtue-based discussions of policy issues can be found in the bioethics literature. Philippa Foote, one of the foremost twentieth-century philosophers in the virtue theory tradition, explored the ethics of euthanasia in an oft-discussed paper, but her goal there was to argue that in the context of a virtue theory, the moral distinction between "allowing someone to die" and "actively causing someone to die" can depend on the circumstances. One of the attractions of virtue theory is that it can allow for a certain flexibility and ambiguity that some find appropriate for moral reasoning. Aristotle famously drew a distinction between moral knowledge and scientific or mathematical knowledge; moral judgments hold "only for the most part." Also, an Aristotelian approach can embrace a rich and varied moral vocabulary.

In the thirteenth century, St. Thomas Aquinas drew on his reading of Aristotle to develop an account of morality known today as "natural law" theory. Aquinas held that the cosmos is divinely and rationally ordered, and that a moral law is part of the cosmic order. Further, it is part of God's plan that everyone can understand the moral law through the use of human reason. One can investigate the natural cosmic order and deduce right moral judgments. Natural law theorists often, therefore, hold that we can learn about morality partly by investigating human nature: What humans are designed (by God) to do can help us understand what they should do. Natural law theory may have influenced some of the scholars who are critical of using medical technology to change human nature. Although rarely explicitly invoked in secular bioethics, natural law theory has a considerable influence on Catholic bioethics.

The natural law account of how the moral law was apprehended by human reason has struck many later philosophers as obscure and unconvincing. The eighteenth-century Scottish Enlightenment philosopher David Hume was reacting partly against natural law theory when he argued that moral judgments are not a matter either of reason or of investigating the world, but instead are derived from what he called "the passions"—what today would be called emotions or attitudes. If you investigate a given case, he argued, you end up only with a set of facts, and it is impossible to derive a moral judgment purely from a set of facts. This point is often abbreviated in the dictum, "no ought from an is." The ought—the moral judgment—is a human response to the case, not part of the case itself.

Many philosophers have taken Hume to be making the metaethical claim that there are no true moral judgments, but only subjective opinions. This position is widely rejected in bioethics. However, Hume's skepticism that a moral judgment could be put on a rock-solid foundation—that one could give a proof of a position such that anyone who can reason and investigate the world would be rationally compelled to accept it—has been more influential (disappointing though it is to many). Also, Hume's view that moral claims cannot be derived purely from factual claims is invoked frequently (although some also reject it, on grounds that there are no purely factual descriptions of a case). A common view of moral reasoning in bioethics is that factual claims and value claims must be articulated more or less independently of each other, and that both are necessary to reach a conclusion.

The great German philosopher Immanuel Kant wrote that Hume "awakened" him from his "dogmatic slumbers." Much of Kant's work in philosophy, however, was devoted to trying to re-create, as best as possible, the foundations that Hume seemed to have destroyed. In moral philosophy, Kant proposed that there was indeed a moral law and that it could be derived from the nature of the rational will itself. Roughly, the law Kant proposed is that one should act only on an intention that one could coherently will that every rational being would act on as well. To lie, for example, is to act on an intention to deceive others, but one could not (Kant wrote) coherently will that everybody would act on that intention, because if that happened, deception itself would be impossible. Deception requires trust, but if deception were universal, trust would be nonexistent. Kant called this law the "categorical imperative." He also offered what he believed was an alternative formulation of it, which was that one should never treat a rational being merely as a tool for achieving some other end; one should always treat a rational being also as an "end in itself"—that is, as having a value beyond any price, since to give something a price is always to see it as something one could sell in order to achieve some other end. From a careful application of these formulations of the categorical imperative, Kant thought, narrower moral rules and specific moral judgments could be derived.

Bioethics is deeply influenced by Kant, although very few bioethicists work by trying to apply the categorical imperative in quite the way Kant envisioned. What has caught on in bioethics is the idea that respect for autonomy provides a core, perhaps the core, moral guide. For Kant, autonomy meant the capacity of a rational being to rule itself and adhere to the categorical imperative. In bioethics, autonomy typically means something a little looser: the capacity of a person to make one's own life decisions (not necessarily always to choose the rational and right thing). Kant's idea that a rational will that has a value beyond price has also influenced bioethics. Human beings are often said to have a special dignity in virtue of being human, and both human beings and parts of human beings, such as organs, are sometimes said to be priceless—in the literal sense of being things that should not be bought and sold.

Kantian moral philosophy is described as deontological, meaning that it is about duties. (Deon means duty, in Greek.) It provides guidance for conduct, rather than character, and it identifies conduct that is required of a person regardless of outcome. A contrasting approach to guiding conduct is found in consequentialist moral theories, the most influential version of which is the utilitarian theory introduced by the British social reformer Jeremy Bentham and refined by the philosopher John Stuart Mill. Consequentialist theories hold that right actions are known by evaluating their outcomes. In utilitarian theory, the morally important outcome is happiness or well-being—"utility," in the parlance utilitarians sometimes adopt. Mill also argued that happiness is typically best promoted by largely promoting individual liberty; individuals largely left to their own devices would discover for themselves the most effective ways of promoting their happiness, and their experimentation and creativity would help others promote their own happiness. The principle Mill set out, in his book *On Liberty*, is known as the harm principle: "the only purpose for which power can be rightfully exercised over any member of a civilized community, against his will, is to prevent harm to others."

Mill has been hugely influential in bioethics. Many accept that, even if good outcomes are not the sole criterion of good conduct, they are certainly very important, and the idea of respect for autonomy as understood in bioethics owes as much to Mill's discussion of liberty as to Kant's categorical imperative. The patients' rights movement is essentially an endorsement of the idea that people ought to be allowed to make decisions for themselves, even when they become patients, and even at the risk of harm to themselves. Physician paternalism is unacceptable. On the other hand, public health policy has often wrestled with the harm principle. Public health policy is often thought to require a kind of paternalism, insofar as the goal is not merely to prevent individuals from harming others but to encourage or require them to do things that are good for themselves.

Moral Reasoning in Bioethics

Bioethics is far from a straightforward application to cases of one or another moral theory, however. Just as the people come to bioethics from many different disciplines, the relevance of moral theory to bioethics is widely disputed. Many in the field who are not philosophers do not explicitly draw on a moral theory, and many also draw on multiple moral theories, according to what seems salient in a particular problem.

One of the most influential uses of theory in bioethics is what is sometimes called the "principlist" approach. In the early 1970s, news broke about a study, begun in 1932 and continued until 1972, in which poor, rural black men with syphilis were monitored by the Public Health Service but never treated, despite the discovery in the 1940s that penicillin was effective against the disease. The study was considered reminiscent of notorious Nazi experiments conducted on Jews and others in concentration camps during World War II, and the federal government responded to the scandal by creating the National Commission for the Protection of Human Subjects of Biomedical and Behavioral Research to lay out guidelines for the ethically acceptable treatment of the subjects of medical research. The National Commission issued a number of recommendations, and then in 1978, in a document called simply the Belmont Report, outlined the underlying ethical principles that the commission members—scholars, religious leaders, and others—had been able to agree on. The three principles identified in the Report—respect for persons, beneficence, and justice—have turned into the basis for much of the work that has been done in bioethics.

The principle of respect for persons is derived from the Kantian idea that the capacity for autonomy, or self-determination, deserves great respect. The Belmont Report drew two conclusions from this principle—that people with autonomy should be allowed to make their own decisions (as long as those decisions do not harm others), and that people who because of age, illness, or other circumstances have less autonomy are entitled to protection. In order to ensure that people decide for themselves whether to participate in medical research, the report goes on to argue, they must be given adequate information about the research and their consent to participate must be explicitly sought. Thus the Report argued for truth-telling about medical research and for obtaining subjects' informed consent to participate in research.

The principle of beneficence is the guidance that, before the patients' rights movement, most doctors regarded as the overriding medical ethical principle. The principle is sometimes said to have two components, first that the doctor should do no harm to the patient (an idea expressed in Latin as Primum non nocere), and second that the doctor should act so as to benefit the patient. Both components are often said to be expressed in the Greek Hippocratic Oath: "I will apply dietetic measures for the benefit of the sick according to my ability and judgment; I will keep them from injustice and harm. . . . Whatever houses I may visit, I will comfort and benefit the sick, remaining free of all intentional injustice."

The National Commission also concluded that medical research should be guided by a principle of justice, which it understood as bearing on the question, "Who ought to receive the benefits of research and bear its burdens?" Arguably, the commission did less well in deciding precisely what justice requires. Instead of going on to identify rules that follow from the principle, it identified five different ways of guiding the allocation of benefits and burdens, ranging from "to each person an equal share" to "to each person according to merit."

The principlist approach was picked up and developed in a highly influential book, now in its sixth edition, titled *Principles of Biomedical Ethics*, by Tom L. Beauchamp and James F. Childress, which has been widely used to discuss moral dilemmas arising in clinical care, extending to medicine generally a framework originally developed to address issues in medical research. An assortment of other ways of thinking about clinical care dilemmas has also been proposed; however, some of them are in deliberate opposition to principlism. The casuistic approach proposed by Albert Jonsen and Stephen Toulmin, for example, argues that ethical guidance starts not with abstract principles but with well-accepted judgments in specific cases, which must then be extended to new cases through analogical reasoning. Clinical ethicists sometimes employ casuistic methodologies designed to encourage people struggling with a specific case to identify a wide range of facts and values that are relevant to a case. Feminist approaches sometimes embrace an ethic of caring, focusing on relationships instead of on individual autonomy.

Bioethical issues outside the contexts of decision making for specific people in medical research and clinical care usually draw on an even wider range of moral philosophical work. For example, in a series of books about the overall goals of medicine and the use of societal resources in medical research, Daniel Callahan, a co-founder of The Hastings Center, has drawn on "communitarianism," a view of moral values that has roots in Aristotelian philosophy, to argue that there should be limits to the use of medicine and the advance of medical research. Communitarianism emphasizes that the well-being of individuals is rooted in the well-being of the community, rather than in unlimited self-determination or the maximization of individual happiness. Debates about public health programs and about health policy—about access to health care and the distribution of health care resources—may deploy either communitarian or broadly utilitarian frameworks. Concerns about selfhood—about agency, authenticity, and dignity, for example—sometimes animate discussions of whether medical science should be used to alter human bodies or behaviors. Yet another way of thinking about the limits of the life sciences could be drawn from environmental ethics (which arguably falls within the ambit of "bioethics" as that term was initially proposed by Van Rensselaer Potter). Environmental ethicists often endorse the idea that not just human autonomy and happiness have value but also nature has value, and that the value of nature ought to constrain what humans can do, using biotechnology or other methods, to naturally occurring species and ecosystems.

Answers and Insights

This book is organized so as to introduce readers to the full range of concerns that have been taken up in bioethics, from clinical dilemmas to questions about the use of biotechnology and just access to health care. It is also intended to canvass both fundamental and philosophical questions about the nature of medical decision making and the values relevant to the development and use of biotechnology, and more practical questions about, for example, the mechanisms for making good decisions at the end of life and for increasing the supply of organs available for transplantation.

Many of these societal problems do not admit of easy answers, and in fact, the title of this book notwithstanding, taking sides on these problems should not always be the goal. Careful exploration of contrasting positions, articulating differences of opinion, and recognizing that both sides may offer important moral insights, are at least the first step in taking sides, and sometimes it may be as far as one can realistically go. Of course, in many bioethical problems, both at the bedside and at the societal level, there is a dilemma that requires answering, one way or another, if only because doing nothing is still to make a decision of sorts. However far we go toward settling on answers, we ought to look for consensus wherever it is available. On some of the issues discussed in this book, some consensus is possible. The legacy of the National Commission for the Protection of Human Subjects of Biomedical and Behavioral Research is that people of different backgrounds can sometimes agree, both on specific recommendations and on the values that inform them. As later presidential bioethics commissions have occasionally discovered, however, the moral questions that led to the emergence of bioethics may uncover intractable controversies.

Internet References . . .

Agency for Healthcare Research and Quality (AHRQ)

The AHRQ website provides research-based information to increase the scientific knowledge needed to enhance consumer and clinical decision making, improve health care quality, and promote efficiency in the organization of public and private systems of health care delivery.

www.ahrq.gov

Bioethics Resources on the Web

Created by the National Institutes of Health Office of Science Policy, this is an excellent starting point and has links to other resources.

http://bioethics.od.nih.gov/

The National Reference Center for Bioethics Literature

Located at the Kennedy Institute of Ethics, Georgetown University, this site has extensive resources on physician–patient relationships and other topics and will perform data researches on request.

http://bioethics.georgetown.edu/

The Hastings Center Bioethics Forum

Among the activities of this bioethics center is the Bioethics Forum, which has timely commentaries on controversial issues.

www.thehastingscenter.org/BioethicsForum/

Center for Adolescent Health and the Law

This site has extensive material about minors' right to consent to medical treatment and access to health care.

www.cahl.org

National Disability Rights Network

This is an organization made up of agencies that work to protect and advocate for individuals with disabilities.

www.napas.org/

Medical Decision Making

*A*s recently as 50 years ago, medical decision making was of concern only to physicians. With their presumed greater knowledge and with patients' best interests at heart, they were entrusted with making life-and-death decisions, as well as ordinary decisions. Ironically, although physicians had greater authority in those times than they do today, they had less ability to treat. As medicine has grown more technologically and scientifically sophisticated, the range of people who have an interest in making decisions—and in some cases, a right to do so—among the medical options has grown. Law and ethics have reaffirmed the status of the patient as the primary decision maker. Nevertheless, many ambiguous and troubling situations remain in implementing patients' wishes. It is not even clear that patients have the moral right to make arbitrary decisions about aspects of their care, especially when their preferences impinge on the rights of others, such as family members, physicians, and other patients. It is even harder, then, when the patient lacks the ability to make such decisions and a surrogate must make decisions on the patient's behalf—yet the cases that require surrogate decision makers can be among the most pressing imaginable. Finally, it is sometimes difficult to decide just which patients lack decision-making ability. This unit explores some of the issues that arise when making medical decisions.

- Is Autonomy Still Central to Medical Ethics?

- May Surrogate Decision Makers Terminate Care for a Person in a Persistent Vegetative State?

- Should Adolescents Be Allowed to Make Their Own Life-and-Death Decisions?

ISSUE 1

Is Autonomy Still Central to Medical Ethics?

YES: **Robert M. Arnold and Charles W. Lidz,** from "Informed Consent: Clinical Aspects of Consent in Health Care," in Stephen G. Post, ed., *Encyclopedia of Bioethics,* vol. 3, 3rd ed. (Macmillan, 2003)

NO: **Onora O'Neill,** from *Autonomy and Trust in Bioethics?* (Cambridge University Press, 2002)

Learning Outcome
After reading this issue, you should be able to:
• Discuss the concepts of autonomy and informed consent, the relationship between them, and how they have been understood and employed in bioethics.

ISSUE SUMMARY

YES: Physician Robert M. Arnold and professor of psychiatry and sociology Charles W. Lidz assert that informed consent in clinical care is an essential process that promotes good communication and patient autonomy despite the obstacles of implementation.

NO: Philosopher Onora O'Neill argues that the most evident change in medical practice in recent decades may be a loss of trust in physicians rather than any growth of patient autonomy. Informed consent in practice, she says, often amounts simply to a right to choose or refuse treatments, not a deeper and more meaningful expression of self-mastery.

Informed consent is undoubtedly one of the best-known and, arguably, one of the least-implemented concepts in modern medicine. Although much of modern medical ethics has ancient roots, the idea of informed consent is relatively recent. Until the mid-twentieth century most medical ethics were firmly based on the obligations of physicians to act for the benefit of their patients.

Information was supposed to be managed carefully in order to protect patients from bad news and to keep them hopeful.

The first "Code of Medical Ethics" of the American Medical Association relied heavily on the work of Thomas Percival, a British physician whose book *Medical Ethics* (1803) played a crucial role in the field for more than a century. Percival believed that the patient's right to the truth was less important than the physician's obligation to benefit the patient. Deception, in the interest of doing good, was thus justified. The patient's consent to treatment, informed or otherwise, is not mentioned in early codes of medical ethics, although on a practical level doctors had to have a patient's permission to perform most procedures.

The modern concept of informed consent came to medical ethics through the courts. The earliest influential decision was *Schloendorff v. New York Hospital* (1914), in which the court ruled that a patient's right to "self-determination" obligated a physician to obtain consent. This case laid the basis for further litigation. The most influential series of decisions occurred in the 1950s and 1960s, when rulings went beyond the obligation to obtain consent to include an explicit duty to disclose information relevant to the patient who is making a decision about consent.

While the earlier cases had been based on the patient's right to be free from unwanted bodily intrusion (legally, "battery"), the court in *Natanson v. Kline* (1960) held that physicians who withheld information while obtaining consent were guilty of negligence. Imposing a legal duty on physicians to inform their patients of the risks, benefits, and alternatives to treatment exposed them to the risk of malpractice suits. Another factor that influenced the ascendance of informed consent in medical treatment was parallel discussions about the ethics of research involving human subjects. Voluntary consent to participate in research was a cornerstone of the Nuremberg Code of 1947, which was issued after the trials of Nazi physicians who had performed lethal experiments on nonconsenting prisoners.

Nevertheless, traditions die hard, and little change was seen in actual practice until the resurgence of interest in medical ethics in the 1970s. In 1972 the case of *Canterbury v. Spence* established a far-reaching patient-centered disclosure standard. The ruling stated, "The patient's right of self-decision can be effectively exercised only if the patient possesses enough information to enable an intelligent choice. . . . Social policy does not accept the paternalistic view that the physician may remain silent because divulgence might prompt the patient to forego needed therapy." In the 1980s and 1990s court cases have focused on individuals who lack the competence to provide informed consent, such as comatose patients, children, and mentally ill persons.

Although the physician's duty to obtain informed consent and the patient's right to information are now firmly established in law and grounded in the ethical principle of respect for persons, medical practice varies considerably. In Stephen G. Post, ed., *Encyclopedia of Bioethics* (2003), Tom L. Beauchamp and Ruth R. Faden, philosophers who have studied informed consent extensively, assert, "The overwhelming impression from the empirical literature and from reported clinical experience is that the actual process of soliciting informed consent often falls short of a serious show of respect for the decisional authority of patients."

The YES and NO selections illustrate two views of the future of informed consent. Robert M. Arnold and Charles W. Lidz reassert the importance of informed consent and offer ways in which the process can be improved in the clinical setting, despite the many obstacles. Onora O'Neill argues that informed consent has not enhanced patient autonomy but has had the opposite effect of lessening patient trust.

YES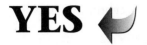

Robert M. Arnold and Charles W. Lidz

Informed Consent: Clinical Aspects of Consent in Health Care

Clinical Aspects of Consent in Healthcare

Decision making is an everyday event in healthcare, not only for doctors and patients, but also for nurses, psychologists, social workers, emergency medical technicians, dentists, and other health professionals. Since the 1960s, however, the cultural ideal of how these decisions should be made has changed considerably. The concept that medical decision making should rely exclusively on the physician's expertise has been replaced by a model in which healthcare professionals share information and discuss alternatives with patients who then make the ultimate decisions about treatment.

The concept of informed consent gained its initial support as part of the general societal trend toward broadening access to decision making during the 1960s. Thus, the initial support for informed consent came from legal and philosophic circles rather than healthcare professionals. In the legal arena, informed consent has been used to develop minimal standards for doctor–patient interactions and clinical decision making (Berg et al.). Although there are some differences by jurisdiction, widely accepted legal standards require that healthcare professionals inform patients of the risks, benefits, and alternatives of all proposed treatments, and then allow the patient to choose among acceptable therapeutic alternatives.

In academia, informed consent has served as a cornerstone for the development of the discipline of bioethics. Based on the importance of autonomy in moral discourse, philosophers have argued that healthcare professionals are obligated to engage patients in discussions regarding the goals of therapy and the alternatives for reaching those goals, and that patients are the final decision makers regarding all therapeutic decisions.

While many physicians would express some support to the concept of shared decision making, this support is largely theoretical and does not seem to have made its way into routine medical practice. Physicians typically think of informed consent as a legal requirement for a signed piece of paper that is at best a waste of time, and at worst a bureaucratic, legalistic interference with their care for patients. Rather than seeing informed consent as a process that promotes good communication and patient autonomy, many healthcare professionals view it as a complex, legally prescribed recitation of risks and benefits that only frightens or confuses patients.

Objections to Informed Consent

There are various objections to informed consent that clinicians often make, and it will be useful to review those objections here.

Consent cannot be truly "informed"   Many practicing clinicians report that their patients are unable to understand the complex medical information necessary for a fully rational weighing of alternative treatments. There is considerable research support for this view. A variety of studies document that patients recall only a small percentage of the information that professionals present to them (Meisel and Roth); that they are not as good decision makers when they are sick as at other times (Sherlock; Cassell, 2001); and that they often make decisions based on medically trivial factors. Informed consent thus appears either to promote uninformed—and thus suboptimal—decisions, or to encourage patients to blindly accept healthcare professionals' recommendations. In either case informed consent appears to be a charade, and a dangerous one at that.

However, the fact that patients often do have difficulty understanding important aspects of medical decisions does not mean that healthcare professionals are the best decision makers about the patient's treatment. Knowledge about medical facts is not enough. Wise house buyers will have a structural engineer check over an old house, but few would be willing to allow the engineer to choose their house for them. Just as structural engineers cannot decide which house a family should buy—because they lack knowledge about the family's pattern of living, personal tastes, and potential family growth—healthcare professionals cannot scientifically deduce the best treatment for a specific patient simply from the medical facts. What matters to individuals about their health depends on their lifestyles, past experiences, and values, so choosing the *optimal therapy* is not a purely objective matter (U.S. President's Commission). Thus, patients and healthcare professionals both contribute essential knowledge to the decision-making process: patients bring their knowledge of their personal situation, goals, and values; and healthcare professionals bring their expertise on the nature of the problem and the technology that may be used to meet the patient's goals (see Brock).

Informed-consent disclosures, even if they are well done, may not lead to what clinicians might consider optimal decisions. Most people make major life decisions, such as whom to marry and which occupation to take up, based on faulty or incomplete information. Patients' lack of understanding of medical information in choosing treatment is probably no worse than their lack of information in choosing a spouse, nor are medical decisions more important than spousal choice. Respecting patient autonomy means allowing individuals to make their own decisions, even if the healthcare professional disagrees with them. The informed-consent process can improve patient decisions, but it cannot be expected to lead to perfect decisions.

Moreover, although sick persons have defects in their rational abilities, so do healthcare professionals. In fact, some of the most famous research on the difficulties individuals have with the rational use of probabilistic data involves physicians (Dawson and Ackes). Health professionals must be careful not to be too pessimistic about patients' ability to become informed decision makers. Patients may not be able to become as technically well-informed as professionals, but they clearly can understand and make decisions based on relevant information. One study, for example, showed that patients' decisions regarding life-sustaining treatment changed when they were given accurate information about the therapy's chance of success and that patients, when given increased information about screening tests for prostate cancer, were less likely to have the test change their decision on having the test (Murphy et al.). Moreover, what seems to be an irrational decision may turn out to be, from the patient's point of view, rational. Thus, a patient may turn down a recommended treatment because of personal experience with surgery or because the long-term benefit is not seen as being worth the short-term risk.

Most important, the difficulty of educating sick persons does not justify unilateral decision making. Rather, it places a special obligation on healthcare professionals to communicate clearly with patients. Using technical jargon, trying to give all of the available information in one visit, and not asking what the patient wants to know is a recipe for confusing even the most intelligent patient. A growing literature deals with informational aides—ranging from question prompt-sheets to giving patients audiotapes of the interaction and formal decision aides—that can be used to promote patient understanding and shared decision-making. New technologies like interactive DVD offer patients the opportunity to participate more fully in shared decision making at their own rate. A limitation of many of these aides is that they are limited helping with specific decisions and need to be updated frequently (Barry). Healthcare professionals also need to become more familiar with different cultural patterns of communication in order to talk with patients from different cultural backgrounds. For example, although a simple, factual discussion of depression and its treatment may be acceptable to most middle-class Americans, it would be seen as inappropriate by a first-generation Vietnamese male, whose culture discourages viewing depression as a disease (Hahn). There is no reason, in principle, why a person who makes decisions at home and work cannot, with help, understand the medical data sufficiently to become involved in medical decisions. Healthcare professionals must learn how best to present that help and involve patients in the decision-making process.

Patients do not wish to be involved in decision making Many healthcare professionals believe that it is unfair to force patients to make decisions regarding their medical care. After all, they argue, patients pay their healthcare professionals to make medical decisions. The empirical literature partially supports the view that patients want professionals to make treatment decisions for them (Steel et al.). For example, in a study of male patients' preferences about medical decision making regarding hypertension, only 53 percent wanted to participate at all in the decision-making process (Strull et al.). More recent data suggest that sicker patients are less interested in information about their disease and more willing to have doctors make decisions (Butow 1997; 2002).

There is no reason to force patients to be involved in decisions if they do not want to be. However, unless the health professional asks, he or she cannot know how involved a patient wants to be. Studies suggest that doctors' ability to predict their patients' interest in information, or their desire to be involved in decision making, is no better than flipping a coin (Butow 1997, 2002). In addition, roughly two-thirds of patients want to be involved in decision making, either by being the primary decision maker (the minority) or in shared decision making with the physician.

Patients may not always want to be involved in decision making, since many have been socialized into believing that "the doctor knows best." This is particularly true for poorer patients. Studies have shown that physicians wrongly assume that because patients with fewer socioeconomic resources ask fewer questions, they do not want as much information. These patients may in fact want just as much information, but they have been socialized into a different way of interacting with healthcare professionals (Waitzkin, 1984).

Patients may choose to allow someone else to make the decision for them. However, when a patient asks, "What would you do if you were me?" the underlying question may be, "As an expert in biomedicine, what alternative do you think will best maximize my values or interest?" If this is the case, the healthcare professional should respond by making a recommendation and justifying it in terms of the patient's values or interests. More frequently, the patient is asking, "If you had this disease, what therapy would you choose?" This question presumes that the professional and patient have the same values, needs, and problems, which is often not the case. Healthcare professionals should respond by pointing this out and emphasizing the importance of the patients' values in the decision-making process.

Although many patients do not want to be actively involved in decision making, they almost always want more information concerning their illness than the healthcare professional gives them. Healthcare professionals should not assume that just because patients do not wish to choose their therapy, they do not want information. Patients may desire information so as to increase compliance or make modifications in other areas of their lives, as well as to make medical decisions.

There are harmful effects of informing patients   Healthcare professionals often justify withholding information from patients because of their belief that informing patients would be psychologically damaging and therefore contrary to the principle of nonmaleficence. Many healthcare professionals, however, overestimate potential psychological harm and neglect the positive effects of full disclosure (Faden et al.). Some discussions that physicians assume are stressful, such as advance care-planning, have been shown to decrease patient anxiety and increase the patient's sense of control. Moreover, bad news can often be communicated in a way that ameliorates the psychological effects of the disclosure (Quill and Townsend). Truth-telling must be distinguished from "truth dumping." Explanation of the care that can be provided, and empathic attention to the patient's fears and uncertainties can often prevent or mitigate otherwise more painful news. Finally, sometimes the harm associated with bad news is unavoidable. It is normal to be sad after finding out that one has an incurable cancer, for example. That does not mean that one should not convey the information, only that it should be done in as sensitively and supportively as possible.

Informed consent takes too much time   Respecting autonomy and promoting patient well-being—the values served through informed consent—are fundamental to good medicine. However, adhering to the ideals of medical practice takes time—time to help patients understand their illness and work through their emotional reactions to stressful information, to discuss each party's preconceptions and to clarify the therapeutic goals, to decide on a treatment plan, and to elicit questions about diagnosis and treatment.

In U.S. healthcare, time is money. As many commentators have noted, physicians are less well reimbursed for talking to patients than for performing invasive tests. This may discourage doctors from spending enough time discussing treatment options with patients. This, along with the pressures of managed care has decreased the average outpatient encounter, allowing even less time for doctor–patient communication. The ultimate justification for spending time to facilitate patient decisions is the same as that for spending any time in medical care: that patients will be better cared for. Moreover, some of the new decision aides, such as question prompts, may in fact decrease the time spent in the patient visit, while simultaneously increasing patient understanding.

Clinical Approaches to Informed Consent

Many of the problems in implementing informed consent result, at least in part, from the way informed consent has been implemented in clinical practice. Informed consent has become synonymous with the *consent form,* a legal invention with a legitimate role in documenting that informed consent has taken place, but hardly a substitute for the discussion process leading to informed consent (Andrews).

A pro forma approach: an event model of informed consent   In many clinical settings, consent begins when *it is time to get consent,* typically just prior to the administration of treatment. The process of getting the patients' consent consists of the recitation by a physician or nurse of the list of material risks and benefits and a request that the patient sign for the proposed treatment. This "conversation" is a very limited one that emphasizes the transfer of information from the physician or nurse to the patient. While it does meet the minimal legal requirements for informed consent efficiently, it does not meet the higher ethical goal of informed consent, which is to empower patients by educating and involving them in their treatment plans. Instead, it imposes an almost empty ritual on an unchanged relationship between provider and patient (Katz).

The procedure just described assumes that care involves a series of discrete, circumscribed decisions. In fact, much of clinical medicine consists of a series of frequent, interwoven decisions that must be repeatedly reconsidered as more information becomes available. When "it is time to get consent," there may be nothing left to decide. Consider the operative consent form obtained the evening prior to an operation. After patients have discussed with their families whether to be admitted to the hospital, rearranged their work and child-care schedules, and undergone a long and painful diagnostic workup, the decision to have surgery seems preordained. The evening before the operation, patients do not seriously evaluate the operation's risks and benefits, so consent is pro forma. No wonder some healthcare professionals feel that *consent* is a waste of time and energy.

The event model for gathering informed consent falls far short of meeting the ethical goal of ensuring patient participation in the decision-making process. Rather than engaging the patient as an active participant in the decision-making process, the patient's role is to agree to or veto the healthcare professionals' recommendations. Little attempt is made to elicit patient preferences and consider how treatment might address them.

A dialogical approach: the process model of informed consent   Fortuately, it is possible to fulfill legal requirements for informed consent while maximizing active patient participation in the clinical setting. An alternative to the event model described above, which sees informed consent as an aberration from clinical practice, the process model attempts to integrate informed consent into all aspects of clinical care (Berg et al). The process model of informed consent assumes that each party has something to contribute to the decision-making process. The physician brings technical knowledge and experience in treating patients with similar problems, while patients bring knowledge about their life circumstances and the ability to assess the effect that treatment may have on them. Open discussion makes it possible for the patient and the physician to examine critically their views and to determine what might be optimal treatment.

The process model also recognizes that medical care rarely involves only one decision made at a single point in time. Decisions about care frequently begin with the suspicion that something is wrong and that treatment may be necessary, and they end only when the patient leaves follow-up care. Decisions involve diagnostic as well as therapeutic interventions. Some decisions are made in one visit, while others occur over a prolonged period of time. Although some interactions between provider and patient involve explicit decisions, decisions are made at each interaction, even if the decision is only to continue treatment. The process model also recognizes that various healthcare professionals may play a role in making sure that the patients' consent is informed. For example, a woman deciding on various breast cancer treatments may talk with an oncologist and a surgeon about the risks of various treatments, with a nurse about the side effects of medication, with a social worker about financial issues in treatment, and with a patient-support group about her husband's reaction to a possible mastectomy.

Ideally, then, informed consent involves shared decision making over a period of time; in a dialogue throughout the course of the patient's relationship with various healthcare professionals. Such a dialogue aims to facilitate patient participation and to strengthen the therapeutic alliance.

Tasks Involved in Informed Consent

Consent is a series of interrelated tasks. First, the patient and professional must agree on the problem that will be the focus of their work together (Eisenthal and Lazare). Most nonemergency consultations involve complex negotiations between healthcare professional and patient regarding the definition of the patient's problem. The patient may see the problem as a routine physical examination for a work release, the need for advice, or the investigation of a physical symptom. If professionals are to respond effectively to the patients' goals, they must find out the reason for the visit. Whereas physicians typically focus on biomedical information and its implications, patients typically view the problem in the context of their social situation (Fisher and Todd). The differences between the patient's perceptions of the problem and the professional's perceptions must be explicitly worked through, since agreement regarding the focus of the interactions will lead to increased patient satisfaction and compliance with further treatment plans (Meichenbaum and Turk).

Even when the professional and patient have agreed on what the problem is, substantial misunderstandings may arise regarding the treatment goals. Patients may expect the medically impossible, or they may expect outcomes based on knowledge of life circumstances about which the physician is unaware. Since assessing the risks and benefits of any treatment option depends on therapeutic goals, the professional and patient must agree on the goals the therapy aims to accomplish.

Finding out what the patient wants is more complicated than merely inquiring, "What do you want?" A patient typically does not come to the professional with well-developed preferences regarding medical therapy except "to get better," with little understanding of what this may involve (Cassell, 1985). As a patient's knowledge and perspective change over the course of an illness, so too may the patient's views regarding the therapeutic goals.

Because clinicians provide much of the medical information needed to ensure that the patient's preferences are grounded in medical possibility, healthcare professionals play a significant role in how a patient's preferences evolve. It is important that they understand that patients may reasonably hold different goals from those their practitioners hold. This is particularly true when they come from different economic strata. For example, a physician's emphasis on the most medically sophisticated care may pale in the light of the patient's financial problems. Therapeutic goals, like the definition of the problem, require ongoing clarification and negotiation.

After agreeing upon the problem and the therapeutic goals, the healthcare professional and the patient must choose the best way to achieve them. If patients have been involved in the prior two steps, the decision about a treatment plan will more likely reflect their values than if they are merely asked to assent to the clinician's strategy.

Healthcare professionals often ask how much information they must supply to ensure that the patient is an informed participant in the decision-making process (Mazur). There is, however, a more important question: Has the information been provided in a manner that the patient can understand? While the law only requires that healthcare professionals inform patients, morally valid consent requires that patients understand the information conveyed. Ensuring patient understanding requires attention to the quality as well as the quantity of information presented (Faden).

A great deal of empirical data has been collected concerning problems with consent forms. These forms have been criticized, for example, as being unintelligible because of their length and use of technical language (Berg et al.). Healthcare professionals thus need to be aware of, and facile in using, a variety of methods to increase patients' comprehension of information, including verbal techniques, written information, and interactive videodiscs (Stanley et al.).

Still, the question of how much information to present remains. The legal standards regarding information disclosure—what a reasonable patient would find essential to making a decision or what a reasonably prudent physician would disclose—are not particularly helpful. Howard Brody has suggested two important features: (1) the physician must disclose the basis on which the proposed treatment or the alternative possible treatments have been chosen; and (2) the patient must be encouraged to ask questions suggested by the physician's reasoning—and the questions need to be answered to the patient's satisfaction (Brody). Healthcare professionals must also inform patients when controversy exists about the various therapeutic options. Similarly, patients should also be told the degree to which the recommendation is based on established scientific evidence rather than personal experience or educated guesses.

Two other factors will influence the amount of information that should be given: the importance of the decision (given the patient's situation and goals) and the amount of consensus within the healthcare professions regarding the agreed-upon therapy. For example, a low-risk intervention, such as giving influenza vaccines to elderly patients, offers a clear-cut benefit with minimal risk. In this case, the professional should describe the intervention and recommend it because of its benefits. A detailed description of the infrequent risks is not needed unless the patient asks or is known to be skeptical of medical interventions. Interventions that present greater risks or a less clear-cut risk-benefit ratio require a longer description—for example, the decision to administer AZT to an HIV (human immunodeficiency virus)-positive, asymptomatic woman with a CD4 cell count of 350. In this situation, the data regarding starting medications are unclear and a patient's preference is critical. In this situation, one would need to talk about the major side effects of the medicines, the burden of taking medicines daily, the immunological benefit of anti-virals, etc. In neither case is a discussion of pathophysiology or biochemistry necessary. It must be emphasized that there is no formula for deciding how much a patient needs to be told or the length of time this will take. The amount of information necessary will depend on the patient's individual situation, values, and goals.

Finally, an adequate decision-making process requires continual updating of information, monitoring of expectations, and evaluation of the patient's progress in reaching the chosen or revised goals. Thus, the final step in informed consent is follow-up. This step is particularly important for patients with chronic diseases for which modifications of the treatment plan are often necessary.

The process model of informed consent has many advantages. Because it assumes many short conversations over time rather than one long interaction, it can be more easily integrated into the professional's ambulatory practice than the event model. It also allows patients to be much more involved in decision making and ensures that treatment is more consistent with their values. Furthermore, the continual monitoring of patients' understanding of their disease, the treatment, and its progress is likely to reduce misunderstandings and increase their investment in, and adherence to, the treatment plan. Thus, the process model of informed consent is likely to promote both patient autonomy and well-being.

Unfortunately, there are situations in which this approach is not very helpful. Some healthcare professionals, anesthesiologists, or emergency medical technicians, for example, are not likely to have ongoing relationships with patients. In emergencies, there is not time for a decision to develop through a series of short conversations. In these cases, informed consent may more closely approximate the event model. However, since most medical care is delivered by primary-care practitioners in an ambulatory setting, the process model of informed consent is more helpful.

Bibliography

Andrews, Lori B. 1984. "Informed Consent Status and the Decision-making Process." *Journal of Legal Medicine* 5(2): 163–217.

Barry, M. 2000. "Involving Patients in Medical Decisions: How Can Physicians Do Better?" *Journal of the American Medical Association* 282(24): 2356–2357.

Berg, Jessica; Appelbaum, Paul S.; Lidz, Charles W.; et al. 2001. *Informed Consent: Legal Theory and Clinical Practice*, 2nd edition. New York: Oxford University Press.

Brock, Dan W. 1991. "The Ideal of Shared Decision Making Between Physicians and Patients." *Kennedy Institute of Ethics Journal* 1(1): 28–47.

Braddock, C. H.; Fihn, S. D.; Levinson, W.; et al. 1997. "How Doctors and Patients Discuss Routine Clinical Decisions: Informed Decision Making in the Outpatient Setting." *Journal of General Internal Medicine* 12(6): 339–345.

Brody, Howard. 1989. "Transparency: Informed Consent in Primary Care." *Hastings Center Report* 19(5): 5–9.

Butow, P. N.; Dowsett, S.; Hagerty, R.; et al. 2002. "Communicating Prognosis to Patients with Metastatic Disease: What Do They Really Want to Know?" *Supportive Care in Cancer* 10(2): 161–168.

Butow, P. N.; Maclean, M.; Dunn, S. M.; et al. 1997. "The Dynamics of Change: Cancer Patients' Preferences for Information, Involvement, and Support." *Annals of Oncology* 8: 857–863.

Cassell, Eric J. 1985. *Talking with Patients.* 2 vols. Cambridge, MA: MIT Press.

Cassell, Eric J. 2001. "Preliminary Evidence of Impaired Thinking in Sick Patients." *Annals of Internal Medicine* 134(12): 1120–1123.

Dawson, Neal V., and Arkes, Hal R. 1987. "Systematic Errors in Medical Decision Making: Judgment Limitations." *Journal of General Internal Medicine* 2(3): 183–187.

Eisenthal, Sherman, and Lazare, Aaron. 1976. "Evaluation of the Initial Interview in a Walk-In Clinic." *Journal of Nervous and Mental Disease* 162(3): 169–176.

Faden, Ruth R. 1977. "Disclosure and Informed Consent: Does It Matter How We Tell It?" *Health Education Monographs* 5(3): 198–214.

Faden, Ruth R.; Beauchamp, Tom L.; and King, Nancy M. P. 1986. *A History and Theory of Informed Consent.* New York: Oxford University Press.

Fisher, Sue, and Todd, Alexandra D., eds. 1983. *The Social Organization of Doctor–Patient Communication.* Washington, D.C.: Center for Applied Linguistics.

Gadow, Sally. 1980. "Existential Advocacy: Philosophic Foundation of Nursing." In *Nursing: Images and Ideals: Opening Dialogue with the Humanities,* ed. Stuart F. Spicker and Sally Gadow. New York: Springer.

Hahn, Robert A. 1982. "Culture and Informed Consent: An Anthropological Perspective." In *Making Health Care Decisions: The Ethical and Legal Implications of Informed Consent in the Patient–Practitioner Relationship,* vol. 2. Washington, D.C.: U.S. President's Commission for the Study of Ethical Problems in Medicine and Biomedical and Behavioral Research.

Katz, Jay. 1984. *The Silent World of Doctor and Patient.* New York: Free Press.

Lidz, Charles W.; Meisel, Alan; Zerubavel, Eviatar; et al., eds. 1984. *Informed Consent: A study of Decision-Making in Psychiatry.* New York: Guilford.

Mazur, Dennis J. 1986. "What Should Patients Be Told Prior to a Medical Procedure? Ethical and Legal Perspectives on Medical Informed Consent." *American Journal of Medicine* 81(6): 1051–1054.

Meichenbaum, Donald, and Turk, Dennis. 1987. *Facilitating Treatment Adherence: A Practitioner's Guidebook.* New York: Plenum Press.

Meisel, Alan, and Roth, Loren H. 1981. "What We Do and Do Not Know About Informed Consent." *Journal of the American Medical Association* 246(21): 2473–2477.

Murphy, Donald J.; Burrows, David; Santilli, Sara; et al. 1994. "The Influence of the Probability of Survival on Patients' Preferences Regarding Cardiopulmonary Resuscitation." *New England Journal of Medicine* 330(8): 545–549.

Quill, Timothy E., and Townsend, Penelope. 1991. "Bad News: Delivery, Dialogue, and Dilemmas." *Archives of Internal Medicine* 151: 463–468.

Sherlock, Richard. 1986. "Reasonable Men and Sick Human Beings." *American Journal of Medicine* 80(1): 2–4.

Stanley, Barbara; Guido, Jeannine; Stanley, Michael; et al. 1984. "The Elderly Patient and Informed Consent: Empirical Findings." *Journal of the American Medical Association* 252(10): 1302–1306.

Steel, David J.; Blackwell, Barry; Gutmann, Mary C.; et al. 1987. "The Activated Patient: Dogma, Dream, or Desideratum." *Patient Education and Counseling* 10(1): 3–23.

Strull, William M.; Lo, Bernard; and Charles, Gerard. 1984. "Do Patients Want to Participate in Medical Decision-Making?" *Journal of the American Medical Association* 252(21): 2990–2994.

U.S. President's Commission for the Study of Ethical Problems in Medicine and Biomedical and Behavioral Research. 1982. *Making Health Care Decisions: A Report on the Ethical and Legal Implications of Informed Consent in the Patient–Practitioner Relationship.* Washington, D.C.: Author.

Waitzkin, Howard. 1984. "Doctor–Patient Communication: Clinical Implications of Social Scientific Research." *Journal of the American Medical Association* 252(17): 2441–2446.

Waitzkin, Howard. 1991. *The Politics of Medical Encounters: How Patients and Doctors Deal with Social Problems.* New Haven, CT: Yale University Press.

West, Candace. 1984. Routine Complications: *Troubles with Talk between Doctors and Patients.* Bloomington: Indiana University Press.

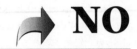

Autonomy and Trust in Bioethics

Contemporary Bioethics

Bioethics is not a discipline, nor even a new discipline; I doubt whether it will ever be a discipline. It has become a meeting ground for a number of disciplines, discourses and organisations concerned with ethical, legal and social questions raised by advances in medicine, science and biotechnology. The protagonists who debate and dispute on this ground include patients and environmentalists, scientists and journalists, politicians and campaigners and representatives of an array of civic and business interests, professions and academic disciplines. Much of the debate is new and contentious in content and flavour; some of it is alarming and some misleading.

The first occasion on which I can remember a discussion of bioethics—we did not then use the word, although it had been coined[1]—was in the mid-1970s at a meeting of philosophers, scientists and doctors in New York City. We were discussing genetically modified (GM) organisms: a topic of breathtaking novelty that was already hitting the headlines. Towards the end of the evening an elderly doctor remarked, with mild nostalgia, that when he had studied medical ethics as a student, things had been easier: the curriculum had covered referrals, confidentiality—and billing. Those simpler days are now very remote. . . .

During [recent] years no themes have become more central in large parts of bioethics, and especially in medical ethics, than the importance of respecting individual rights and individual autonomy. These are now the dominant ethical ideas in many discussions of topics ranging from genetic testing to geriatric medicine, from psychiatry to *in vitro* fertilisation, from beginning to end of life problems, from medical innovation to medical futility, from heroic medicine to hospices. In writing on these and many other topics, much time and effort has gone into articulating and advancing various conceptions of respect for persons, and hence for patients, that centre on ensuring that their rights and their autonomy are respected. Respect for autonomy and for rights are often closely identified with medical practice that seeks individuals' informed consent to all medical treatment, medical research or disclosure of personal information, and so with major changes in the acceptable relationships between professionals and patients. Medical practice has moved away from paternalistic traditions, in which professionals were seen as the proper judges of patients' best interests. Increased recognition and respect of patients' rights and insistence on the ethical importance of securing their consent are now viewed as standard and obligatory ways of securing respect for patients' autonomy.[2] . . .

We might expect the increasing attention paid to individual rights and to autonomy to have increased public trust in the ways in which medicine, science and biotechnology are practised and regulated. Greater rights and autonomy give individuals greater control over the ways they live and increase their capacities to resist others' demands and institutional pressures. Yet amid widespred and energetic efforts to respect persons and their autonomy and to improve regulatory structures, public trust in medicine, science and biotechnology has seemingly faltered. The loss of trust is a constant refrain in the claims of campaigning groups and in the press. . . .

Trust and Autonomy in Medical Ethics

[The] traditional model of the trusting doctor–patient relationship has been subject to multiple criticisms for many years. Traditional doctor–patient relationships, it has been said on countless occasions, have in fact nearly always been based on asymmetric knowledge and power. They institutionalise opportunities for abuse of trust. Doctor–patient relationships were viewed as relationships of trust only because a paternalistic view of medicine was assumed, in which the dependence of patients on professionals was generally accepted. The traditional doctor–patient relationship, so its critics claim, may have been one of trust, but not of reasonable trust. Rather, they claimed, patients who placed trust in their doctors were like children who initially must trust their parents blindly. Such trust was based largely on the lack of any alternative, and on inability to discriminate between well-placed and misplaced trust.

If there was one point of agreement about necessary change in the early years of contemporary medical ethics, it was that this traditional, paternalistic conception of the doctor–patient relationship was defective, and could not provide an adequate context for reasonable trust. A more adequate basis for trust required patients who were on a more equal footing with professionals, and this meant that they would have to be better informed and less dependent. The older assumption that relations of trust are in themselves enough to safeguard a weaker, dependent party was increasingly dismissed as naive. The only trust that is well placed is given by those who understand what is proposed, and who are in a position to refuse or choose in the light of that understanding. We can look at the same image with a less innocent eye, and see it as raising all these questions about the traditional doctor–patient relationship. In this second way of seeing the picture the doctor dominates: the white coat and intimidating office are symbols of her professional authority; the patient's anxious and discontented expression reveals how little this is a relationship of trust.

These considerations lie behind many discussions of supposedly better models of the doctor–patient relationship, in which patients are thought of as equal partners in their treatment, in which treatment is given only with the informed consent of patients, in which patient satisfaction is an important indicator of professional adequacy, in which patients are variously seen as consumers, as informed adults and are not infantilised or treated paternalistically and in which the power of doctors is curbed.[3] In this more sophisticated approach to trust, autonomy is seen as a precondition of genuine trust. Here, as one writer puts it, 'informed consent is the modern clinical ritual of trust',[4] a ritual of trust that embeds it in properly institutionalised respect for patient autonomy. So we can also read the image in the frontispiece in a third, more optimistic, way as combining patient autonomy with mutual trust in the new, recommended, respecting way. What we now see is a relationship between equals: the patient too is a professional, dressed in a suit and sitting like an equal at the desk; the patient has heard a full explanation and is being offered a consent form; he is deciding whether to give his fully informed consent. Trust is properly combined with patient autonomy.

This revised model of doctor–patient interaction demands more than a simple change of attitude on the part of doctors, or of patients. It also requires huge changes in the terms and conditions of medical practice and ways of ensuring that treatment is given only where patients have consented. Informed consent has not always been so central to doctor–patient relationships, which were traditionally grounded in doctors' duties not to harm and to benefit. Informed consent came to be seen as increasingly important in part because of legal developments, especially in the USA, and in part because of its significance for research on human subjects, and the dire abuse of research subjects by Nazi doctors. The first principle of the Nuremberg Doctors' Code of 1947 states emphatically that subjects' consent must be 'voluntary, competent, informed and comprehensive'.[5] Only later did the thought emerge clearly that consent was also central to clinical practice, and that patient autonomy or self-determination should not be subordinated to doctors' commitments to act for their patients' benefit or best interest. Yet despite the enormous stress laid on individual autonomy and patient rights in recent years, this heightened concern for patient autonomy does not extend throughout medicine: public health, and the treatment of those unable to consent are major domains of medical practice that cannot easily be subjected to requirements of respecting autonomy and securing informed consent.

From the patient's point of view, however, the most evident change in medical practice of recent decades may be loss of a context of trust rather than any growth of autonomy. He or she now faces not a known and trusted face, but teams of professionals who are neither names nor faces, but as the title of one book aptly put it, *strangers at the bedside*.[6] These strangers have access to large amounts of information that patients give them in confidence. Yet to their patients they remain strangers—powerful strangers. They are the functionaries of medical institutions whose structures are opaque to most patients, although supposedly designed to secure their best interest, to preserve confidentiality and to respect privacy. Seen 'from the patient's point of view every development in the post World War II period distanced the physician and the hospital from the patient, disrupting social connection and serving the bonds of trust'.[7]

From the practitioner's point of view, too, the situation has losses as well as gains. The simplicities of the Hippocratic oath and of other older professional codes have been replaced by far more complex professional codes, by more formal certification of competence to perform specific medical interventions, by enormous increases in requirements for keeping records and by many exacting forms of professional accountability.[8] In medicine, as in most other forms of professional life and public service, and 'audit society' has emerged.[9] The doctor now faces the patient knowing that he or she must comply with explicit standards and codes, that many aspects of medical practice are regulated, that compliance is monitored and that patients who are not properly treated may complain—or even sue.

These new relationships may live up to their billing by replacing traditional forms of trust with a new and better basis for trust. The new structures may provide reasons for patients to trust even if they do not know their doctors personally, and do not understand the details of the rules and codes that constrain doctors' action. Supposedly they can feel reassured that the power of doctors is now duly regulated and constrained, that doctors will act with due respect and that they can seek redress where doctors fail. Although traditional trust has vanished with the contexts in which it arose, a more acceptable basis for reasonable trust has been secured, which anchors it in professional respect for patients' rights. Supposedly the ideals of trust and autonomy have been reshaped and are now compatible. . . .

The Triumph of Informed Consent

Yet what does the supposed triumph of autonomy in medical ethics amount to? . . .

By insisting on the importance of informed consent we *make* it *possible* for individuals to choose autonomously, however that it is to be construed. But we in no way guarantee or require that they do so. Those who insist on the importance of informed consent in medical practice typically say nothing about individuality or character, about self-mastery, or reflective endorsement, or self-control, or rational reflection, or second-order desires, or about any of the other specific ways in which autonomous choices supposedly are to be distinguished from other, mere choices.

In short, the focus of bioethical discussions of autonomy is not on patient autonomy or individual autonomy of any distinctive sort. What is rather grandly called 'patient autonomy' often amounts simply to a right to choose or refuse treatments on offer, and the corresponding obligations of practitioners not to proceed without patients' consent. Of course, some patients may use this liberty to accept or refuse treatment with a high degree of reflection and individuality, hence (on some accounts) with a high degree of individual or personal autonomy. But this need not generally be the case. Requirements for informed consent are relevant to specifically autonomous choice only because they are relevant to choice of all sorts. What passes for patient autonomy in medical practice is operationalised by practices of informed consent: the much-discussed triumph of autonomy is mostly a triumph of informed consent requirements.

This minimalist interpretation of individual or personal autonomy in medical ethics in fact fits rather well with medical practice. When we are ill or injured we often find it hard to achieve any demanding version of individual autonomy. We are all too aware of our need and ignorance, and specifically that we need help from others whose expertise, control of resources and willingness to assist is not guaranteed. A person who is ill or injured is highly vulnerable to others, and highly dependent on their action and competence. Robust conceptions of autonomy may seem a burden and even unachievable for patients; mere choosing may be hard enough. And, in fact, the choices that patients are required to make typically quite limited. It is not as if doctors offer patients a smorgasbord of possible treatments and interventions, a variegated menu of care and cure. Typically a diagnosis is followed with an indication of prognosis and suggestions for treatment to be undertaken. Patients are typically asked to choose from a smallish menu—often a menu of one item—that others have composed and described in simplified terms. This may suit us well when ill, but it is a far cry from any demanding exercise of individual autonomy.

It is probably a considerable relief to many patients that they are not asked to muster much in the way of individual autonomy. When we are ill or injured we often lack the skills or energy for demanding cognitive tasks. Our highest priority is to get help from others and in particular from others with relevant skills and knowledge. The traditional construction of doctor–patient relations as relations of trust, as quasi-personal, as guided by professional concern for the patient's best interests makes sense to many patients because (if achievable) it would secure what they most need. The point and the context of the older, trust-centred model of doctor–patient relationships are not at all obscure.

However, at a time at which the real relations between doctors and patients are no longer personal relationships, nor even one-to-one relationships, but rather relationships between patients and complex organisations staffed by many professionals, the older personal, trust-based model of doctor–patient relationships seems increasingly obsolete. Contemporary relations between professionals and patients are constrained, formalised and regulated in many ways, and may erode patients' reasons for trusting. The very requirements to record and file medical information, for example, while intended to control information and protect patients, can inhibit doctors' abilities to communicate freely. Doctors, like many other professionals, find themselves pressed to be accountable rather than to be communicative, to conform to regulations rather than to enter relations of trust. As layers of regulation and control are added with the aim of protecting dependent, ignorant and vulnerable patients, as professionals are disciplined by multiple systems of accountability backed by threats of litigation on grounds of professional negligence in case of failure to meet these requirements, relations between patients and professionals are inevitably reshaped. Much is demanded of informed consent requirements if they are to substitute for forms of trust that are no longer achievable (or perhaps were never widely achieved, and still less widely warranted), and safeguard the interests of patients who find strangers at their bedsides. . . .

Notes

1. The Kennedy Institute in Washington DC was founded in 1971 with the full name 'The Joseph and Rose Kennedy Institute for the Study of Human Reproduction and Bioethics'. See W.T. Reich, 'The Word 'Bioethics': Its Birth and the Legacies of Those Who 'Shaped It', *Kennedy Institute of Ethics Journal,* 4, 1994, 319–35.

2. For a highly informative account of these changes, . . . see Ruth Faden and Tom Beauchamp, *A History and Theory of Informed Consent,* Oxford University Press, 1986; for a sociological perspective see Paul Root Wolpe, 'The Triumph of Autonomy in American Bioethics: A Sociological View', in Raymond DeVries and Janardan Subedi, eds., *Bioethics and Society: Constructing the Ethical Enterprise,* Prentice-Hall, 1998, 38–59.

3. R.A. Hope and K.W.M. Fulford, 'Medical Education: Patients, Principles, Practice Skills', in R. Gillon, ed., *Principles of Health Care Ethics,* John Wiley & Sons, 1993.

4. Wolpe, 'The Triumph of Autonomy', 48.

5. See Faden and Beauchamp, *A History and Theory of Informed Consent;* Ulrich Tröhler and Stella Reiter-Theil, *Ethics Codes in Medicine: Foundations and Achievements of Codification Since 1947,* Ashgate; Lori B. Andrews, 'Informed Consent Statutes and the Decision-Making Process', *Journal of Legal Medicine,* 30, 163–217; World Medical Association, Declaration of Helsinki, 2000; see institutional bibliography.

6. David J. Rothman, *Strangers at the Bedside: A History of How Law and Ethics Transformed Medical Decision-Making,* Basic Books, 1991. Rosamond Rhodes and James J. Strain, 'Trust and Transforming Healthcare Institutions', *Cambridge Journal of Healthcare Ethics,* 9, 2000, 205–17.

7. Rothman, *Strangers at the Bedside.*

8. Nigel G.E. Harris, 'Professional Codes and Kantian Duties', in Ruth Chadwick, ed., *Ethics and the Professions,* Amesbury, 1994, 104–15.

9. Michael Power, *The Audit Explosion,* Demos, 1994 and *The Audit Society: Rituals of Verification,* Oxford University Press, 1994.

EXPLORING THE ISSUE

Is Autonomy Still Central to Medical Ethics?

Critical Thinking and Reflection

1. How can one tell when a medical decision is made well? What, in your view, is the criterion for good medical decision making?
2. Do all medical decisions involve autonomy and informed consent in the same way, or do different kinds of decisions involve them in different ways?
3. Both YES and NO selections register concerns with how informed consent has been put into practice and the effect it has had on medicine. Describe and compare their concerns.
4. What do you think is the most important attribute for a doctor who is closely involved with difficult medical decisions? What is that doctor's role?

Is There Common Ground?

A number of scholars have argued that although the concept of informed consent, and the principle underlying it of respect for patient autonomy, is undeniably central to Western values, informed consent cannot do quite the work that bioethicists have sometimes hoped. Eric Cassell argues, for example, that the experience of illness impairs patient's ability to make decisions, that the doctor's task is not merely to supply information to the patient but to support and guide the patient, and that the overriding consideration is the patient's well-being (*The Nature of Healing: The Modern Practice of Medicine* (Oxford University Press, 2012)). In a book on medical decision making in the context of cancer, Rebecca Dresser and a group of other prominent medical ethicists discuss their own experiences as patients and the limits of seemingly central concepts like patient autonomy. Dresser notes, for example, that she needed her doctor to persuade her to accept an intervention that she, trying to act entirely autonomously, had been refusing (*Malignant: Medical Ethicists Confront Cancer* [Oxford University Press, 2012]). This general kind of approach to medical decision making is also sometimes known as "shared decision making."

Other constraints on informed consent are also accepted. If the patient lacks decision-making capacity, then the patient will not be able to give informed consent and other standards must be found. See issues 2 and 6. In addition, many commentators have pointed out that patient autonomy is also limited by the physician's autonomy. Patients have a right not to be treated in ways they do not want, but they do not always have a right to get precisely the treatment they do want. See issues 8 and 11.

Additional Resources

The most comprehensive account of informed consent is *A History and Theory of Informed Consent* by Ruth L. Faden, Tom L. Beauchamp, and Nancy M. P. King (Oxford University Press, 1986). Another useful volume, particularly in terms of psychiatric treatment, is *Informed Consent: Legal Theory and Clinical Practice* by Paul S. Appelbaum, Charles W. Lidz, and Alan Meisel (Oxford University Press, 1987). Jay Katz's *The Silent World of Doctor and Patient* (Free Press, 1984; paper edition 2002, Johns Hopkins University Press) is an insightful discussion of the reasons physicians may be reluctant to disclose information to their patients. See also, Jessica W. Berg, Paul S. Appelbaum, Charles W. Lidz, and Lisa S. Parker, *Informed Consent: Legal Theory and Clinical Practice*, 2nd ed. (Oxford University Press, 2001), and Terrance C. McConnell, *Inalienable Rights: The Limits of Consent in Medicine and the Law* (Oxford University Press, 2000).

Two articles in the *Journal of the American Medical Association* (September 13, 1995)—"Western Bioethics on the Navajo Reservation," by Joseph A. Carrese and Lorna A. Rhodes, and "Ethnicity and Attitudes Toward Patient Autonomy," by Leslie J. Blackhall—suggest that disclosing negative information and involving patients in decision making may be contrary to the beliefs of certain ethnic populations.

For further elaboration of Onora O'Neill's critique of informed consent, see Neil C. Manson and Onora O'Neill, *Rethinking Informed Consent in Bioethics* (Cambridge University Press, 2007). *The Ethics of Consent: Theory and Practice*, edited by Franklin Miller and Alan Wertheimer, brings together expert views on informed consent in many fields beyond bioethics (Oxford University Press, 2009).

ISSUE 2

May Surrogate Decision Makers Terminate Care for a Person in a Persistent Vegetative State?

YES: **Jay Wolfson**, from *A Report to Governor Jeb Bush and the 6th Judicial Circuit in the Matter of Theresa Marie Schiavo* (December 2003)

NO: **Tom Koch**, from "The Challenge of Terri Schiavo: Lessons for Bioethics," *Journal of Medical Ethics* (2005)

Learning Outcomes

After reading this issue, you should be able to:

- Explain the concept of surrogate decision making and how it is related to patient autonomy.
- Explain artificial nutrition and hydration and its relationship to medical treatment.
- Discuss the concerns that those from a disability rights perspective have about surrogate decision making.

ISSUE SUMMARY

YES: Jay Wolfson, a lawyer and the special guardian ad litem appointed for Theresa Marie Schiavo, explains the clinical and legal considerations that justified removal of Ms. Schiavo's feeding tube, causing her to die.

NO: Tom Koch, an independent writer and researcher, holds that helping a person die cannot be said to benefit the person and that questions of personhood and sanctity of life gave reason to help her live.

Most medical decisions require the informed consent of the patient. Often, however, patients are incapable of giving informed consent, either because of an illness or an underlying condition like dementia, or because of the effects of treatment itself. In these cases, decisions must be made by a surrogate decision maker, that is, a person who makes decisions on behalf of the incapacitated person. A surrogate decision maker is either somebody designated by the patient to fill that role or a close family member or friend who knows the patient well and can be trusted to represent the patient's interests.

Some of the most difficult and controversial surrogate decision-making cases involve patients diagnosed as being in a persistent vegetative state, or PVS. Patients in a vegetative state show no evidence that they have any awareness of themselves or their surroundings. They do not respond to stimuli purposefully. To be diagnosed as being in a PVS, a patient must have been in a vegetative state for at least 1 month. In a 2010 study that used functional magnetic resonance imaging (fMRI) to study the brains of people in a PVS, some people who showed no outward signs of consciousness showed imaging findings associated with consciousness, but what these findings actually meant was not clear.

Unfortunately, it is possible to linger in a vegetative state for many years, even for decades. If that happens, and if the patient had never prepared a legal document known as an advance directive to explicitly identify his or her wishes for medical care in these circumstances, then a surrogate decision maker may have to decide what kind of medical care is appropriate, including whether to discontinue medical care altogether. When making these decisions, surrogate decision makers are supposed to follow a legal doctrine known as substituted judgment, which instructs them to try to determine what the patient would have wanted done. In Missouri and New York, surrogate decision makers must rely on the patient's own formal statements about his or her wishes, but in other states that accept substituted judgment, they can consider other evidence about the patient's wishes as well, such as conversations that they remember having with the patient.

One question that commonly arises about surrogate decision making has to do with what counts as "medical care." A patient in a PVS is incapable of swallowing and must therefore be given "artificial nutrition and hydration," typically through a tube placed into the stomach. Most legal and medical commentators hold that artificial nutrition and hydration is medical care, and that if the surrogate decision maker decides that stopping treatment is appropriate, then the feeding tube may be withdrawn. Some people believe, however, that artificial nutrition and hydration is just a matter of giving a person a meal, not of providing medical care.

Another common question is whether the medical diagnosis of PVS is reliable. An Internet search will quickly turn up stories of people who were thought to be in a PVS but turn out to be misdiagnosed. Indeed, some people who have been declared to be in a PVS are actually in what has been described as a "minimally conscious state": they demonstrate some awareness of self and surroundings, and magnetic resonance imaging (MRI) shows that their brains sometimes activate in response to stimuli, but their mental state fluctuates and can be very hard to distinguish from a vegetative state.

The difficulty of distinguishing PVS from a minimally conscious state complicates the medical decision making that must be made about them. First, of course, careful diagnostic work is needed to determine whether the patient is in a PVS or a minimally conscious state. The patient's prognosis will depend on the circumstances of the case. Recovery from a correctly diagnosed PVS is exceedingly rare, and after 12 months in a PVS, the condition is considered permanent. There are scattered cases of people in a minimally conscious state recovering, but many have no hope of meaningful recovery.

Once the patient's medical condition is established as well as possible, the surrogate must face the decisions about what treatments are appropriate. In the YES selection, legal scholar Jay Wolfson explains why medical care, including artificial nutrition and hydration, could be withdrawn from a patient in a PVS. Wolfson has wrestled with the decisions personally: In 2003, he was appointed guardian ad litem for Theresa Marie Schiavo, a woman who was in a PVS and whose husband believed that treatment should be withdrawn. In the NO selection, Tom Koch, an independent writer, lecturer, and researcher who has studied medical decision making concerning people with disabilities, explains why many people believed the decision to withdraw medical treatment from Schiavo was unacceptable.

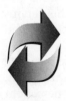

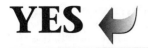

YES

Jay Wolfson

A Report to Governor Jeb Bush and the 6th Judicial Circuit in the Matter of Theresa Marie Schiavo

Introduction

Sometimes good law is not enough, good medicine is not enough, and all too often, good intentions do not suffice. Sometimes, the answer is in the process, not the presumed outcome. We must be left with hope that the right thing will be done well.

We are, each of us, standing in Theresa Marie Schiavo's shoes. Each of us is profoundly affected by the decisions that have and will be made in this case. Advocates of privacy rights and death with dignity, and advocates of right to life and rights of the disabled provide the compelling definitional parameters of this matter.

On 31 October 2003, pursuant to the requirements of Florida H.B. 35-E (Chapter 2003-418, Laws of Florida) and the order of the Hon. David Demers, Chief Judge, Florida 6th Judicial Circuit, a Guardian Ad Litem was appointed for a period of thirty days with the following charge:

> "... make a report and recommendations to the Governor as to whether the Governor should lift the stay that he previously entered. The report will specifically address the feasibility and value of swallow tests for this ward and the feasibility and value of swallow therapy. Additionally, the report will include a thorough summary of everything that has taken place in the trial court and the appellate court concerning this case."
>
> ... The Guardian Ad Litem's efforts have been to deduce and represent the best wishes and best interests of Theresa Schiavo. In that no express, written advance directive existed, determining what Theresa's wishes might be require a combination of substituted judgment, reasonable person considerations, and an aggressive, objective assessment of the massive legal and clinical record that has been compiled over thirteen years. ...

A Report to Governor Jeb Bush and the 6th Judicial Circuit in the Matter of Theresa Marie Schiavo, December 2003.

Historical Facts in Theresa Marie Schiavo's Case

. . . On the tragic early morning of 25 February 1990, Theresa collapsed in the hallway of her apartment, waking [her husband] Michael, who called Theresa's family and 911. The lives of Theresa, Michael and the Schindlers were to change forever.

Theresa suffered a cardiac arrest. During the several minutes it took for paramedics to arrive, Theresa experienced loss of oxygen to the brain, or anoxia, for a period sufficiently long to cause permanent loss of brain function. Despite heroic efforts to resuscitate, Theresa remained unconscious and slipped into a coma. She was intubated, ventilated and trached, meaning that she was given life-saving medical technological interventions, without which she surely would have died that day. . . .

Theresa spent two and a half months as an inpatient at Humana Northside Hospital, eventually emerging from her coma state, but not recovering consciousness. On 12 May 1990, following extensive testing, therapy and observation, she was discharged to the College Park skilled care and rehabilitation facility. Forty-nine days later, she was transferred again to Bayfront Hospital for additional, aggressive rehabilitation efforts. In September of 1990, she was brought home, but following only three weeks, she was returned to the College Park facility because the "family was overwhelmed by Terry's care needs."

On 18 June 1990, Michael was formally appointed by the court to serve as Theresa's legal guardian, because she was adjudicated to be incompetent by law. Michael's appointment was undisputed by the parties.

The clinical records within the massive case file indicate that Theresa was not responsive to neurological and swallowing tests. She received regular and intense physical, occupational and speech therapies.

Theresa's husband, Michael Schiavo, and her mother, Mary Schindler, were virtual partners in their care of and dedication to Theresa. There is no question but that complete trust, mutual caring, explicit love and a common goal of caring for and rehabilitating Theresa, were the shared intentions of Michael Shiavo and the Schindlers. . . .

On 19 July 1991 Theresa was transferred to the Sable Palms skilled care facility. Periodic neurological exams, regular and aggressive physical, occupational and speech therapy continued through 1994.

Michael Schiavo, on Theresa's and his own behalf, initiated a medical malpractice lawsuit against the obstetrician who had been overseeing Theresa's fertility therapy. In 1993, the malpractice action concluded in Theresa and Michael's favor, resulting in a two element award: More than $750,000 in economic damages for Theresa, and a loss of consortium award (non economic damages) of $300,000 to Michael. The court established a trust fund for Theresa's financial award, with SouthTrust Bank as the Guardian and an independent trustee. This fund was meticulously managed and accounted for and Michael Schiavo had no control over its use. There is no evidence in the record of the trust administration documents of any mismanagement of Theresa's estate, and the records on this matter are excellently maintained.

After the malpractice case judgment, evidence of disaffection between the Schindlers and Michael Schiavo openly emerged for the first time. The Schindlers petitioned the court to remove Michael as Guardian. They made allegations that he was not caring for Theresa, and that his behavior was disruptive to Theresa's treatment and condition.

Proceedings concluded that there was no basis for the removal of Michael as Guardian. Further, it was determined that he had been very aggressive and attentive in his care of Theresa. . . .

By 1994, Michael's attitude and perspective about Theresa's condition changed. During the previous four years, he had insistently held to the premise that Theresa could recover and the evidence is incontrovertible that he gave his heart and soul to her treatment and care. This was in the face of consistent medical reports indicating that there was little or no likelihood for her improvement.

In early 1994 Theresa contracted a urinary tract infection and Michael, in consultation with Theresa's treating physician, elected not to treat the infection and simultaneously imposed a "do not resuscitate" order should Theresa experience cardiac arrest. When the nursing facility initiated an intervention to challenge this decision, Michael cancelled the orders. Following the incident involving the infection, Theresa was transferred to another skilled nursing facility.

Michael's decision not to treat was based upon discussions and consultation with Theresa's doctor, and was predicated on his reasoned belief that there was no longer any hope for Theresa's recovery. It had taken Michael more than three years to accommodate this reality and he was beginning to accept the idea of allowing Theresa to die naturally rather than remain in the non-cognitive, vegetative state. . . .

The Evolution of the Law about Dying and Nutrition in Florida

Our society is at a legal, political, biotechnological, bioethical and spiritual crossroad. Theresa Schiavo is alternately depicted as a living, loving person, capable of interacting at a level of cognition with her family and deserving of the right to continue to live—and as a tragically and profoundly brain damaged person, who earlier expressed a desire never to find herself in a circumstance analogous to waking up in a coffin—and being there forever. But she cannot speak to us now. So we must rely upon the auspices of good law and good medicine and the good intentions of those who marshal these arts in order to do our best to do the right thing well for Theresa Schiavo.

During the early 1970s the States began to revise their Probate Codes. There were many reasons for this, including a rapidly aging population, larger numbers of aged persons in the population, people living longer, new and advancing medical technologies that enhanced, extended and affected life, and changing values and orientations about death, dying and the medical-decision processes. These matters have been seriously addressed through a combination of inquiries and actions by church leaders, legislators, medical scientists, and the courts, as all have sought to respond to emerging issues such as those in the Quinlan, Cruzan, Browning, and now the Schiavo cases.

States cooperated with the federal Administration on Aging to address legislative and policy challenges surfacing around these matters. A particularly important topic related to medical technology and its use in the care, treatment and maintenance of patients, is when, who and by what means "artificial" life support and other medical interventions should or could be removed or never withheld in the first place.

Today, most states would afford an adult person the right to deny most health care treatments. But if the patient is a minor, unconscious, in a coma, in a vegetative state, or unable to communicate personal wishes and intentions, there are serious moral, ethical and legal questions that demanded attention. There had been inconsistencies, even within states, as to how decisions regarding termination or removal or withholding a procedure were made. There was also a long standing, well accepted recognition that the relationship between the patient and the physician—the sacred trust—served as the foundation for how and where and when many of these decisions would be made. Often, physicians, in consultation with family members and the patient have done what was deemed to be in best interests of the patient, given the physician's medical opinion and the express, known or believed intentions of the patient.

To reduce ambiguities, many states began to encourage and accept written advance directives as the basis for decisions regarding end of life treatment. Living wills, durable powers of attorney for health care and health care surrogate documents, stating a person's explicit intentions regarding end of life care, became increasingly accepted and even formalized into the statutory framework of most states. A written expression was deemed to be an important element in this process to avoid the possibility of confusion or uncertainty with respect to a person's intention regarding their health and medical care.

Throughout the 1980s and 1990s, Florida lawmakers struggled with how they would provide individuals with the prerogatives for establishing their wishes regarding end of life decisions, while at the same time, protecting against perceived and actual abuses and assisted suicides. Among the most sensitive of issues is this regard has been the withdrawal of artificial life support in the form of nutrition and hydration. The idea of withholding or withdrawing these has created significant debates within and across religious, philosophical and political groups and interests. But the topic has been addressed at great lengths by each of these groups, and there is surprising consensus in principle and even in practice.

The current, generally accepted applications to terminal illness or persistent vegetative state define artificial feeding as artificial life support that may be withheld or withdrawn. In 1989, the Florida Legislature permitted the withdrawal of artificial nutrition and hydration under very specific circumstances. In 1999, following extensive bipartisan efforts, life-prolonging procedures were redefined as "any medical procedure, treatment, or intervention, including artificially provided sustenance and hydration, which sustains, restores, or supplants a spontaneous vital function." It is noteworthy that the general principle of artificial nutrition as artificial life support that may be removed in terminal and even vegetative state conditions is reflected in nearly all state's laws and within the guidelines of end of life care enunciated by the American Conference of Catholic Bishops and other religious denominations.

These general principles are in no way intended to encourage or condone suicide or assisted suicide. But they reflect the acceptance of artificial nutrition as artificial life support that may be withdrawn or withheld as a matter of public policy, when these decisions capture the intentions of the person and with the premise that people should not be required to remain "artificially alive", or to have their natural peaceful deaths postponed and prolonged if they would otherwise choose not to, and that they should be allowed to die with dignity, and return, if their beliefs so accommodate, to God.

When written advance directives are not available, and the affected person is incompetent and unable to communicate, a decision to discontinue nutrition and hydration is especially challenging. But Florida law, as reflected in F.S. 765, and as interpreted through *In re Guardianship of Browning,* 568 So. 2d 4 (Fla. 1990), provides for a substituted judgment basis for such decisions and/or the presentation of clear and convincing evidence to demonstrate the intentions of the person.

It has been suggested that in the case of incapacitated persons, particularly those who have not expressed an advance directive, the "clear and convincing" evidence standard for establishing the intent to discontinue artificial life support is insufficient and incongruous. The insufficiency, it is argued, is because of the possibility of using information that is not accurate, complete or even honest. The incongruity is related to the "beyond a reasonable doubt" standard that serves as the basis for decisions to convict and then execute capitol felons.

If persons unable to speak for themselves have decisions made on their behalf by guardians or family members, the potential for abuse, barring clear protections, could lead to a "slippery slope" of actions to terminate the lives of disabled and incompetent persons. And it is not difficult to imagine bad decisions being made in order to make life easier for a family or to avoid spending funds remaining in the estate on the maintenance of a person.

There is, of course, the other side of that slippery slope, which would be to keep people in a situation they would never dream of: unable to die, unable to communicate, dependent for everything, and unaware, being maintained principally or entirely through state resources—and for reasons that may relate to guilt, fear, needs or wants of family members, rather than what the person's best wishes might otherwise have been.

And there is the chillingly practical, other public policy matter of the cost of maintaining persons diagnosed in persistent vegetative states and terminal conditions alive for potentially indefinite periods of time—at what inevitably becomes public expense. Here the "reasonable person" standard, with respect to how one would want to be treated were they in Theresa's shoes affects the discussion. This is not easy stuff, and should not be.

In withholding or withdrawing life support, or in keeping a person alive, there is the risk of transposing intentions and values. The reasoned, even substituted judgment decisions of guardians or loved ones may be based upon either a "quality of life determination", or the desires of family members. This remains a risk in a system that does not require an explicit, advance directive. . . .

Cruzan and the Role of States in Guidelines for Medical Decisions

. . . Not all states deploy the specific guidelines and measures adopted by Florida. Many states refuse to accept anything but advance, written directives of the person as a basis for removal of artificial life support. Florida has chosen to employ guidelines that include surrogate decisions by the bona fide legal guardian and/or clear and convincing evidence as to the intentions of the person.

In Theresa's case, evidence regarding her intentions consisted of admitted hearsay regarding conversations between Theresa and her spouse and spousal relatives. The context and nature of this hearsay were deemed sufficiently probative, competent and reliable to serve as a basis for admission, and was determined to be sufficiently clear and convincing. The court then served as proxy decision maker, essentially assuming the role of legal guardian. The privacy interests of the person, as established in the Florida Constitution, and as articulated with specificity in *Browning* . . . served as the legitimate legal bases for the court's conclusions to withdraw life support consistent with Florida Statute, 765.

Evidence regarding the persistent vegetative state consisted of highly credible medical testimony and documentation reflecting both early and recently performed neurological examinations and a case history that included early swallowing studies conducted multiple times nearly ten years ago.

The Swallowing Test and Neurological Function

The review of the medical and clinical evidence in the case goes directly to the issues of the feasibility and value of swallowing tests and swallowing therapy, and to the relationship between neurological function and swallowing food and liquid.

Three independent sets of swallowing tests were performed early in Theresa's medical treatment: 1991, 1992 and 1993. Each of these determined that Theresa was not able to swallow without risk of aspiration (and consequent infection).

Swallowing tests and swallowing therapy address many of the core issues in contention. If Theresa can swallow, then she can take nutrition and hydration orally, and it is argued that she would not elect to stop eating. But to orally eat and drink, Theresa must possess cognitive capacity beyond mere reflex, or she will not only fail to ingest, but could easily aspirate substances into her lungs and be subjected to infections and subsequent death. . . .

Early in Theresa's care, neurological examinations were performed to assess her cognitive capacity. Competent medical practitioners determined that

Theresa was in what has been consistently defined as a persistent vegetative state—a finding that throughout the litigation was not disputed by either side. Quite recently, the Schindlers have disputed that Theresa is in a persistent vegetative state, and in the alternative, they have argued that even if she is, she deserves to live and be maintained via artificial nutrition and hydration. . . .

A particularly disarming aspect of persons diagnosed with persistent vegetative state is that they have waking and sleeping cycles. When awake, their eyes are often open, they make noises, they appear to track movement, they respond to deep pain, and appear startled by loud noises. Further, because the autonomic nervous system those brain related functions are not affected, they can often breathe (without a respirator) and swallow (saliva). But there is no purposeful, reproducible, interactive, awareness. There is some controversy within the scientific medical literature regarding the characterization and diagnosis of persons in a persistent vegetative state. Highly competent, scientifically based physicians using recognized measures and standards have deduced, within a high degree of medical certainty, that Theresa is in a persistent vegetative state. This evidence is compelling.

Terri is a living, breathing human being. When awake, she sometimes groans, makes noises that emulate laughter or crying, and may appear to track movement. But the scientific medical literature and the reports this GAL obtained from highly respected neuro-science researchers indicate that these activities are common and characteristic of persons in a persistent vegetative state.

In the month during which the GAL conducted research, interviews and compiled information, he sought to visit with Theresa as often as possible, sometimes daily, and sometimes, more than once each day. During that time, the GAL was not able to independently determine that there were consistent, repetitive, intentional, reproducible interactive and aware activities. When Theresa's mother and father were asked to join the GAL, there was no success in eliciting specific responses. Hours of observed videotape recordings of Theresa offer little objective insight about her awareness and interactive behaviors. There are instances where she appears to respond specifically to her mother. But these are not repetitive or consistent. There were instances during the GAL's visits, when responses seemed possible, but they were not consistent in any way.

This having been said, Theresa has a distinct presence about her. Being with Theresa, holding her hand, looking into her eyes and watching how she is lovingly treated by Michael, her parents and family and the clinical staff at hospice is an emotional experience. It would be easy to detach from her if she were comatose, asleep with her eyes closed and made no noises. This is the confusing thing for the lay person about persistent vegetative states.

Theresa's neurological tests and CT scans indicate objective measures of the persistent vegetative state. These data indicate that Theresa's cerebral cortex is principally liquid, having shrunken due to the severe anoxic trauma experienced thirteen years ago. The initial oxygen deprivation caused damage that could not be repaired, and the brain tissue in that area continued to devolve. It is noteworthy to recall that from the time of her collapse, and for more than three years, Theresa did receive active physical, occupational, speech and even recreational therapy. There is evidence early in her records of care that she said "no" during physical therapy session. That behavior did not recur and was not further referenced.

In recent months, individuals have come forward indicating that there are therapies and treatments and interventions that can literally regrow Theresa's functional, cerebral cortex brain tissue, restoring part or all of her functions. There is no scientifically valid, medically recognized evidence that this has been done or is possible, even in rats, according to the president of the American Society for Neuro-Transplantation. It is imaginable that some day such things may be possible; but holding out such promises to families of severely brain injured persons today may be a profound disservice.

In the observed circumstances, the behavior that Theresa manifests is attributable to brain stem and forebrain functions that are reflexive, rather than cognitive. And the substantive difference according to neurologists and neurosurgeons is that reflexive activities of this nature are neither conscious nor aware activities. And without cognition, there is no awareness. (Descartes addressed this in his proposition that it is our awareness, our consciousness that defines our being: "Cogito, ergo sum". This logic would imply that unless we are aware and conscious, we cease to be.)

By all measures in the literature, Theresa has beaten the odds in terms of surviving her persistent vegetative state condition. While younger persons fare better than older victims, life spans rarely, according to the American Academy of Neurology, exceed ten years following the onset of the condition. Persons who have been comatose have worse outcomes than those who have not. But Theresa has also far outlived any documented periods from which persons in persistent vegetative states have emerged in any functional capacity. The reasonable degree of medical certainty associated with her diagnosis and prognosis is very high. . . .

Summary of Guardian Ad Litem Recommendations

. . .

1. Should the Governor lift the stay that he previously entered relative to Theresa Schiavo's feeding tube?

   a. Yes. The Governor should lift the stay, if valid, independent scientific medical evidence clearly indicates that Theresa has no reasonable medical hope of regaining any swallowing function and/or if there is no evidence of cognitive function and no hope of improvement.

   b. No. The Governor should not lift the stay if valid, independent scientific medical evidence clearly indicates that Theresa has a reasonable medical hope of regaining any swallowing function and/or if there is evidence of cognitive function with or without hope of improvement.

  2. Is there feasibility and value in swallowing tests and swallowing therapy given the totality of circumstances?

  a. Yes. There is feasibility and value in swallowing tests and swallowing therapy being administered if the parties agree in advance as to how the results of these tests will be used with respect to the decision about Theresa's future. If the parties do not agree in advance as to how the tests will be used, then the court must be prepared to once again make a final judgment on the matter. Given the history of the case, this would not, in and of itself, assure a resolution, and is not, therefore, deemed either feasible or of value to Theresa Schiavo without prior agreement.

The GAL concludes from the medical records and consultations with medical experts that the scope and weight of the medical information within the file concerning Theresa Schiavo consists of competent, well-documented information that she is in a persistent vegetative state with no likelihood of improvement, and that the neurological and speech pathology evidence in the file support the contention that she cannot take oral nutrition or hydration and cannot consciously interact with her environment.

The GAL concludes that the trier of fact and the evidence that served as the basis for the decisions regarding Theresa Schiavo were firmly grounded within Florida statutory and case law, which clearly and unequivocally provide for the removal of artificial nutrition in cases of persistent vegetative states, where there is no advance directive, through substituted/proxy judgment of the guardian and/or the court as guardian, and with the use of evidence regarding the medical condition and the intent of the parties that was deemed, by the trier of fact to be clear and convincing. . . .

We remain in Theresa Schiavo's shoes.

Tom Koch 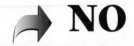 **NO**

The Challenge of Terri Schiavo: Lessons for Bioethics

Definitions

Since her collapse in 1990, Mrs Schiavo had been assumed to be in a "persistent vegetative state," legally defined in a Florida statute as a "permanent and irreversible condition of unconsciousness" from which no recovery is possible.[1] Withdrawal of nutrition and hydration permitting a "natural" death was therefore appropriate in a "terminal condition" like Mrs Schiavo's where end-of-life protocols are legally permitted in Florida statutes for "end-stage" cases.[2]

Those seeking Mrs Schiavo's continuance argued, however, her condition was only "end-stage" and "terminal" when hydration and nutrition were removed. Her life might have continued for years had her care continued. In this construction withdrawal of hydration and nutrition is active euthanasia neither warranted clinically nor to be accepted ethically. Simply, advocates of her continued care reject the argument that cessation of life support, prohibited in all other situations, is acceptable when physical or cognitive limits are defined as extreme.

More concretely, some challenge the diagnosis of persistent vegetative state itself as uncertain and open to challenge. This argument is given weight in a series of clinical studies published in recent years. Shewmon,[3] for example, argues that contrary to standard definitions we cannot state categorically that the vegetative state is defined by a total loss of cortical function. Others studying patients diagnosed as vegetative—a term many critiques reject as demeaning[4] have found that between 12% and 34% of patients diagnosed as persistently vegetative are at least minimally conscious and may respond to therapy.[5]

Suffering and "Quality of Life"

For some bioethicists the niceties of these distinctions are largely irrelevant. A person in Mrs Schiavo's obviously limited state is "suffering" from an unacceptably minimal "quality of life" that may be "naturally" ended by the withdrawal of hydration and nutrition. In such situations euthanasia is permissible, and in Helga Kuhse's words, "doctors should be permitted to give death a helping hand."[6]

If all cerebral function had ceased Mrs Schiavo could not have been suffering, however. And if she had been even minimally conscious then death

From *Journal of Medical Ethics*, Vol. 31, No. 7, July 1, 2005, pp. 376–378. Copyright © 2005 by Institute of Medical Ethics. Reprinted by permission of BMJ Publishing Group via Rightslink.

by starvation and thirst would themselves have caused suffering that cannot, critics say, be supported. The doctor's "helping hand", encouraged by some bioethicists, seen from this perspective is malicious. To assume there is no "benefit" to continuation because treatment will be "futile"—with no curative value[7]—imposes upon the patient a doctor's frustration at being unable to do anything but maintain his or her patient in a limited state.

Further, arguing that Mrs Schiavo's quality of life was insupportable, and death therefore preferable to continuation, conjures for some the eugenic arguments famously argued by Binding and Hoche in 1920s Germany,[8] and more generally by US eugenicists from Haiselden to Mr Justice Oliver Wendell Holmes in the famous US Supreme Court decision *Buck v Bell* (for a comprehensive review of this history see Pernick, 1996[9]).

This critique empowers a radically different reading of not simply appropriate behaviour in the Schiavo case but in a range of situations—genetic, neurological, and post-traumatic injury—involving those with physical and cognitive limits. From this perspective the battle over Terri Schiavo's continuance was a special case within a far broader field of dispute over the legitimate rights of restricted persons and the broader duty for their continuing care. The importance of this challenge, and the strength of its argument, is signalled by US Congressional and state legislative involvement in this case. To the extent law reflects the ethics of a population, arguments in this case signal the rise of an ethical and moral construct strongly opposed to accepted standards of practice currently codified in law and the bioethics literature. For those who argue Mrs Schiavo's continuance, and by extension that of others in physically or cognitively limited states, legislatures are the appropriate place to seek longer term relief, replacing codes informed by one ethical perspective with another.

Personhood

Perhaps the central issue in ethics and law is what we mean by personhood within the circle of protected life. Among Mrs Schiavo's supporters, and more generally within some disability communities, personhood is not an existential attribute based upon cognitive or physical abilities but a communal attribute whose meaning is grounded in one's relationship to others.[10] In this construction Mrs Schiavo was a person equal to others because her parents said she was and her continuance had been mandated by their historically anchored, unwavering commitment to that relationship's continuance.

The argument finds some support in the literature of medical ethics and bioethics. The enduring popularity of Oliver Sacks's work—from *Awakenings*[11] to *An Anthropologist on Mars*[12]—is based in large part on his insistence that even the most extreme neurological conditions deny neither personhood nor the duty to care. In this construct the sustaining relation need not be reciprocal to be respected. "I see how you love her", Sacks says to the father of an autistic artist.[13] "Does she love you, too?" The answer, one Sacks obviously accepts as sufficient, is: "She loves us as much as she can."

Stephen G Post implies a similar valuation when he considers a Cleveland man who lovingly maintains his persistently unconscious wife. "Even the

PVS conditions does not disqualify a loved one from equal moral standing. . . . It further suggests that the concept of quality of life might be replaced by the quality of lives, including family members."[14] The result is a duty to care for the person the family member perceives as a person-in-relation.

The distance between this definition of the person and one of the person as a discrete, existential being lies at the heart of a now famous exchange between disability rights lawyer Harriet McBryde Johnson and Princeton University bioethicist Peter Singer.[15] She described a family's caring at home for a persistently unconscious teenager as "beautiful", an act that Singer thought somewhat "weird". The gulf between their ethical frames was sufficiently severe to prevent either from clearly arguing the primary values and resulting constructs that resulted in the apparently aesthetic judgements.[16]

It may be this sense of personhood as a shared rather than discrete quality that fuelled the extraordinary public demonstration of support for Terri Schiavo's survival. For those protesting the withdrawal of hydration and nutrition, the act of demonstration served in itself as affirmation of Mrs Schiavo's personhood and thus her place within the protected circle of the state's "life interest" in its citizens. The unprecedented political involvement of the Florida State Legislature and the US Congress in the Schiavo case is, from this perspective, wholly appropriate. Where else in a democracy do citizens turn when they believe current policy and law are inappropriate, prejudicial, and unethical? When courts cannot offer redress the logical next step is to seek legislation that will alter the laws in a manner that permits future judicial support.

Sanctity of Life

The central concern of Mrs Schiavo's supporters appears to be that physical continuance is lexicographically a primary value violated by the discontinuation of her nutrition and hydration. That many who so argued in the Florida case did so from a religious perspective is neither surprising nor relevant. The operative law and ethic in North America, as it is in Europe, is at heart Judeo-Christian. The "sanctity of life" argument espoused by many in this case has deep roots in that tradition as well as a long secular tradition.

Peter Singer's famous declaration that "after ruling our thoughts and our decisions about life and death for nearly two thousand years, the traditional western ethic [of life sanctity] has collapsed" was clearly premature.[17] The Schiavo case signals a resurgence of this collapsed ethic as a lexicographically superior, primary value, one in which the default remains life sanctity irrespective of "quality". Whether those arguing a "culture of care", will do so uniformly and realistically—embracing the increased taxation a fully caring culture assuredly would require, for example—is a separate if important issue.

Conclusion

The story of the public debate surrounding Terri Schiavo should impress upon laypersons and professionals alike the uncertainty of the context in which issues of continuation and termination are argued ethically. Nobody knows what Mrs Schiavo would have wanted. She left no advance directive and in its absence her husband says one thing and her parents another. While the husband is the typical surrogate in this case his status has been challenged for a decade by her parents. Similarly, we do not know to an absolute certainty her cognitive status. Was she "minimally conscious" or permanently unconscious? In either case we do not know to an absolute certainty whether or not she sensed any discomfort from dehydration and starvation, or anything else. Our neurology is insufficient to make a definitive determination.

These uncertainties pale before the greater one: What is the ethical frame in which such cases should be judged? Bioethicists who assume the facts are clear and the frame for their application self-evident dismiss the concerns of those who coherently argue from a different ethical framework. The result will be to marginalise their own position, assuring their status as non-participants in the ethical, moral, legal, and political debates this case generally promotes.

Time to redefine the ethical principles of care for restricted people.

References

1. Florida Statute 765.101 s4; 12 a and b; 17.
2. Drager P. Terri Schiavo: Facts. manipulation . . . innuendo . . . bias . . . truth. American Society for Bioethics and the Humanities Annual Meeting, Montreal, PQ, 22–26 October 2003.
3. Shewmon AD. Critical analysis of conceptual domains of the vegetative state: sorting fact from fancy. Neurol Rehab2004;**19**:343–7.
4. Koch T. The difference that difference makes: bioethics and the challenge—disability. J Med Philos2004;29:703.
5. Schoenle PW, Witzke W. How vegetative is the vegetative state? Preserved semantic processing in VS patients—evidence from n 400 event-related potentials. Neurol Rehabil2004;**19**:329–34 Andrews K, Murphy R, Littlewood C, Misdiagnosis of the vegetative state: retrospective study in a rehabilitation unit. BMJ 1996;**313**:13–16; Childs NL, Mercer WN, Childs HW. Accuracy of diagnosis of persistent vegetative state. Neurology1993;**43**:1465–7.
6. Kuhse H. Voluntary euthanasia and other medical end-of-life decisions: doctors should be permitted to give death a helping hand. In: Thomasma DC, Kushner T, eds. Birth to Death: Science and Bioethics. New York: Cambridge University Press, 1996:247–58.
7. Jecker N, Schneiderman LJ. Stopping futile medical treatment: ethical issues. In: Thomasma DC, Kushner T, eds. Birth to Death: Science and Bioethics. New York: Cambridge University Press, 1996, 169–76; at 170.
8. Binding K, Hoche A. 1920. Permitting the destruction of unworthy life: its extent and form, In: Wright W, Deer P, Salmonon R, eds. Trans Issues in Law and Medicine1992;**8**:231–68.
9. Pernick MS. The Black Stork: Eugenics and the death of "defective" babies in American medicine and motion pictures since 1915. New York: Oxford University Press, 1996.

10. Koch T, Singer P. Point counterpoint: the ideology of normalcy: the ethics of difference. J Disabil Policy Studies. 2005, in press.

11. Sacks O. Awakenings (1983) revised edn. New York: Harper Collins, 1990.

12. Sacks O. An Anthropologist on Mars. New York: Knopf, 1995.

13. See reference 17: p. 210.

14. Post SG. The moral challenge of Alzheimer disease. Baltimore, MD: Johns Hopkins Press, 1995:197–8.

15. Koch T. The difference that difference makes (see reference 3); Koch T. Disability and difference: balancing social and physical constructions, J Med Ethics. 2001;**27**: 370–6; Koch T. Life quality vs. the "quality of life": Assumptions underlying prospective quality of life instruments in health care planning. Soc Sci Med2000;**51**:419–28.

16. Lantos J. Johnson, Singer, Almodovar, and the aesthetics of bioethics. ASBH Exchange. 2003;6: 1, 2, 7,.

17. Singer P. Rethinking Life and Death: The Collapse of Our Traditional Ethics. New York: St, Martin's Griffin 1005:1.

EXPLORING THE ISSUE

May Surrogate Decision Makers Terminate Care for a Person in a Persistent Vegetative State?

Critical Thinking and Reflection

1. Would you want your surrogates to keep you alive if you were in a persistent vegetative state? What account of personhood and the value of life would you give as part of an explanation for that view?
2. If someone you love ended up in a PVS and you were asked to be the surrogate decision maker, what sort of evidence could you give to justify your views about what that person would have wanted done?
3. Express Tom Koch's concerns about the Schiavo case in your own words. Can you envision ways of responding constructively to Koch's concerns while still allowing surrogate decisions to withdraw medical treatment?

Is There Common Ground?

The case of Terri Schiavo garnered more media attention and political involvement than did the similar case of Nancy Cruzan, 30 years earlier. Cruzan's family was united in their effort to remove her feeding tube. In contrast, Schiavo's husband Michael began efforts to remove her feeding tube in 1998, declaring that this was his wife's wish should she be in a permanent nonresponsive condition, but her parents, Robert and Mary Schindler, vehemently opposed this action. The case was tried in the legal system and in the court of public opinion through extensive media coverage and political actions. In the end, Michael Schiavo prevailed and the feeding tube was removed.

Perhaps the best hope for reaching common ground in cases like that of Terri Schiavo is the realization that MRI might to some degree allow us to "see" into the brain of people with PVS and at least in some cases gain some confirmation of the diagnosis that otherwise must depend on close observation of the patient's behavior. At the same time, as some commentators have pointed out, it would be easy for family members and physicians to misinterpret the possible MRI results. An article in *New England Journal of Medicine* suggested that MRI might not only show that the brains of some patients now diagnosed as being in a PVS in fact respond to stimuli, but also even allow family and physicians to communicate with some of those minimally responsive patients—that we could ask them to answer yes to a question by imagining

41

that they are playing tennis, for example. But other commentators argue that we are a long way from knowing how to interpret the MRIs, and that meaningful communication with a patient would require much more than activation of different brain areas in response to yes–no questions.

Additional Resources

In March 2006, three books were published presenting different sides of the controversy: Michael Schiavo and Michael Hirsh published *Terri: The Truth* (Dutton); "Terri's Family" (her parents, brother, and sister) published *A Life That Matters: The Legacy of Terri Schiavo—A Lesson for Us All* (Warner Books); and Arthur L. Caplan, James J. McCartney, and Dominic A. Sisti published *The Case of Terri Schiavo: Ethics at the End of Life* (Prometheus).

For the ground-breaking work on the use of MRIs with patients in PVS, see M.M. Monti et al., "Willful Modulation of Brain Activity in Disorders of Consciousness," *New England Journal of Medicine* (vol. 362, 2010, pp. 579–589). For a critical discussion of this work, see J. Andrew Billings, Larry R. Churchill, and Richard Payne, "Severe Brain Injury and the Subjective Life," *Hastings Center Report* (vol. 40, no. 3, 2010, pp. 17–21).

Jay Wolfson has described his experience with Theresa Schiavo in a number of moving articles and essays. See Jay Wolfson, "Erring on the Side of Theresa Schiavo: Reflections of the Special Guardian ad Litem," *Hastings Center Report* (vol. 35, no. 3, 2005, pp. 16–19), and "The Basis for Decisions to End Life. The Schiavo Dilemma: An Essay by the Special Guardian Ad Litem," *Clinical Interventions in Aging* (vol. 1, no. 1, 2006, pp. 3–6).

ISSUE 3

Should Adolescents Be Allowed to Make Their Own Life-and-Death Decisions?

YES: **Robert F. Weir and Charles Peters**, from "Affirming the Decisions Adolescents Make About Life and Death," *Hastings Center Report* (November–December 1997)

NO: **Lainie Friedman Ross**, from "Health Care Decisionmaking by Children" *Hastings Center Report* (November–December 1997)

Learning Outcomes

After reading this issue, you should be able to:

- Describe how the concepts of autonomy and informed consent apply to pediatric and adolescent decision making.
- Discuss the concepts of competence and decision-making capacity and the ability of parents to make decisions in their children's best interests.

ISSUE SUMMARY

YES: Ethicist Robert F. Weir and pediatrician Charles Peters assert that adolescents with normal cognitive and developmental skills have the capacity to make decisions about their own health care. Advance directives, if used appropriately, can give older pediatric patients a voice in their care.

NO: Pediatrician Lainie Friedman Ross counters that parents should be responsible for making their child's health care decisions. Children need to develop virtues, such as self-control, that will enhance their long-term, not just immediate, autonomy.

$\mathbf{A}$ patient is brought to the emergency room after an accident. The physicians believe that he will die if he does not receive a blood transfusion, but the patient says that he is a Jehovah's Witness and will not accept blood. A cancer patient has undergone months of debilitating therapy with discouraging results; she says that she does not want any more treatment. These patients have the right to refuse treatment because they are adults. What if they were 15 or 16 years old? Would they have the same rights or could their wishes be overruled?

If there is one Golden Rule of contemporary bioethics, it is that competent adults are legally and ethically empowered to make health care decisions for themselves. Competent in this context means able to understand the choices and the consequences of decisions made. People base these decisions on values and preferences, personal experiences, religious beliefs, the availability of alternatives, level of pain and suffering, economic consequences, or any combination of these and other factors.

Except in unusual situations, parents are presumed to be in the best position to make these decisions for their children. Children, especially young children, are assumed to have neither the cognitive skills nor the mature judgment to make complex choices that may have far-reaching health consequences. Parents share the consequences of the decision, so they make it with the best interests of their children and themselves in mind.

But adolescents are neither children nor fully mature adults. Where do they fit in this scheme? There are differences of opinion of how to define adolescence. Depending on the definition, adolescence may begin as young as 10 and end as late as 21. Legally the age of 18 defines the end of adolescence. However, that may not be an appropriate boundary for health care decision making. Those who support the idea that young people of a certain age should make their own health care decisions tend to call them "adolescents"; those who are critical of this view tend to call them "children" or "minors." In general adolescents have achieved a degree of emotional and intellectual maturity that surpasses that of young children. Still, they may be unable to appreciate long-term consequences of their actions.

In making health care decisions for children and adolescents, an alliance among the patient, parents, and physicians sometimes develops. Together they choose among alternative plans for treatment or, in the case of terminal illness, palliative care instead of aggressive treatment. However, parents, adolescents, and physicians do not always agree.

The YES and NO selections present two opposing views on whether adolescents should make their own life-and-death decisions. Robert F. Weir and Charles Peters argue for adolescent capacity and autonomy. They summarize an expanding body of professional literature to indicate that, with a few exceptions, adolescents are capable of making major health decisions and giving informed consent. Lainie Friedman Ross argues against the 1995 American Academy of Pediatrics recommendations that give children a greater voice in their care. She contends that it is the parents' right and responsibility to make decisions that enhance their children's long-term autonomy.

YES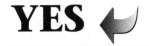

Robert F. Weir and
Charles Peters

Affirming the Decisions Adolescents Make About Life and Death

Some Illustrative Cases

Scott Rose was a talented adolescent who loved poetry, music, writing, and acting. Unfortunately, he had Nezelof syndrome, a cellular immunodeficiency disease similar to the condition of the famous "bubble boy" in Houston. Scott refused to remain in a similar enclosure, preferring to live as normal a life as his condition permitted. At the age of fourteen, with his lungs deteriorating and his suffering increasing, Scott decided that he could accept no more life-sustaining treatment. Against his physician's wishes but with tacit approval from his family, Scott died by disconnecting himself from the ventilator that was keeping him alive in a community hospital in Oklahoma.

C.G. was a fifteen-year-old with end-stage cystic fibrosis. During the last year of his life, he was hospitalized four times in a critical care unit for pneumonia and respiratory distress. He repeatedly expressed fear that his life would end in a slow, agonizing death. He realized that he was dying and stated that he did not want to "smother" or die on a ventilator. On his last admission, he experienced increasing respiratory distress and became disoriented as his carbon dioxide rose. However, his parents were adamant, insisting to the attending physician that "everything possible" be done to keep C.G. alive, including prolonged intubation and mechanical ventilation.

Benito Agrela was born with an enlarged liver and spleen. He received a liver transplant when he was eight years old, had a second liver transplant when he was fourteen, and then stopped taking his medication several months after the second transplant because he could not tolerate its side effects. When the Florida Department of Social Services discovered that he was not taking his antirejection medications, they forcibly removed him from his parents' home and admitted him to a transplant floor of a Miami hospital. After he refused further treatment, his case was taken to court; the circuit court judge spent several hours with Benito and his physicians, then ruled that Benito had a legal right to refuse the medications and return home. Before his death at the age of fifteen, Benito said: "I should have the right to make my own decision. I know the consequences, I know the problems."

M.C. was ten years old when she was diagnosed with acute lymphoblastic leukemia. During two years of chemotherapy, she maintained excellent grades,

From *Hastings Center Report,* Vol. 27, No. 6, November/December 1997, pp. 29–40. Copyright © 1997 by The Hastings Center. Reprinted by permission of Wiley-Blackwell via Rightslink.

joined a swim team, and demonstrated, according to her teachers, "a particularly mature and far-reaching perspective on her life." Then the leukemia relapsed. Following discussions with a health care team and her parents, she decided that a partially matched, related donor bone marrow transplant was her best chance for continued life. Before she received the transplant, at the age of thirteen, she told her parents and others that she did not want to "grow up to be a vegetable," did not want to be supported on "a lot of machines," and did not want to be a psychological or financial burden on the family. Two months after the transplant, she was diagnosed as having an Epstein Barr virus-associated lymphoproliferative disorder. Despite aggressive treatment efforts in a pediatric ICU, her condition did not improve. Four days later the ventilator sustaining her life was withdrawn, at the request of her family and in keeping with her previously expressed wishes.

B.C. was a sixteen-year-old adolescent who was diagnosed with cystic fibrosis shortly after birth. Over the years, both his medical condition and his relationship with his parents deteriorated. He watched several friends with cystic fibrosis die, and mentioned on several occasions that he did not want to be placed on a ventilator. Nevertheless, even as his pulmonary tests deteriorated rapidly, his parents refused to discuss death with him, or any decisions that might need to be made about limiting life-sustaining treatment, the possibility of do-not-resuscitate status, or his preferences about treatment options. When he was soon thereafter admitted, unresponsive, following an unsuccessful suicide attempt, his parents requested that no life-sustaining measures be employed. They forbade the medical staff from discussing this matter with B.C., even when he became sufficiently alert to communicate.

Our reason for presenting these cases is simple. Every day, in hospitals throughout this country, adolescent patients cope with chronic conditions, struggle to survive with life-threatening illnesses, and think about the burdens of continued existence compared with the prospect of death. Sometimes, as indicated by Scott Rose and Benito Agrela, these adolescent patients conclude that death is preferable to the suffering they are experiencing, decide to refuse further life-sustaining interventions, and carry out that decision in spite of opposition from physicians and/or parents. Other times, as in the case of M.C., parents and physicians carry out the decision to abate life-sustaining treatment, knowing it to be consistent with the adolescent patient's wishes. Yet other times, as in the cases of C.G. and B.C., parents request, and physicians carry out, a plan of care that has not been discussed with the adolescent patient and may be completely contrary to his or her expressed wishes.

Such cases reflect the considerable uncertainty that sometimes surrounds the medical management of these patients. Do most adolescents have the capacity to make major decisions about their lives and health, even when they are hospitalized? Do only *some* adolescents have this decisionmaking capacity and, if so, what kinds of lines need to be drawn in terms of adolescent decisional abilities? Do adolescents have the right not only to *assent*, but also to *consent*—and to refuse to consent—to recommended medical treatment or participation in research studies? . . .

Adolescents as Capable Decisionmakers

An expanding body of professional literature indicates that adolescents, with some exceptions, are capable of making major health decisions and giving informed consent, whether in a clinical or research setting. An increasing number of professionals in developmental psychology, pediatrics, biomedical ethics, and health law agree that a fundamental reorientation toward adolescents—in clinical medicine, in research settings, and in the law—is necessary to increase adult acceptance of the important decisions that many adolescents now seem capable of making for themselves.

Numerous studies can be cited to make the basic point. Almost twenty years ago, a comprehensive analysis of the literature in developmental psychology by Thomas Grisso and Linda Vierling indicated that "generally minors below the ages of 11–13 do not possess many of the cognitive capacities one would associate with the psychological elements of 'intelligent' consent."[1] By contrast, the authors stated that there "is little evidence that minors of age 15 and above as a group are any less competent to provide consent than are adults." On the basis of their literature analysis, they concluded that "minors are entitled to have some form of consent or dissent regarding the things that happen to them in the name of assessment, treatment, or other professional activities that have generally been determined unilaterally by adults in the minor's interest." Similar conclusions came from an empirical study reported by Lois Weithron and Susan Campbell.[2]

In the pediatric literature, Sanford Leikin surveyed the findings of developmental psychologists, mainly those of Jean Piaget, and applied them to the issue of minors' assent or dissent to medical treatment. He observed that while cognitive development cannot always be equated with chronological age, good evidence exists "that, by age 14 years, many minors attain the cognitive developmental stage associated with the psychological elements of rational consent." As to other adolescent ages, he concluded that "minors between 11 and 14 years of age appear to be in a transition period . . . [and] there appear to be no psychological grounds for the general assumption that minors 15 years of age or older cannot provide competent consent."[3]

In a subsequent publication Leikin addressed the question of how parents and physicians should respond to the decisions made by adolescents to withhold or withdraw life-sustaining treatment. In large part, he argued, it depends on the psychological development of the adolescent in question and that person's ability to make "authentic choices" guided by logical thought patterns, a physiologic understanding of illness, and a willingness to make decisions independent of authority figures (a willingness, he pointed out, not usually found in adolescents less than fourteen or fifteen years of age).[4] Other writers agree.[5] . . .

Legal Developments

Even if most adolescents between age fourteen and seventeen increasingly are regarded as having the capacity to make health decisions for themselves, and even if leading pediatric groups have for over twenty years called for an expansion of adolescent rights in health care settings, important questions about the law remain. . . .

Traditionally, state laws reflected the view that adolescents and other legal minors under the age of twenty-one were incapable of understanding, deliberating about, and making decisions regarding important health care choices. The power to make such decisions was vested in parents, legal guardians, or someone standing in *loco parentis* to a child. Any physician who might have provided nonemergency medical care to a legal minor without parental consent risked being charged with civil battery (performing treatment without consent), even if there was no charge of malpractice.[6]

Legal minors and personal health decisions.   During the past three decades, this view of legal minors has changed in a number of ways. One important change involves the age of majority. Until 1971, the standard age of majority was twenty-one, with a perennial debate focusing on the differences in age required for voting compared with the age required for being drafted into the military. That debate stopped with the passage of the 26th amendment to the Constitution in 1971, thereby permitting persons aged between eighteen and twenty to vote in federal elections. Most state legislatures subsequently lowered the age of majority to eighteen, thus granting legal adulthood to millions of persons who previously could not vote, make contractual obligations, or consent to medical treatment apart from their parents.[7]

Another change in the law involves the creation of exceptional legal categories for some adolescents to make personal health decisions. Two such categories are common among the states. Some adolescents, depending on the state, are legally recognized as *emancipated minors* on the basis of marriage, parenthood, military service, consent of parents (for example, adolescents who are "thrown away" by parents after family conflicts), judicial order of emancipation, or financial independence. Some state statutes (such as in Arizona, Idaho, Massachusetts, Montana, Nevada, North Carolina, Oregon, and Texas) specifically grant emancipated minors the right to consent to medical treatment.

Other adolescents are legally recognized in some jurisdictions as *mature minors* for the purpose of making health decisions because of their individual ability to understand the nature and purposes of recommended medical treatment. The "mature minor rule" recognizes that some adolescents are sufficiently mature to make their own decisions about recommended medical treatment and, when necessary, to go against their parents' views regarding the treatment. Physicians who carry out these decisions seem to run little legal risk, since there are no reported judicial decisions over the past twenty-five years in which parents have recovered damages for the medical treatment of an adolescent over the age of fifteen without parental consent.[8]

A third change in the law pertains to *minor treatment statutes* according to which states permit legal minors to consent to certain types of medical care. These statutes usually specify certain health problems for which legal minors can seek medical treatment without parental consent, precisely because the nature of the health problems is such that some adolescents would probably choose to go without medical treatment rather than seek their parents' consent for the treatment. Such statutes are typically limited to treatment for sexually transmitted diseases, pregnancy and pregnancy prevention (including abortion in some states, but not sterilization), alcohol and other drug abuse, and in some states, psychiatric problems.

Legal minors, end-of-life decisions, and state legislatures. Despite these changes, most state legislatures have not addressed the issue of treatment refusal by adolescents, especially in circumstances in which a refusal of life-sustaining treatment is likely to result in the adolescent's death. Thus, even though forty-seven states have living will statutes (the exceptions are Massachusetts, Michigan, and New York) and forty-eight states have surrogate decisionmaking statutes that include end-of-life decisions (the exceptions are Alabama and Alaska), the legislative statutes in thirty-eight states and the District of Columbia do not specifically address end-of-life decisions made by legal minors.[9]

Most state legislatures seem to think that adolescents either do not die in clinical settings, or are incapable of making informed consent or informed refusal decisions about treatment options, must be protected from their own lack of judgment, or simply should not be permitted to give legally binding advance directions regarding life-sustaining treatments and surrogate decisionmakers. If a given adolescent does not qualify for emancipation under state law, does not live in one of the three states (Alaska, Arkansas, and Mississippi) having a mature-minor statute, and is unable or unwilling for some reason to go through a judicial hearing to be designated a mature minor, he or she is left with only three options: (1) persuading parents and physicians to act according to the adolescent's expressed views on life-sustaining treatment, (2) persuading parents to execute an advance directive on the patient's behalf (in the seven states having this legal option), or (3) acquiescing to the views of legal adults (namely, parents and physicians) regarding the medical circumstances under which the remaining portion of life is to be lived. . . .

Advance Directives and Moral Persuasion

Most adolescents who want to participate in the decisionmaking process connected with their medical conditions, especially in regard to decisions about life-sustaining medical interventions, have chronic conditions that often deteriorate over time: certain kinds of cancer, cystic fibrosis, AIDS, complicated types of heart disease, and so on. Having experienced years of physical and psychological suffering, gone through multiple hospitalizations and numerous treatments, probably experienced depression, and probably observed the suffering and dying of several hospitalized friends with similar medical problems, these adolescent patients are frequently mature beyond their chronological years. They have had, at the very least, multiple opportunities to think about the inescapable suffering that characterizes their lives, the features of life that make it worth continuing, the benefits and burdens that accompany medical treatment, and the prospect of death. At least some of these adolescents want to give voice to their values, provide directions for parents, physicians, and nurses regarding end-of-life care, and be assured that their wishes and preferences will be respected and carried out should their medical conditions deteriorate to the point that they will no longer be able to communicate their deeply felt views.

How parents, physicians, nurses, and other health professionals respond to these adolescents' desires for control and self-determination at the end of life is vitally important. These adults, individually and collectively, may simply *choose not to* listen. Alternatively, parents, physicians, and other adults involved in these cases may think that these personal life-and-death decisions are *primarily matters of law,* quite apart from the wishes and preferences expressed by individual patients. If so, the attending physician will likely check with hospital legal counsel, who will report on relevant statutory and case law and give legal advice that, understandably, will be protective of the hospital's legal interests. . . .

There is a third alternative. Parents, physicians, and other adults involved in these cases may regard the thoughtful comments, the verbalized reflections on the meaning of life and death, and the communicated choices regarding treatment options by *at least some* (perhaps most) adolescents with life-threatening conditions as *efforts of moral persuasion,* quite apart from what the law may or may not say.[10] Parents may reluctantly conclude that their son or daughter has suffered enough, seen enough, and communicated enough to convince them that however much they may want their child to live, he or she has the moral right to make end-of-life decisions that, when carried out, will result in death. Physicians, nurses, and other health care professionals also may be convinced.

Advance directives can help meet this goal, especially if the use of such directives becomes an acceptable part of the informed consent process in pediatric medicine. Enabling at least some adolescent patients—patients with chronic, life-threatening conditions—to communicate their decisions about treatment options through oral or written advance directives would also provide a measure of legal protection for physicians. Pediatricians, family practice physicians, and other physicians having such cases would be more able to document the specific end-of-life treatment decisions made by these patients, the maturity and decisionmaking capacity of individual patients, and the conversations about consenting to or refusing life-sustaining treatment that had taken place with the patients and their parents.

References

1. Thomas Grisso and Linda Vierling, "Minors' Consent to Treatment: A Developmental Perspective," *Professional Psychology* 9 (August 1978): 412–427, at 420.

2. Lois A. Weithorn and Susan B. Campbell, "The Competency of Children and Adolescents to Make Informed Treatment Decisions," *Child Development* 53 (1982): 1589–98.

3. Sanford L. Leikin, "Minors' Assent or Dissent to Medical Treatment," *Journal of Pediatrics* 102 (1983): 173.

4. Sanford L. Leikin, "A Proposal Concerning Decisions to Forgo Life-Sustaining Treatment for Young People," *Journal of Pediatrics* 108 (1989): 17–22, at 20; Leikin, "The Role of Adolescents in Decisions Concerning Their Cancer Therapy," *Cancer Supplement* 71 (15 May 1993): 3342–46.

5. For example, C. E. Lewis, "A Comparison of Minors' and Adults' Pregnancy Decisions," *American Journal of Orthopsychiatry* 50 (1980): 446–53; Richard H. Nicholson, ed., *Medical Research with Children* (Oxford: Oxford University Press, 1986), p. 140–52; Angela Holder, *Legal Issues in Pediatrics and Adolescent Medicine,* 2d ed. (New Haven: Yale University Press, 1985), p. 133.

6. Sarah D. Cohn, "The Evolving Law of Adolescent Health Care," *Clinical Issues 2* (1991): 201–7, at 201; Angela R. Holder, "Disclosure and Consent Problems in Pediatrics," *Law, Medicine & Health Care* 16 (1988): 219–28; Steven M. Selbst, "Treating Minors Without Their Parents," *Pediatric Emergency Care* 1 (1985): 168–73.

7. Richard A. Leiter, ed., *National Survey of State Laws* (Detroit: Gale Research Inc., 1993), pp. 279–91.

8. Angela R. Holder, "Children and Adolescents: Their Right to Decide about Their Own Health Care," in *Children and Health Care: Moral and Social Issues,* ed. Loretta Kopelman and John C. Moskop (Boston: Kluwer Academic Publishers, 1989), p. 163.

9. Information from Choice in Dying, New York, 1995.

10. Robert F. Weir, "Advance Directives as Instruments of Moral Persuasion," in *Medicine Unbound,* ed. Robert H. Blank and Andrea L. Bonnicksen (New York: Columbia University Press, 1994), pp. 171–87.

Lainie Friedman Ross 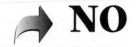 **NO**

Health Care Decisionmaking by Children

In pediatrics, the doctor-patient relationship traditionally has included three parties: the physician, the child, and his or her parents. Parents were not merely surrogate decisionmakers on the grounds of child incompetence, but rather, parents were believed to have both a right and a responsibility to partake in their child's medical decisions.[1] In this [selection] I will examine the evolving position regarding the role of the child in the decisionmaking process as advocated by the American Academy of Pediatrics (AAP). I will offer both moral and pragmatic arguments why I believe this position is misguided.

Recommendations of the American Academy of Pediatrics

In 1995, the AAP published its recommendations for the role of children in health care decisionmaking. The AAP recommended that the child's voice be given greater weight as the child matured. The AAP categorized children as (1) those who lack decisionmaking capacity; (2) those with a developing capacity; and (3) those who have decisionmaking capacity for health care decisions.[2]

For children who lack decisionmaking capacity, the AAP recommended that their parents should make decisions unless their decisions are abusive or neglectful. When children have developing decisionmaking capacity, the physician should seek parental permission and the child's assent. In many cases, the child's dissent should be binding, or at minimum, the physician should seek third-party mediation for parent-child disagreement. Although the child who dissents to life-saving care can be overruled, attempts should be made to persuade the child to assent for "coercion in diagnosis or treatment is a last resort." When children have decisionmaking capacity, the AAP concluded that the children should give informed consent for themselves and their parents should be viewed as consultants.

A major problem with the AAP recommendations is that it assumes decisionmaking capacity can be defined and measured, although the AAP offers no guidance as to what this definition is or how to test for it. Instead, the AAP recommends individual assessment of decisionmaking capacity in each case. However, since there are no criteria on which to base maturity or decisionmaking capacity, the decision of whether to respect a child's decision is dependent upon the judgment of the particular pediatrician—a judgment he or she has no training to make.

My main concern with the AAP recommendations, however, is what should be done when parents and children disagree on health care decisions: according to the AAP, if there is parental-child disagreement and the child is judged to have decisionmaking authority, the child's decision should be binding. If the child has developing capacity, various mechanisms to resolve the conflict should be attempted. They propose:

> short term counseling or psychiatric consultation for patient and/or family, "case management" or similar multidisciplinary conference(s), and/or consultation with individuals trained in clinical ethics or a hospital based ethics committee. In rare cases of refractory disagreement, formal legal adjudication may be necessary.

I will ignore the difficulties in determining whether a minor has decision-making capacity and assume that some minors are competent to make at least some health care decisions. If autonomy is based solely on competency, then competent children should have decisionmaking autonomy in the health care setting. It is my view, however, that even if children are competent, there is a morally significant difference between competent minors and adults. Competency is a necessary but not a sufficient condition on which to base respect for a minor's health care decisionmaking autonomy.

Competency of Children

The psychological literature divides the process of giving informed consent into three components: the patient's consent is informed (made knowingly), is competent (made intelligently), and is voluntary.[3] Although a survey of the literature reveals scant empirical data, existing data suggest that most health care decisions made by adults and children do not fulfill these three components.[4] The data also suggest that adults and older children do not significantly differ in their consent skills.[5] If competency is the only criterion on which respect for autonomy in health care is based, then this difference in treatment cannot be justified.

No test has been developed that uniformly distinguishes all competent individuals from incompetent individuals. Given that competency is context-specific, it is doubtful whether such a test could be developed. And even if a nonculturally biased, objective test could be devised, individual testing of every potential patient would exact a high price in terms of efficiency, privacy, and respect for autonomy. Instead, adults have traditionally been presumed competent and children have been presumed incompetent. That is, respect for autonomy in health care uses both a threshold concept of competency and an age-standard.

To some extent the age-standard is arbitrary as there are individuals above the line (older than the legal age of emancipation) who are incompetent and individuals below the line (younger than the legal age of emancipation) who are competent. But the statutes are not capricious: in general, individuals above the line are more likely to be competent than individuals below it.

Autonomy of Children

One reason to limit the child's present-day autonomy is based on the argument that parents and other authorities need to promote the child's life-time autonomy. Given the value that is placed on self-determination, it makes sense to grant adults autonomy provided that they have some threshold level of competency. Respect is shown by respecting their present project pursuits. But respect for a threshold of competency in children places the emphasis on present-day autonomy rather than on a child's life-time autonomy. Children need a protected period in which to develop "enabling virtues"—habits, including the habit of self-control, which advance their life-time autonomy and opportunities. Although many adults would also benefit from developing their potentials and improving their skills and self-control, at some point (and it is reasonable to use the age of emancipation as the proper cut-off), the advantages of self-determination outweigh the benefits of further guidance and its potential to improve life-time autonomy.

A second reason to limit the child's present-day autonomy is the fact that the child's decisions are based on limited world experience and so her decisions are not part of a well-conceived life plan. Again, many adults have limited world experience, but children have a greater potential for improving their knowledge base and for improving their skills of critical reflection and self-control. . . . By protecting the child from his own impetuosity, his parents help him obtain the background knowledge of the world and the capacities that will allow him to make decisions that better promote his life plans. His parents' attempt to help him flourish may not be achieved, but that does not invalidate their attempt.

A third reason childhood competency should not necessarily entail respect for a child's autonomy is the significant role that intimate families play in our lives. Elsewhere, I have argued that when the family is intimate, parents should have wide discretion in pursuing family goals, goals which may compete and conflict with the goals of particular members.[6] In general, parental autonomy promotes the interests and goals of both children and parents. It serves the needs and interests of the child to have autonomous parents who will help him become an autonomous individual capable of devising and implementing his own life plan. It serves the adults' interest in having and raising a family according to their own vision of the good life. These interests do not abruptly cease when the child becomes competent. If anything, now parents have the opportunity to inculcate their beliefs through rational discourse, instead of through example, bribery, or force.

There are also pragmatic reasons to permit parents to override the present-day autonomy of competent children. First, one can argue for a determination of competency that allows unusually mature children to be emancipated. The problem, as I have already mentioned, is that no such test exists. Second, one can acknowledge that it is best if parents recognize their child's maturity and treat them accordingly, but deny that this justifies granting competent children legal emancipation. Many parents respect their mature child's decisions voluntarily. Laura Purdy remarks: "It is plausible to think that children's maturity is not completely unrelated to parental good sense."[7] Child liberationists may object because a voluntary approach only encourages parents to respect their children's autonomy, but it does not legally enforce it. However, the voluntary approach is more consistent with a policy to limit the state's role in intrafamilial decisions, which is important for the family's ability to flourish.

Health Care Rights in Context

A final argument against respecting the health care decisions of minors is based on placing the notion of health care rights in context. Most individuals who support health care decisionmaking for children view it as an exception and do not seek to emancipate children in other spheres. But why should a child who is competent to make major health care decisions not have the right to make other types of decisions? That is, if a fourteen-year-old is competent to make life-and-death decisions, then why can't this fourteen-year-old buy and smoke cigarettes? Participate in interscholastic football without his parents' consent? Or even drop out of school? . . .

What would it mean to endorse equal rights for children? It is a radical proposal with wide repercussions.[8] It would mean that children could make binding contracts, and that there would be the dissolution of child labor laws, mandatory education, statutory rape laws, and child neglect statutes. As such, it would give children rights for which they are ill-prepared and deny them the protection they need from predatory adults. It would leave children even more vulnerable than they presently are.

Endorsement of child liberation would make a child's membership in a family voluntary. For example, Howard Cohen argues that children should be allowed to change families, either because the child's parents are abusive, or because a neighbor or wealthy stranger offers him a better deal.[9] Such freedom ignores the important role that continuity and permanence play in the parent-child relationship—a significance the child may not yet appreciate.[10] . . .

The Family as the Locus of Decisionmaking

One of my major concerns with the AAP's recommendations is their willingness to involve third-parties in the decisionmaking process. My concern is that these decisions undermine the family. Physicians provide only for the child's transient medical needs; his parents provide for all of his needs and are responsible for raising the child in such a way that he becomes an autonomous responsible adult. Goldstein and colleagues at Yale University's Child Study Center expressed their concern that health care professionals sometimes forget where their professional responsibilities end, and described the harm that we do when we think we can replace parents.[11] By deciding that the child's decision should be respected over the parents' decision, physicians are replacing the parents' judgment that the decision should be overridden with their judgment that the child's decision should be respected. To do so makes this less an issue of respecting the child's autonomy, and more about deciding who knows what is best for the child. In general, parents are the better judge as they have a more vested interest in their child's well-being and are responsible for the day-to-day decisions of child-rearing. It behooves physicians to be humble as they are neither able nor willing to take over this daily function.

I do not mean to suggest that children, particularly mature children, should be ignored in the decisionmaking process. Diagnostic tests and treatment plans should be explained to children to help them understand what is being done to them and to garner, when possible, their cooperation. Parents should include their children in the decisionmaking process both to get their active support and to help them learn how to make such decisions. However, when there is parental-child disagreement, the child's decision should not be decisive nor should health care providers, as I have argued, seek third-party mediation. Rather, as I have already argued, there are both moral and pragmatic reasons why the parents should have final decisionmaking authority.

References

1. Allen Buchanan and Dan Brock, *Deciding for Others: The Ethics of Surrogate Decision Making* (New York: Cambridge University Press, 1989).

2. American Academy of Pediatrics, Committee on Bioethics, "Informed Consent, Parental Permission, and Assent in Pediatric Practice," *Pediatrics* 95 (1995): 314–17.

3. Thomas Grisso and Linda Vierling, "Minor's Consent to Treatment: A Developmental Perspective," *Professional Psychology* 9, no. 3 (1978): 412–27.

4. Paul S. Appelbaum, Charles W. Lidz, and Alan Meisel, *Informed Consent: Legal Theory and Clinical Practice* (New York: Oxford University Press, 1987); Stanley Milgram, *Obedience to Authority: An Experimental View* (New York: Harper and Row, 1974).

5. Grisso and Vierling, "Minor's Consent to Treatment."

6. Lainie Friedman Ross, *Health Care Decision Making for Children,* unpublished manuscript, 1996.

7. Laura M. Purdy, *In Their Best Interest? The Case Against Equal Rights for Children* (New York: Cornell University Press, 1992).

8. Richard Farson, "A Child's Bill of Rights," in *Justice: Selected Readings,* ed. Joel Feinberg and Hyman Gross (Belmont, Calif.: Dickenson Publishing Co. 1977).

9. Howard Cohen, *Equal Rights for Children* (Totowa, N.J.: Rowman and Littlefield, 1980); John Harris, "The Political Status of Children," in *Contemporary Political Philosophy,* ed. Keith Graham (Cambridge, Mass.: Cambridge University Press, 1982), pp. 35–55.

10. Joseph Goldstein, Anna Freud, and Albert J. Solnit, *Before the Best Interests of the Child* (New York: The Free Press, 1979).

11. Joseph Goldstein et al., *In the Best Interest of the Child* (New York: The Free Press, 1986).

EXPLORING THE ISSUE

Should Adolescents Be Allowed to Make Their Own Life-and-Death Decisions?

Critical Thinking and Reflection

1. What do you think are the criteria relevant to determining whether a person is competent? If someone demonstrates competence to make some major decisions, does that mean that the person should also be deemed competent to make health care decisions?
2. Are all health care decisions the same? Could a person be justifiably considered competent to make some decisions but not others?
3. Ross argues that a child's autonomy should be considered limited even if the child is competent to make decisions. How would you describe Ross's account of autonomy? What does she mean by "lifetime autonomy" and "a well-conceived life plan"?
4. Why does Ross think that the family's role in shaping decisions for the child should not be eclipsed by the child's autonomy? How would Weir and Peters respond?

Is There Common Ground?

Prominent legal cases continue to show a wide divide in thinking about adolescents' capacity to make their own health care decisions. In August 2006, Starchild Abraham Cherrix, a 16-year-old Virginia adolescent with Hodgkin's disease, a form of cancer, was granted the right to pursue a course of Hoxsey therapy instead of chemotherapy. Hoxsey therapy is an alternative form of herbal therapy that is illegal in the United States but is available in Mexico. The case was settled out of court at the start of what was to be a 2-day hearing. In this case, Starchild Abraham's parents supported his decision to forego the second round of chemotherapy that his doctors recommended. As of June 2008, when Abraham turned 18, he was free of Hodgkin's disease and no longer had to report his blood test results to a court. "Abraham's law," passed in Virginia, gives teenagers and their parents the right to refuse doctor-recommended treatments for life-threatening ailments.

In Washington State, Dennis Lindberg, 14, died in November 2007, 3 weeks after a court granted his right to refuse blood transfusions for leukemia because of his Jehovah's Witness religious beliefs. His biological parents opposed the court's decision, but it was supported by his aunt, a Jehovah's Witness, and uncle, who had taken over his care because his birth parents were addicted to drugs.

Some scholars have suggested that children and young adults who have chronic health conditions such as diabetes, and who, therefore, must learn to make decisions about their health needs on a regular basis, are particularly likely to develop a capacity to do so.

Additional Resources

A recent special issue of *Journal of Medicine and Philosophy* contains several articles on pediatric decision making. See *Journal of Medicine and Philosophy* (vol. 35, no. 5, 2010).

For a commentary opposing the court decision in the case of Dennis Lindberg, see Rosamond Rhodes, "Death or Damnation: An Adolescent's Treatment Refusal," www.thehastingscenter.org/BioethicsForum

For a discussion of children's decision-making capacity for chronic conditions, particularly diabetes, see Priscilla Alderson, Katy Sutcliffe, and Katherine Curtis, "Children's Competence to Consent to Medical Treatment," *Hastings Center Report* (vol. 36, no. 6, 2006, pp. 25–34).

Three earlier cases are discussed in Isabel Traugott and Ann Alpers, "In Their Own Hands: Adolescents' Refusals of Medical Treatment," *Archives of Pediatric and Adolescent Medicine* (September 1, 1997). Although published in 1985, *Legal Issues in Pediatrics and Adolescent Medicine* by Angela Roddey Holder (Yale University Press) is still a classic text. She supports the right of competent adolescents to make treatment decisions. Other documents supporting this position are the 1995 statement of the American Academy of Pediatrics (cited in the selection by Ross) and "Health Care Decision Making Guidelines for Minors" (Midwest Bioethics Center, 1995). Hillary Rodham Clinton also supports children's rights in several articles, including "Children's Rights: A Legal Perspective," *Children's Rights: Contemporary Perspectives*, edited by Patricia A. Vardin and Ilene N. Brody (Teachers College Press, 1979). Among those critical of the movement to grant children and adolescents more decision-making authority is Laura M. Purdy, *In Their Best Interests? The Case Against Equal Rights for Children* (Cornell University Press, 1992). In "Minor Rights and Wrongs," *Journal of Law, Medicine & Ethics* (Summer 1996), Michelle Oberman urges particular concern about cases in which adolescents refuse life-sustaining treatment.

In *The Adolescent "Alone": Decision Making in Health Care in the United States* (Cambridge University Press, 1999), Jeffrey Blustein, Nancy N. Dubler, and Carol Levine present a series of papers and case studies concerning adolescents who do not have a parent or surrogate in their lives to help them make health care decisions.

A useful resource for thinking about competence generally is Thomas Grisso and Paul S. Appelbaum, *Assessing Competence to Consent to Treatment: A Guide for Physicians and Other Health Professionals* (New York: Oxford University Press, 2000).

Internet References . . .

National Hospice and Palliative Care Organization

This organization's Web site has information about each state's advance directive rules as well as aspects of care of dying people. See especially the Caring Connections program on the site.

www.nhpco.org

Euthanasia and Physician-Assisted Suicide: All Sides of the Issues

This site offers a general overview of the controversy concerning physician-assisted suicide as well as statistics and a list of Web sites that represent both sides of the debate.

www.religioustolerance.org/euthanas.htm

U.S. Catholic Conference of Bishops

Essays and other resources on this site set out the Catholic position against physician-assisted suicide.

**www.usccb.org/issues-and-action/human-life-and-dignity/
assisted-suicide/**

End-of-Life Dilemmas

*W*hat are the ethical responsibilities associated with death? Doctors are sworn "to do no harm," but this proscription is open to many different interpretations. Death is a natural event that can, in some instances, be hastened to put an end to suffering. Is it ethically necessary to prolong life at all times under all circumstances? Medical personnel as well as families often face this agonizing question. The right of an individual to decide his or her own fate may conflict with society's interest in maintaining the value of human life. Even when doctors uphold the value of human life, however, they should surely strive to help their patients die with as little pain and suffering as possible. But what does that mean? How far may doctors go to bring about a "good" death? This unit examines some of these anguishing questions.

- Have Advance Directives Failed?
- Is "Palliative Sedation" Ethically Different from Active Euthanasia?
- Should Physicians Be Allowed to Assist in Patient Suicide?

ISSUE 4

Have Advance Directives Failed?

YES: **Angela Fagerlin and Carl E. Schneider,** from "Enough: The Failure of the Living Will," *Hastings Center Report* (March–April 2004)

NO: **Susan E. Hickman et al.,** from "Hope for the Future: Achieving the Original Intent of Advance Directives," *Hastings Center Report* (November–December 2005)

Learning Outcomes

After reading this issue, you should be able to:

- Discuss the challenges of anticipating and making decisions about one's own health care needs at the end of life.
- Describe the concepts of advance directives, living wills, health care durable powers of attorney, and physician orders for life-sustaining treatment.

ISSUE SUMMARY

YES: Psychologist Angela Fagerlin and law professor Carl E. Schneider believe not only that living wills have failed to live up to their advocates' expectations but also that these expectations were unrealistic from the start.

NO: Susan E. Hickman, Bernard J. Hammes, Alvin H. Moss, and Susan W. Tolle, multidisciplinary specialists in end-of-life care, recognize the limitations of traditional advance directives but argue that newer processes of introducing advance directives can achieve their original aims.

Since ancient times people have drawn up wills to determine what should be done with their property, or who should take custody of their children, after they die. In 1969 Luis Kutner, a law professor, proposed a "living will," a document that would determine the course of medical treatment should the signer become unable to express his or her wishes. A typical living will states,

"If I am permanently unconscious or there is no reasonable expectation for my recovery from a serious incapacitating or lethal illness or condition, I do not wish to be kept alive by artificial means." The proposal came at a time when the public was just beginning to be aware of the use of machines to keep people breathing and their hearts beating even though there was no possibility of regaining consciousness. In 1975, the Karen Ann Quinlan case, involving a young, permanently unconsciousness woman on a ventilator, focused ethical and legal attention on the unwanted use of medical technology.

In 1976, following the Quinlan case, California enacted the nation's first law approving the use of living wills. Nearly every state in the United States followed suit. Sometimes called "natural death acts," these laws and the wills they approved were so vaguely worded and so difficult to interpret that they were hardly ever effective in achieving their goals. It was difficult, for example, to determine what was meant by "reasonable expectation," "artificial means," or even "lethal illness."

In 1983 the President's Commission for the Study of Ethical Problems in Medicine and Biomedical and Behavioral Research recommended an alternative approach. Rather than signing a document that specified certain treatments that should be forgone, patients were encouraged to name a person who would make health care decisions in their place.

There are several types of advance directives. They can be formally written and legally authorized, or they can be informal communications with family members or health care providers. Much of the legal wrangling about withdrawal of life supports has turned on whether or not the patient expressed such desires while competent. The case of Nancy Cruzan, which eventually went to the U.S. Supreme Court, is one example. The parents of this young Missouri woman, who was permanently unconscious after an automobile accident, sued the state to have her life supports removed, claiming that this is what Nancy herself would have wanted. The state argued that there was no clear and convincing evidence that Nancy would have made the same decision. In 1990 the U.S. Supreme Court ruled that states had an interest in preserving life and could require a high standard of evidence of the patient's expressed preference for withdrawing treatment. The case then went back to the Missouri courts, which this time found the evidence convincing and agreed to allow withdrawal of life support.

To add to the weight of the Supreme Court's decision, in 1991 Congress passed the Patient Self-Determination Act (PSDA), which requires all health care providers reimbursed by Medicare to inform patients about their right to sign advance directives. By this measure Congress intended to promote the use of advance directives in hospitals and nursing homes where elderly patients are often treated.

Despite legislative and judicial approval of advance directives and widespread public opinion supporting them, such documents are still rarely signed by competent patients, and even when signed they are still rarely consulted or implemented. Studies have documented barriers such as lack of appropriate communication and physicians' disregard of the wishes expressed in the directives.

The YES and NO selections address the status and future of advance directives from the vantage point of more than 30 years' experience. Angela Fagerlin and Carl E. Schneider want to call halt to the attempt to get people to sign living wills (not health care proxies) because they believe that despite vigorous attempts, the policy has not produced results. Susan E. Hickman and colleagues argue that the original intent of advance directives—to enable patients to gain control over their terminal care—can be achieved by newer, more successful models.

YES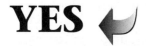

Angela Fagerlin and
Carl E. Schneider

Enough: The Failure of the Living Will

By their fruits ye shall know them.

Enough. The living will has failed, and it is time to say so.

We should have known it would fail: A notable but neglected psychological literature always provided arresting reasons to expect the policy of living wills to misfire. Given their alluring potential, perhaps they were worth trying. But a crescendoing empirical literature and persistent clinical disappointments reveal that the rewards of the campaign to promote living wills do not justify its costs. Nor can any degree of tinkering ever make the living will an effective instrument of social policy.

As the evidence of failure has mounted, living wills have lost some of their friends. We offer systematic support for their change of heart. But living wills are still widely and confidently urged on patients, and they retain the allegiance of many bioethicists, doctors, nurses, social workers, and patients. For these loyal advocates, we offer systematic proof that such persistence in error is but the triumph of dogma over inquiry and hope over experience.

A note about the scope of our contentions: First, we reject only living wills, not durable powers of attorney. Second, there are excellent reasons to be skeptical of living wills on principle. For example, perhaps former selves should not be able to bind latter selves in the ways living wills contemplate.[1] And many people do and perhaps should reject the view of patients, their families, and their communities that informs living wills.[2] But we accept for the sake of argument that living wills desirably serve a strong version of patients' autonomy. We contend, nevertheless, that living wills do not and cannot achieve that goal.

And a stipulation: We do not propose the elimination of living wills. We can imagine recommending them to patients whose medical situation is plain, whose crisis is imminent, whose preferences are specific, strong, and delineable, and who have special reasons to prescribe their care. We argue on the level of public policy: In an attempt to extend patients' exercise of autonomy beyond their span of competence, resources have been lavished to make living wills routine and even universal. This policy has

From *Hastings Center Report*, March/April 2004. Copyright © 2004 by The Hastings Center. Reprinted by permission of Wiley-Blackwell.

not produced results that recompense its costs, and it should therefore be renounced.

Living wills are a bioethical idea that has passed from controversy to conventional wisdom, from the counsel of academic journals to the commands of law books, from professors' proposal to professional practice. Advance directives generally are embodied in federal policy by the Patient Self-Determination Act, which requires medical institutions to give patients information about their state's advance directives. In turn, the law of every state provides for advance directives, almost all states provide for living wills, and most states "have at least two statutes, one establishing a living will type directive, the other establishing a proxy or durable power of attorney for health care."[3] Not only are all these statutes very much in effect, but new legislative activity is constant. Senators Rockefeller, Collins, and Specter have introduced bills to "strengthen" the PSDA and living wills,[4] and state legislatures continue to amend living will statutes and to enact new ones.

Courts and administrative agencies too have become advocates of living wills. The Veterans Administration has proposed a rule to encourage the use of advance directives, including living wills.[5] Where legislatures have not granted living wills legal status, some courts have done so as a matter of common law, and where legislatures have granted them legal status, courts have cooperated with eager enthusiasm.[6] Living wills have assumed special importance in states that prohibit terminating treatment in the absence of strong evidence of the patient's wishes.[7] One supreme court summarized a common theme: "[A] written directive would provide the most concrete evidence of the patient's decisions, and we strongly urge all persons to create such a directive."[8]

The grandees of law and medicine also give their benediction to the living will. The AMA's Council on Ethical and Judicial Affairs proclaims: "Physicians should encourage their patients to document their treatment preferences or to appoint a health care proxy with whom they can discuss their values regarding health care and treatment."[9] The elite National Conference of Commissioners on Uniform State Laws continues to promulgate the Uniform Health-Care Decisions Act, a prestigious model statute that has been put into law in a still-growing number of states. Medical journals regularly admonish doctors and nurses to see that patients have advance directives, including living wills.[10] Bar journals regularly admonish lawyers that their clients—*all* their clients—need advance directives, including living wills.[11] Researchers demonstrate their conviction that living wills are important by the persistence of their studies of patients' attitudes toward living wills and ways of inveigling patients to sign them.

Not only do legislatures, courts, administrative agencies, and professional associations promote the living will, but other groups unite with them. The Web abounds in sites advocating the living will to patients.[12] The web site for our university's hospital plugs advance directives and suggests that it "is probably better to have written instructions because then everyone can read them and understand your wishes."[13]

Our own experience in presenting this paper is that its thesis provokes some bioethicists to disbelief and indignation. It is as though they simply cannot bear to believe that living wills might not work. How can anything so intuitively right be proved so infuriatingly wrong? And indeed, bioethicists continue to investigate ways the living will might be extended (to deal with problems of the mentally ill and of minors, for example) and developed for other countries.

Although some sophisticated observers have long doubted the wisdom of living wills,[14] proponents have tended to respond in one of three ways, all of which preserve an important role for living wills. First, proponents have supposed that the principal problem with living wills is that people just won't sign them. These proponents have persevered in the struggle to find ways of getting more people to sign up.[15]

Second, proponents have reasserted the usefulness of the living wills. For example, Norman Cantor, distinguished advocate of living wills, acknowledges that "(s)ome commentators doubt the utility or efficacy of advance directives," (by which he means the living will), but he concludes that "these objections don't obviate the importance of advance directives."[16] Other proponents are daunted by the criticisms of living wills but offer new justifications for them. Linda Emanuel, another eminent exponent of living wills, writes that "living wills can help doctors and patients talk about dying" and can thereby "open the door to a positive, caring approach to death."[17]

Third, some proponents concede the weaknesses of the living will and the advantages of the durable power of attorney and then propose a durable power of attorney that incorporates a living will. That is, the forms they propose for establishing a durable power of attorney invite their authors to provide the kinds of instructions formerly confined to living wills.[18]

None of these responses fully grapples with the whole range of difficulties that confound the policy promoting living wills. In fairness, this is partly because the case against that policy has been made piecemeal and not in a full-fledged and full-throated analysis of the empirical literature on living wills.

In sum, the law has embraced the principle of living wills and cheerfully continues to this moment to expound and expand that principle. Doctors, nurses, hospitals, and lawyers are daily urged to convince their patients and clients to adopt living wills, and patients hear their virtues from many other sources besides. Some advocates of living wills have shifted the grounds for their support of living wills, but they persist in believing that they are useful. The time has come to investigate those policies and those hopes systematically. That is what this article attempts.

We ask an obvious but unasked question: What would it take for a regime of living wills to function as their advocates hope? First, people must have living wills. Second, they must decide what treatment they would want if incompetent. Third, they must accurately and lucidly state that preference. Fourth, their living wills must be available to people making decisions for a patient. Fifth, those people must grasp and heed the living will's instructions. These conditions are unmet and largely unmeetable.

Do People Have Living Wills?

At the level of principle, living wills have triumphed among the public as among the princes of medicine. People widely say they want a living will, and living wills have so much become conventional medical wisdom "that involvement in the process is being portrayed as a duty to physicians and others."[19] Despite this, and despite decades of urging, most Americans lack them.[20] While most of us who need one have a property will, roughly 18 percent have living wills.[21] The chronically or terminally ill are likelier to prepare living wills than the healthy, but even they do so fitfully.[22] In one study of dialysis patients, for instance, only 35 percent had a living will, even though all of them thought living wills a "good idea."[23]

Why do people flout the conventional wisdom? The flouters advance many explanations.[24] They don't know enough about living wills,[25] they think living wills hard to execute,[26] they procrastinate,[27] they hesitate to broach the topic to their doctors (as their doctors likewise hesitate).[28] Some patients doubt they need a living will. Some think living wills are for the elderly or infirm and count themselves in neither group.[29] Others suspect that living wills do not change the treatment people receive; 91 percent of the veterans in one study shared that suspicion.[30] Many patients are content or even anxious to delegate decisions to their families, [31] often because they care less what decisions are made than that they are made by people they trust. Some patients find living wills incompatible with their cultural traditions.[32] Thus in the large SUPPORT and HELP studies, most patients preferred to leave final resuscitation decisions to their family and physician instead of having their own preferences expressly followed (70.8% in HELP and 78.0% in SUPPORT). "This result is so striking that it is worth restating: not even a third of the HELP patients and hardly more than a fifth of the SUPPORT patients "would want their own preferences followed."[33]

If people lacked living wills only because of ignorance, living wills might proliferate with education. But studies seem not to "support the speculations found in the literature that the low level of advance directives use is due primarily to a lack of information and encouragement from health care professionals and family members."[34] Rather, there is considerable evidence "that the elderly's action of delaying execution of advance directives and deferring to others is a deliberate, if not an explicit, refusal to participate in the advance directives process."[35]

The federal government has sought to propagate living wills through the Patient Self-Determination Act,[36] which essentially requires medical institutions to inform patients about advance directives. However, "empirical studies demonstrate that: the PSDA has generally failed to foster a significant increase in advance directives use; it is being implemented by medical institutions and their personnel in a passive manner; and the involvement of physicians in its implementation is lacking."[37] One commentator even thinks "the PSDA's legal requirements have become a ceiling instead of a floor."[38]

In short, people have reasons, often substantial and estimable reasons, for eschewing living wills, reasons unlikely to be overcome by persuasion.

Indeed, persuasion seems quickly to find its limits. Numerous studies indicate that without considerable intervention, approximately 20 percent of us complete living wills, but programs to propagate wills have mixed results.[39] Some have achieved significant if still limited increases in the completion of living wills,[40] while others have quite failed to do so.[41]

Thus we must ask: If after so much propaganda so few of us have living wills, do we really want them, or are we just saying what we think we ought to think and what investigators want to hear?

Do People Know What They Will Want?

Suppose, counterfactually, that people executed living wills. For those documents to work, people would have to predict their preferences accurately. This is an ambitious demand. Even patients making contemporary decisions about contemporary illnesses are regularly daunted by the decisions' difficulty. They are human. We humans falter in gathering information, misunderstand and ignore what we gather, lack well-considered preferences to guide decisions, and rush headlong to choice.[42] How much harder, then, is it to conjure up preferences for an unspecifiable future confronted with unidentifiable maladies with unpredictable treatments?

For example, people often misapprehend crucial background facts about their medical choices. Oregon has made medical policy in fresh and controversial ways, has recently had two referenda on assisted suicide, and alone has legalized it. Presumably, then, its citizens are especially knowledgeable. But only 46 percent of them knew that patients may legally withdraw life-sustaining treatment. Even experience is a poor teacher: "Personal experience with illness . . . and authoring an advance directive . . . were not significantly associated with better knowledge about options."[43]

Nor do people reliably know enough about illnesses and treatments to make prospective life-or-death decisions about them. To take one example from many, people grossly overestimate the effectiveness of CPR and in fact hardly know what it is.[44] For such information, people must rely on doctors. But doctors convey that information wretchedly even to competent patients making contemporaneous decisions. Living wills can be executed without even consulting a doctor,[45] and when doctors are consulted, the conversations are ordinarily short, vague, and tendentious. In the Tulsky study, for example, doctors only described either "dire scenarios . . . in which few people, terminally ill or otherwise, would want treatment" or "situations in which patients could recover with proper treatment."[46]

Let us put the point differently. The conventional—legal and ethical wisdom—insists that candidates for even a flu shot give "informed consent." And that wisdom has increasingly raised the standards for disclosure.[47] If we applied those standards to the information patients have before making the astonishing catalog of momentous choices living wills can embody, the conventional wisdom would be left shivering with indignation.

Not only do people regularly know too little when they sign a living will, but often (again, we're human) they analyze their choices only superficially before placing them in the time capsule. An ocean of evidence affirms that answers are shaped by the way questions are asked. Preferences about treatments are influenced by factors like whether success or failure rates are used,[48] the level of detail employed,[49] and whether longor short-term consequences are explained first.[50] Thus in one study, "201 elderly subjects opted for the intervention 12% of the time when it was presented negatively, 18% of the time when it was phrased as in an advance directive already in use, and 30% of the time when it was phrased positively. Seventy-seven percent of the subjects changed their minds at least once when given the same case scenario but a different description of the intervention."[51]

If patients have trouble with contemporaneous decisions, how much more trouble must they have with prospective ones? For such decisions to be "true," patients' preferences must be reasonably stable. Surprisingly often, they are not. A famous study of eighteen women in a "natural childbirth" class found that preferences about anesthesia and avoiding pain were relatively stable before childbirth, but at "the beginning of active labor (4–5 cm dilation) there was a shift in the preference toward avoiding labor pains. . . . During the transition phase of labor (8–10 cm) the values remained relatively stable, but then . . . the mothers' preferences shifted again at postpartum toward avoiding the use of anesthesia during the delivery of her next child."[52] And not only are preferences surprisingly labile, but people have trouble recognizing that their views have changed.[53] This makes it less likely [that] they will amend their living wills as their opinions develop and more likely that their living wills will treasonously misrepresent their wishes.

Instability matters. The healthy may incautiously prefer death to disability. Once stricken, competent patients can test and reject that preference. They often do.[54] Thus Wilfrid Sheed "quickly learned [that] cancer, even more than polio, has a disarming way of bargaining downward, beginning with your whole estate and then letting you keep the game warden's cottage or badminton court; and by the time it has tried to frighten you to death and threatened to take away your very existence, you'd be amazed at how little you're willing to settle for."[55]

At least sixteen studies have investigated the stability of people's preferences for life-sustaining treatment.[56] A meta-analysis of eleven of these studies found that the stability of patients' preferences was 71 percent (the range was 57 percent to 89 percent).[57] Although stability depended on numerous factors (including the illness, the treatment, and demographic variables), the bottom line is that, over periods as short as two years, almost one-third of preferences for life-sustaining medical treatment changed. More particularly, illness and hospitalization change people's preferences for life-sustaining treatments.[58] In a prospective study, the desire for life-sustaining treatment declined significantly after hospitalization but returned almost to its original level three to six months later.[59] Another study concluded that the "will to live is highly unstable among terminally ill cancer patients."[60] The authors thought their findings "perhaps not surprising, given that only 10–14% of individuals who survive a suicide attempt commit suicide during the next 10 years, which suggests that a desire to die is inherently changeable."

The consistent finding that interest in life-sustaining treatment shifts over time and across contexts coincides tellingly with research charting people's struggles to predict their own tastes, behavior, and emotions even over short periods and under familiar circumstances.[61] People mispredict what poster they will like,[62] how much they will buy at the grocery store,[63] how sublimely they will enjoy an ice cream,[64] and how they will adjust to tenure decisions.[65] And people "miswant" for numerous reasons.[66] They imagine a different event from the one that actually occurs, nurture inaccurate theories about what gives them pleasure,[67] forget they might outwit misery, concentrate on salient negative events and ignore offsetting happier ones,[68] and misgauge the effect of physiological sensations like pain.[69] Given this rich stew of research on people's missteps in predicting their tastes generally, we should expect misapprehensions about end-of-life preferences. Indeed, those preferences should be especially volatile, since people lack experience deciding to die.

Can People Articulate What They Want?

Suppose, *arguendo,* that patients regularly made sound choices about future treatments and write living wills. Can they articulate their choices accurately? This question is crucially unrealistic, of course, because the assumption is false. People have trouble reaching well-considered decisions, and you cannot state clearly on paper what is muddled in your mind. And indeed people do, for instance, issue mutually inconsistent instructions in living wills.[70]

But assume this difficulty away and the problem of articulation persists. In one sense, the best way to divine patients' preferences is to have them write their own living wills to give surrogates the patient's gloriously unmediated voice. This is not a practical policy. Too many people are functionally illiterate,[71] and most of the literate cannot express themselves clearly in writing. It's hard, even for the expert writer. Furthermore, most people know too little about their choices to cover all the relevant subjects. Hence living wills are generally forms that demand little writing. But the forms have failed. For example, "several studies suggest that even those patients who have completed AD forms . . . may not fully understand the function of the form or its language."[72] Living wills routinely baffle patients with their

> "syntactic complexity, concept density, abstractness, organization, coherence, sequence of ideas, page format, length of line of print, length of paragraph, punctuation, illustrations, color, and reader interest." Unfortunately, most advance directive forms . . . often have neither a reasonable scope nor depth. They do not ask all the right questions and they do not ask those questions in a manner that elicits clear responses.[73]

Doctors and lawyers who believe their clients are all above average should ask them what their living will says. One of us (CES) has tried the experiment. The modal answer is, in its entirety: "It says I don't want to be a vegetable."

No doubt the forms could be improved, but not enough to matter. The world abounds in dreadfully drafted forms because writing complex instructions for the future is crushingly difficult. Statutes read horribly because their authors are struggling to (1) work out exactly what rule they want, (2) imagine all the circumstances in which it might apply, and (3) find language to specify all those but only those circumstances. Each task is ultimately impossible, which is why statutes explicitly or implicitly confide their enforcers with some discretion and why courts must interpret—rewrite—statutes. However, these skills and resources are not available to physicians or surrogates.

One might retort that property wills work and that living wills are not that far removed from property wills. But wills work as well as they do to distribute property because their scope is—compared to living wills—narrow and routinized. Most people have little property to distribute and few plausible heirs. As property accumulates and ambitions swell, problems proliferate. Many of them are resolvable because experts—lawyers—exclusively draft and interpret wills. Lawyers have been experimenting for centuries with testamentary language in a process which has produced standard formulas with predictable meanings and standard ways of distributing property into which testators are channeled. Finally, if testators didn't say it clearly enough in the right words and following the right procedures, courts coolly ignore their wishes and substitute default rules.

The lamentable history of the living will demonstrates just how recalcitrant these problems are. There have been, essentially, three generations of living wills. At first, they stated fatuously general desires in absurdly general terms. As the vacuity of overgenerality became clear, advocates of living wills did the obvious: Were living wills too general? Make them specific. Were they "one size fits all"? Make them elaborate questionnaires. Were they uncritically signed? "Require" probing discussions between doctor and patient. However, the demand for specificity forced patients to address more questions than they could comprehend. So, generalities were insufficiently specific and insufficiently considered. Specifics were insufficiently general and perhaps still insufficiently considered. What was a doctor—or lawyer—to do? Behold the "values history," a disquisition on the patient's supposed overarching beliefs from which to infer answers to specific questions.[74] That patients can be induced to trek through these interminable and imponderable documents is unproved and unlikely. That useful conclusions can be drawn from the platitudes they evoke is false. As Justice Holmes knew, "General propositions do not decide concrete cases."[75]

The lessons of this story are that drafting instructions is harder than proponents of living wills seem to believe and that when you move toward one blessing in structuring these documents, you walk away from another. The failure to devise workable forms is not a failure of effort or intelligence. It is a consequence of attempting the impossible.

Where Is the Living Will?

Suppose that, *mirabile dictu*, people executed living wills, knew what they will want, and could say it. That will not matter unless the living will reaches the people responsible for the incompetent patient. Often, it does not. This should be no surprise, for long can be the road from the drafter's chair to the ICU bed.

First, the living will may be signed years before it is used, and its existence and location may vanish in the mists of time.[76] Roughly half of all living wills are drawn up by lawyers and must somehow reach the hospital, and 62 percent of patients do not give their living will to their physician. [77] On admission to the hospital, patients can be too assailed and anxious to recall and mention their advance directives.[78] Admission clerks can be harried, neglectful, and loath to ask patients awkward questions.

Thus when a team of researchers reviewed the charts of 182 patients who had completed a living will before being hospitalized, they found that only 26 percent of the charts accurately recorded information about those directives,[79] and only 16 percent of the charts contained the form. And in another study only 35 percent of the nursing home patients who were transferred to the hospital had their living wills with them.[80]

Will Proxies Read It Accurately?

Suppose, *per impossibile,* that patients wrote living wills, correctly anticipated their preferences, articulated their desires lucidly, and conveyed their document to its interpreters. How acutely will the interpreters analyze their instructions? Living wills are not self-executing: someone must decide whether the patient is incompetent, whether a medical situation described in the living will has arisen, and what the living will then commands.

Usually, the patient's intimates will be central among a living will's interpreters. We might hope that intimates already know the patient's mind, so that only modest demands need be made on their interpreting skills. But many studies have asked such surrogates to predict what treatment the patient would choose.[81] Across these studies, approximately 70 percent of the predictions were correct—not inspiring success for life-and-death decisions.

Do living wills help? We know of only one study that addresses that question. In a randomized trial, researchers asked elderly patients to complete a disease- and treatmentbased or a value-based living will.[82] A control group of elderly patients completed no living will. The surrogates were generally spouses or children who had known the patient for decades. Surrogates who were not able to consult their loved one's living will predicted patients' preferences about 70 percent of the time. Strikingly, surrogates who consulted the living will did no better than surrogates denied it. Nor were surrogates more successful when they discussed living wills with patients just before their prediction.

What is more, a similar study found that primary care physicians' predictions were similarly unimproved by providing them with patients' advance directives.[83] On the other hand, emergency room doctors (complete strangers) given a living will more accurately predicted patients' preferences than ER doctors without one.[84]

Do Living Wills Alter Patient Care?

Our survey of the mounting empirical evidence shows that none of the five requisites to making living wills successful social policy is met now or is likely to be. The program has failed, and indeed is impossible.

That impossibility is confirmed by studies of how living wills are implemented, which show that living wills seem not to affect patients' treatments. For instance, one study concluded that living wills "do not influence the level of medical care overall. This finding was manifested in the quantitatively equal use of diagnostic testing, operations, and invasive hemodynamic monitoring among patients with and without advance directives. Hospital and ICU lengths of stay, as well as health care costs, were also similar for patients with and without advance directive statements."[85] Another study found that in thirty of thirty-nine cases in which a patient was incompetent and the living will was in the patient's medical record, the surrogate decisionmaker was not the person the patient had appointed.[86] In yet a third study, a quarter of the patients received care that was inconsistent with their living will.[87]

But all this is normal. Harry Truman rightly predicted that his successor would "sit here, and he'll say, 'Do this! Do that!' And nothing will happen. Poor Ike—it won't be a bit like the army. He'll find it very frustrating." (Of course, the army isn't like the army either, as Captain Truman surely knew.) Indeed, the whole law of bioethics often seems a whited sepulchre for slaughtered hopes, for its policies have repeatedly fallen woefully short of their purposes. Informed consent is a "fairytale."[88] Programs to increase organ donation have persistently disappointed. Laws regulating DNR orders are hardly better. Legal definitions of brain death are misunderstood by astonishing numbers of doctors and nurses. And so on.[89]

But why don't living wills affect care?[90] Joan Teno and colleagues saw no evidence "that a physician unilaterally decided to ignore or disregard an AD." Rather, there was "a complex interaction of . . . three themes." First (as we have emphasized), "the contents of ADs were vague and difficult to apply to current clinical situations." The imprecision of living wills not only stymies interpreters, it exacerbates their natural tendency to read documents in light of their own preferences. Thus "(e)ven with the therapy-specific AD accompanied by designation of a proxy and prior patient–physician discussion, the proportion of physicians who were willing to withhold therapies was quite variable: cardiopulmonary resuscitation, 100%; administration of artificial nutrition and hydration, 82%; administration of antibiotics, 80%; simple tests, 70%; and administration of pain medication, 13%."[91]

Second, the Teno team found that "patients were not seen as 'absolutely, hopelessly ill,' and thus, it was never considered the time to invoke the AD." Living wills typically operate when patients become terminally ill, but neither doctors nor families lightly conclude patients are dying, especially when that means ending treatment. And understandably. For instance, "on the day before death, the median prognosis for patients with heart failure is still a 50% chance to live 6 more months because patients with heart failure typically die quickly from an unpredictable complication like arrhythmia or infection."[92]

So by the time doctors and families finally conclude the patient is dying, the patient's condition is already so dire that treatment looks pointless quite apart from any living will. "In all cases in which life-sustaining treatment was withheld or withdrawn, this decision was made after a trial of life-sustaining treatment and at a time when the patient was seen as 'absolutely, hopelessly ill' or 'actively dying.' Until patients crossed this threshold, ADs were not seen as applicable." Thus "it is not surprising that our previous research has shown that those with ADs did not differ in timing of DNR orders or patterns of resource utilization from those without ADs."[93]

Third, "family members or the surrogate designated in a [durable power of attorney] were not available, were ineffectual, or were overwhelmed with their own concerns and did not effectively advocate for the patient." Family members are crucial surrogates because they should be: patients commonly want them to be; they commonly want to be; they specially cherish the patient's interests. Doctors ordinarily assume families know the patient's situation and preferences and may not relish responsibility for life-and-death decisions, and doctors intent on avoiding litigation may realize that the only plausible plaintiffs are families. The family, however, may not direct attention to the advance directive and may not insist on its enforcement. In fact, surrogates may be guided by either their own treatment preferences or an urgent desire to keep their beloved alive.[94]

In sum, not only are we awash in evidence that the prerequisites for a successful living wills policy are unachievable, but there is direct evidence that living wills regularly fail to have their intended effect. That failure is confirmed by the numerous convincing explanations for it. And if living wills do not affect treatment, they do not work.

Do Living Wills Have Beneficial Side Effects?

Even if living wills do not effectively promote patients' autonomy, they might have other benefits that justify their costs. There are three promising candidates.

First, living wills might stimulate conversation between doctor and patient about terminal treatment. However, at least one study finds little association between patients' reports of executing an advance directive and their reports of such conversations.[95] Nor do these conversations, when they occur, appear satisfactory.[96] James Tulsky and colleagues asked experienced clinicians who had relationships with patients who were over sixty-five or seriously ill to "discuss advance directives in whatever way you think is appropriate" with them. Although the doctors knew they were being taped, the conversations were impressively short and one-sided: The median discussion "lasted 5.6 minutes (range, 0.9 to 15.0 minutes.) Physicians spoke for a median of 3.9 minutes (range, 0.6 to 10.9 minutes), and patients spoke for the remaining 1.7 minutes (range, 0.3 to 9.6 minutes). . . . Usually, the conversation ended without any specific follow-up plan." The "(p)atients' personal values, goals for care, and reasons for treatment preferences were discussed in 71% of cases and were explicitly elicited by 34% of physicians." But doctors commonly "did not explore the reasons for patient's preferences and merely determined whether they wanted specific interventions."[97]

Nor were the conversations conspicuously informative: "Physicians used vague language to describe scenarios, asking what patients would want if they became 'very, very sick' or 'had something that was very serious.' . . ." Further, "[v]arious qualitative terms were used loosely to describe outcome probabilities." In addition, these brief conversations considered almost exclusively the two ends of the continuum—the most hopeless and the most hopeful cases. Conversations tended to ignore "the more common, less clear-cut predicaments surrounding end-of-life care." True, the patients all thought "their physicians 'did a good job talking about the issues,'" but this only suggests that patients did not understand how little they were told.

The second candidate for beneficial side effect arises from evidence that living wills may comfort patients and surrogates. People with a living will apparently gain confidence that their surrogates will understand their preferences and will implement them comfortably, and the surrogates concur.[98] Improved satisfaction with decisions was also a rare positive effect of the SUPPORT study (which devoted enormous resources to improving end-of-life decisions and care but made dismayingly little difference).[99] In another study, living wills reduced the stress and unhappiness of family members who had recently withdrawn life support from a relative.[100] But even if living wills make patients and surrogates more confident and comfortable, those qualities are apparently unrelated to the accuracy of surrogates' decisions. Thus we are left with the irony that one of the best arguments for a tool for enhancing people's autonomy is that it deceives them into confidence.

Third, because living wills generally constrain treatment, they might reduce the onerous costs of terminal illness. Although several studies associated living wills with small decreases in those costs,[101] several studies have reached the opposite conclusion.[102] The old Scotch verdict, "not proven," seems apt.

The Costs

There is no free living will, and the better (or at least more thorough and careful) the living will, the more it costs. Living wills consume patient's time and energy. When doctors or lawyers help, costs soar. On a broader view, Jeremy Sugarman and colleagues estimated that the Patient Self-Determination Act imposed on all hospitals a start-up cost of $101,569,922 and imposed on one hospital (Johns Hopkins) initial costs of $114,528.[103] These figures omit the expenses, paid even as we write and you read, of administering the program. And this money has bought only *pro forma* compliance.

These are real costs incurred when over 40 million people lack health insurance and when we are spending more of our gross domestic product on health care than comparable countries without buying commensurately better health. If programs to promote and provide living wills showed signs of achieving the goals cherished for them, we would have to decide whether their valuable but incalculable rewards exceeded their diffuse but daunting costs.

However, since those programs have failed, their costs plainly outweigh their benefits.

What Is To Be Done?

Living wills attempt what undertakers like to call "pre-need planning," and on inspection they are as otiose as the mortuary version. Critically, empiricists cannot show that advance directives affect care. This is damning, but were it our only evidence, perhaps we might not be weary in well doing: for in due season we might reap, if we faint not. However, our survey of the evidence suggests that living wills fail not for want of effort, or education, or intelligence, or good will, but because of stubborn traits of human psychology and persistent features of social organization.

Thus when we reviewed the five conditions for a successful program of living wills, we encountered evidence that not one condition has been achieved or, we think, can be. First, despite the millions of dollars lavished on propaganda, most people do not have living wills. And they often have considered and considerable reasons for their choice. Second, people who sign living wills have generally not thought through its instructions in a way we should want for life-and-death decisions. Nor can we expect people to make thoughtful and stable decisions about so complex a question so far in the future. Third, drafters of living wills have failed to offer people the means to articulate their preferences accurately. And the fault lies primarily not with the drafters; it lies with the inherent impossibility of living wills' task. Fourth, living wills too often do not reach the people actually making decisions for incompetent patients. This is the most remediable of the five problems, but it is remediable only with unsustainable effort and unjustifiable expense. Fifth, living wills seem not to increase the accuracy with which surrogates identify patients' preferences. And the reasons we surveyed when we explained why living wills do not affect patients' care suggest that these problems are insurmountable.

The cost-benefit analysis here is simple: If living wills lack detectable benefits, they cannot justify any cost, much less the considerable costs they now exact. Any attempt to increase their incidence and their availability to surrogates must be expensive. And the evidence suggests that broader use of living wills can actually disserve rather than promote patients' autonomy: If, as we have argued, patients sign living wills without adequate reflection, lack necessary information, and have fluctuating preferences anyway, then living wills will not lead surrogates to make the choices patients would have wanted. Thus, as Pope suggests, the "PSDA, rather than promoting autonomy has 'done a disservice to most real patients and their families and caregivers.' It has promoted the execution of uninformed and under-informed advance directives, and has undermined, not protected, self-determination."[104]

If living wills have failed, we must say so. We must say so to patients. If we believe our declamations about truth-telling, we should frankly warn patients how faint is the chance that living wills can have their intended effect. More broadly, we should abjure programs intended to cajole everyone into signing living wills. We should also repeal the PSDA, which was passed with arrant and arrogant indifference to its effectiveness and its costs and which today imposes accumulating paperwork and administrative expense for paltry rewards.[105]

Of course we recognize the problems presented by the decisions that must be made for incompetent patients, and our counsel is not wholly negative. Patients anxious to control future medical decisions should be told about durable powers of attorney. These surely do not guarantee patients that their wishes will blossom into fact, but nothing does. What matters is that powers of attorney have advantages over living wills. First, the choices that powers of attorney demand of patients are relatively few, familiar, and simple. Second, a regime of powers of attorney requires little change from current practice, in which family members ordinarily act informally for incompetent patients. Third, powers of attorney probably improve decisions for patients, since surrogates know more at the time of the decision than patients can know in advance. Fourth, powers of attorney are cheap; they require only a simple form easily filled out with little advice. Fifth, powers of attorney can be supplemented by legislation (already in force in some states) akin to statutes of intestacy. These statutes specify who is to act for incompetent patients who have not specified a surrogate. In short, durable powers of attorney are—as these things go—simple, direct, modest, straightforward, and thrifty.

In social policy as in medicine, plausible notions can turn out to be bad ideas. Bad ideas should be renounced. Bloodletting once seemed plausible, but when it demonstrably failed, the course of wisdom was to abandon it, not to insist on its virtues and to scrounge for alternative justifications for it. Living wills were praised and peddled before they were fully developed, much less studied. They have now failed repeated tests of practice. It is time to say, "enough."

Disclaimer

This report and its conclusions are the opinions of the authors and do not necessarily represent those of the Department of Veterans Affairs.

References

1. R. Dresser, "Missing Persons: Legal Perceptions of Incompetent Patients," *Rutgers Law Review* 46 (1994): 609–695.

2. J. Lynn, "Why I Don't Have a Living Will," *Law, Medicine & Health Care* 19, nos. 1-2 (1991): 101–104.

3. C.P. Sabatino, "End-of-Life Legal Trends," *ABA Commission on Legal Problems of the Elderly 2*, (2000).

4. Health Care Assurance of 2001. S. 26. 107th Congress ed; 2001; The Advance Planning and Compassionate Care Act of 1999. S. 628. 106th Congress ed; 1999.

5. 38 CFR Part 17 RIN. 2900-AJ28. November 2, 1998.

6. Knight v. Beverly Health Care. 820 S2d 92; 2001.

7. See *Conservatorship of Wendland*, where the California Supreme Court construed the state's Health Care Decisions Law as "requiring clear and convincing evidence of a conscious conservatee's wish to justify with-

holding life-sustaining treatment" but held that decision did not affect patients who had left "formal directions for health care." 28 P.3d 151; 2001.

8. In re Martin. 538 NW2d 399; Mich 1995.

9. Council on Ethical and Judicial Affairs of the American Medical Association, *Surrogate Decision Making* E8.081. http://www.ama-assn.org

10. P.J. Aitken, "Incorporating Advance Care Planning into Family Practice," *American Family Physician,*" 59 (1999): 605–620; A.O. Calvin and A.P. Clark, "How Are You Facilitating Advance Directives in Your Clinical Nurse Specialist Practice?" *Clinical Nurse Specialist* 16, no. 6 (2002): 292–94.

11. A document that "[g]ives person responsible for making medical decisions greater information, specificity and insight about your specific health-care related decisions, wishes, and objectives" is "A MUST FOR NEARLY EVERYONE" (P. A. Meints, "A Trust and Estate Planning Questionnaire for Families with Minor Children," *The Practical Tax Lawyer* 16, no. 1, [2001]: 33). Providing living wills has also become a pro bono activity. "Wills on Wheels was established by a committee of paralegals and consulting attorneys determined to provide . . . low-income adults with simple wills and living wills" (J.M. Price, "pro Bono and Paralegals: Helping to Make a Difference" *Colorado Lawyer* (September 30, 2000), 55–56.

12. See www.aarp.org/confacts/programs/endoflife.html.

13. The form's critical paragraph reads; "My desires concerning medical treatment are—." Then it leaves fourteen bland lines the patient may fill in. Available at www.med.umich.edu/1libr/aha/umlegal04.htm.

14. R. Dresser, "Precommitment: A Misguided Strategy for Securing Death with Dignity," *Texas Law Review* 81 (2003): 1823–1847.

15. A.R. Eiser and M.D. Weiss, "The Underachieving Advance Directive: Recommendations for Increasing Advance Directive Completion," *American Journal of Bioethics* 1 (2001): 1–5.

16. N.L. Cantor, "Twenty-five Years after Quinlan: A Review of the Jurisprudence of Death and Dying," *Journal of Law, Medicine & Ethics* 29 (2001): 182–96.

17. L. Emanuel, "Living Wills Can Help Doctors and Patients Talk about Dying," *Western Journal of Medicine* 173 (2000): 368.

18. For example, the form provided by a consortium of the American Bar Association, the American Medical Association, and the American Association of Retired Persons "combines and expands the traditional Living Will and Health Care Power of Attorney into a single, comprehensive document" (http://www.ama-assn.org/public/booklets/livgwill.htm).

19. D.M. High, "Why Are Elderly People Not Using Advance Directives?" *Journal of Aging and Health* 5, no. 4 (1993): 497–515.

20. L.L. Emanuel, "Advance Directives for Medical Care; Reply." *NEJM* 325 (1991): 1256; N.L. Cantor, "Making Advance Directives Meaningful," *Psychology, Public Policy, and Law* 4, no. 3 (1998): 629–52; D.M. Cox and G.A. Sachs, "Advance Directives and the Patient Self-Determination Act," *Clinics in Geriatric Medicine* 10 (1994): 431–43; G.A.D. Havens, "Differences in the Execution/Nonexecution of Advance Directives by Community Dwelling Adults," *Research in Nursing and Health* 23 (2000): 319–33;

D.M. High, "Advance Directives and the Elderly: A Study of Intervention Strategies to Increase Use," *Gerontologist* 33, no. 3 (1993): 342–49; S.H. Miles, R. Koepp, and E.P. Weber, "Advance End-of-Life Treatment Planning: A Research Review," *Archives of Internal Medicine* 156, no. 10 (1996): 1062–1068; S.R. Steiber, "Right to Die: Public Balks at Deciding for Others," *Hospitals* 61 (1987): 572; J. Teno et al., "Do Advance Directives Provide Instructions that Direct Care? SUPPORT Investigators. Study to Understand Prognoses and Preferences for Outcomes and Risks of Treatment," *Journal of the American Geriatrics Society* 45, no. 4 (1997): 508–512.

21. Emanuel, "Advance Directives for Medical Care; Reply."

22. Miles, Koepp, and Weber, "Advance End-of-Life Treatment Planning"; J.L. Holley et al., "Factors Influencing Dialysis Patients' Completion of Advance Directives," *American Journal of Kidney Diseases* 30, no. 3 (1997): 356–60; L.C. Hanson and E. Rodgman, "The Use of Living Wills at the End of Life: A National Study," *Archives of Internal Medicine* 156, no. 9 (1996): 1018–1022; J.M. Teno et al., "Do Advance Directives Provide Instructions that Direct Care? SUPPORT Investigators. Study to Understand Prognoses and Preferences for Outcomes and Risks of Treatment," *Journal of the American Geriatrics Society* 45, no. 4 (1997): 508–512.

23. Holley et al., "Factors Influencing Dialysis Patients' Completion of Advance Directives."

24. Cox and Sachs, "Advance Directives and the Patient Self-Determination Act"; Miles, Koepp, and Weber, "Advance End-of-Life Treatment Planning"; D.M. High, "All in the Family: Extended Autonomy and expectations in Surrogate Health Care Decision-Making," *Gerontologist* 28 (suppl) (1988): 46–51.

25. L.L. Emanuel and E.J. Emanuel, "The Medical Directive: A New Comprehensive Advance Care Document," *JAMA* 261 (1989): 3288–93.

26. High, "Advance Directives and the Elderly"; J.M. Roe et al., "Durable Power of Attorney for Health care: A Survey of Senior Center Participants," *Archives of Internal Medicine* 152 (1992): 292–96.

27. High, "Why Are Elderly People Not Using Advance Directives?"; Roe et al., "Durable Power of Attorney for Health care."

28. High, "Why Are Elderly People Not Using Advance Directives?"; Roe et al., "Durable Power of Attorney for Health care"; E.J. Emanuel, L.L. Emanuel, and D. Orentlicher, "Advance Directives," *JAMA* 266 (1991): 2563–63; G.A. Sachs, C.B. Stocking, and S.H. Miles, "Empowerment of the older patient? A Randomized, Controlled Trial to Increase Discussion and Use of Advance Directives," *Journal of the American Geriatrics Society* 40, no. 3 (1992): 269–73; L.L. Brunetti, S.D. Carperos, and R.E. Westlund, "Physicians' Attitudes towards Living Wills and Cardiopulmonary Resuscitation," *Journal of General Internal Medicine* 6 (1991): 323–29; T.E. Finucane et al., "Planning with Elderly Outpatients for Contingencies of Severe Illness: A Survey and Clinical Trial," *Journal of General Internal Medicine* 3, no. 4 (1988): 322–25; B. Lo, G.A. McLeod, and G. Saika, "Patient Attitudes to Discussing Life-sustaining Treatment," *Archives of Internal Medicine* 146, no. 8 (1986): 1613–15; R. Yamada et al., "A Multimedia Intervention on Cardiopulmonary Resuscitation and Advance Directives," *Journal of General Internal Medicine* 14 (1999): 559–63.

29. Cox and Sachs, "Advance Directives and the Patient Self-Determination Act"; L.L. Emanuel and E. Emanuel, "Advance Directives," *Annals of Internal Medicine* 116 (1992): 348–49; B.B. Ott, "Advance Directives: The Emerging Body of Research," *American Journal of Critical Care* 8 (1999): 514–19.

30. J. Sugarman, M. Weinberger, and G. Samsa, "Factors Associated with Veterans' Decisions about Living Wills," *Archives of Internal Medicine* 152 (1992): 343–47.

31. Cox and Sachs, "Advance Directives and the Patient Self-Determination Act"; Holley et al., "Factors Influencing Dialysis Patients' Completion of Advance Directives," High, "All in the Family"; Roe et al., "Durable Power of Attorney for Health care"; Ott, "Advance Directives"; N.A. Hawkins et al., "Do Patients Want to Micro-manage Their Own Deaths? Process Preferences, Values and Goals in End-of-Life Medical Decision Making," Unpublished manuscript. P.B. Terry et al., "End-of-Life Decision Making: When Patients and Surrogates Disagree," *Journal of Clinical Ethics* 10, no. 4 (1999): 286–93.

32. J. Carrese and L. Rhodes, "Western Bioethics on the Navajo Reservation: Benefit or Harm?" *JAMA* 274 (1995): 826–29; L.J. Blackhall et al., "Ethnicity and Attitudes toward Patient Autonomy," *JAMA* 274 (1995): 820–25.

33. C.M. Puchalski et al., Patients Who Want their Family and Physician to Make Resuscitation Decisions for Them: Observations from SUPPORT and HELP; *JAGS* 48 (2000): S84.

34. High, "Why Are Elderly People Not Using Advance Directives?"

35. Ibid.

36. Patient Self-Determination Act of 1990. of the Omnibus Reconsiliation Act of 1990.

37. J.L. Yates and H.R. Glick, "The Failed Patient Self-Determination Act and Policy Alternatives for the Right to Die," *Journal of Aging and Social Policy* 29 (1997): 29, 31.

38. M.T. Pope, "The Maladaptation of Miranda to Advance Directives: A Critique of the Implementation of the Patient Self-Determination Act," *Health Matrix* 9 (1999): 139.

39. Cox and Sachs, "Advance Directives and the Patient Self-Determinaction Act."

40. J. Hare and C. Nelson, "Will Outpatients Complete Living Wills? A Comparison of Two Interventions," *Journal of General Internal Medicine* 6 (1991): 41–46.

41. Yamada et al., "A Multimedia Intervention on Cardiopulmonary Resuscitation and Advance Directives"; G.A. Sachs, S.H. Miles, and R.A. Levin, "Limiting Resuscitation: Emerging Policy in the Emergency Medical System," *Annals of Internal Medicine* 114 (1991): 151–54.

42. C.E. Schneider, *The Practice of Autonomy: Patients, Doctors, and Medical Decisions* (New York: Oxford University Press, 1998).

43. M.J. Silveira et al., "Patient's Knowledge of Options at the End of Life: Ignorance in the Face of Death," *JAMA* 284 (2000): 2483, 2486–87.

44. Yamada et al., "A Multimedia Intervention on Cardiopulmonary Resuscitation and Advance Directives"; S.H. Miles, "Advanced Directives to Limit Treatment: The Need for Portability," *Journal of the American Geriatrics Society* 35, no. 1 (1987): 74–76; K.M. Coppola et al., "Perceived Benefits and Burdens of Life-Sustaining Treatments: Differences among Elderly Adults, Physicians, and Young Adults," *Journal of Ethics, Law, and Aging* 4, no. 1 (1998): 3–13.

45. Roe et al., "Durable Power of Attorney for Health care."

46. J.A. Tulsky et al., "Opening the Black Box: How Do Physicians Communicate about Advance Directives?" *Annals of Internal Medicine* 129 (1998): 441, 444.

47. C.E. Schneider and M. Farrell, *Information, Decisions, and the Limits of Informed Consent* (New York: Oxford University Press, 2000).

48. B.J. McNeil et al., "On the Elicitation of Preferences for Alternative Therapies," *NEJM* 306 (1982): 1259–62.

49. T.R. Malloy et al., "The Influence of Treatment Descriptions on Advance Medical Directive Decisions," *Journal of the American Geriatrics Society* 40, no. 12 (1992): 1255–60; D.J. Mazur and D.H. Hickman, "Patient Preferences: Survival versus Quality-of-Life Considerations," *Journal of General Internal Medicine* 8, no. 7 (1993): 374–77; D.J. Mazur and J.F. Merz, "How Age, Outcome Severity, and Scale Influence General Medicine Clinic Patients' Interpretations of Verbal Probability Terms" (See comments), *Journal of General Internal Medicine* 9 (1994): 268–71.

50. Miles, Koepp, and Weber, "Advance End-of-Life Treatment Planning."

51. Ott, "Advance Directives." pp. 514, 517.

52. J.J. Christensen-Szalanski, "Discount Functions and the Measurement of Patients' Values: Women's Decisions during Childbirth," *Medical Decision Making* 4, no. 1 (1984): 47–58.

53. R.M. Gready et al., "Actual and Perceived Stability of Preferences for Life-Sustaining Treatment," *Journal of Clinical Ethics* 11, no. 4 (2000): 334–46.

54. A. Upadya et al, "Patient, Physician, and Family Member Understanding of Living Wills," *American Journal of Respiratory and Critical Care Medicine* 166 (2002): 1433.

55. W. Sheed, *In Love with Daylight: A Memoir of Recovery* (New York: Simon and Schuster, 1995): 14.

56. Gready et al., "Actual and Perceived Stability of Preferences for Life-Sustaining Treatment"; J.T. Berger and D. Majerovitz, "Stability of Preferences for Treatment among Nursing Home Residents," *Gerontologist* 28, no. 2 (1998): 217–23; S. Carmel and E. Mutran, "Stability of Elderly Persons' Expressed Preferences regarding the Use of Life-Sustaining Treatments," *Social Science and Medicine* 49, no. 3 (1999): 303–311; M. Danis et al., "Stability of Choices about Life-Sustaining Treatments," *Annals of Internal Medicine* 120, no. 7 (1994): 567–73; P.H. Ditto et al., "A Prospective Study of the Effects of Hospitalization on Life-Sustaining Treatment Preferences: Context Changes Choices," Unpublished manuscript; P.H. Ditto et al., "The Stability of Older Adults' Preferences for Life-Sustaining Medical Treatment," Unpublished manuscript; E.J. Emanuel, "Commentary on Discussions about Life-Sustaining Treatments," *Journal of Clinical Ethics* 5, no. 3 (1994): 250–51; L.L. Emanuel et al., "Advance Directives: Stability

of Patients' Treatment Choices," *Archives of Internal Medicine* 154 (1994): 209–217; M.A. Everhart and R.A. Pearlman, "Stability of Patient Preferences regarding Life-Sustaining Treatments," *Chest* 97 (1990): 159–64; L. Ganzini et al., "The Effect of Depression Treatment on Elderly Patients' Preferences for Life-Sustaining Medical Therapy," *American Journal of Psychiatry* 151, no. 11 (1994): 1631–36; N. Kohut et al., "Stability of Treatment Preferences: Although Most Preferences Do Not Change, Most People Change Some of their Preferences," *Journal of Clinical Ethics* 8, no. 2 (1997): 124–35; M.D. Silverstein et al., "Amyotrophic Lateral Sclerosis and Life-Sustaining Therapy: Patients' Desires for Information, Participation in Decision Making, and Life-Sustaining Therapy," *Mayo Clinic Proceedings* 66 (1991): 906–913; J.S. Weissman et al., "The Stability of Preferences for Life-Sustaining Care among Persons with AIDS in the Boston Health Study," *Medical Decision Making* 19 (1999): 16–26; K.M. Coppola et al., "Are Life-Sustaining Treatment Preferences Stable over Time? An Analysis of the Literature," unpublished manuscript.

57. Coppola et al., "Are Life-Sustaining Treatment Preferences Stable over Time?"

58. Danis et al., "Stability of Choices about Life-Sustaining Treatments"; Ditto et al., "A Prospective Study of the Effects of Hospitalization"; Weissman et al., "The Stability of Preferences for Life-Sustaining Care."

59. Ditto et al., "A Prospective Study of the Effects of Hospitalization."

60. H.M. Chochinov et al., "Will to Live in the Terminally Ill," *Lancet* 354 (1999): 816, 818.

61. D.T. Gilbert and T.D. Wilson, "Miswanting: Some Problems in the Forecasting of Future Affective States," in *Feeling and Thinking: The Role of Affect in Social Cognition,* ed. J.P. Forgas (New York: Cambridge University Press, 2000): 178–97; C.H. Griffith 3rd et al., "Knowledge and Experience with Alzheimer's Disease: Relationship to Resuscitation Preference," *Archives of Family Medicine* 4, no. 9 (1995): 780–84; T.M. Osberg and J.S. Shrauger, "Self-prediction: Exploring the Parameters of Accuracy," *Journal of Personality and Social Psychology* 51, no. 5 (1986): 1044–57.

62. Griffith 3rd et al., "Knowledge and Experience with Alzheimer's Disease."

63. Gilbert and Wilson, "Miswanting."

64. D. Kahneman and J. Snell, "Predicting a Changing Taste: Do People Know What They Will Like?" *Journal of Behavioral Decision Making* 5, no. 3 (1992): 187–200.

65. Gilbert and Wilson, "Miswanting."

66. Ibid.

67. G. Loewenstein and D. Schkade, "Wouldn't It Be Nice? Predicting future feelings," in *Hedonic Psychology: Scientific Approaches to Enjoyment, Suffering and Wellbeing,"* ed. N. Schwartz and D. Kahneman (New York: Russell Sage Foundation, 1997).

68. D. Schkade, Does Living in California Make People Happy? A Focusing Illusion in Judgements of Life Satisfaction," *Psychological Science* 9 (1998): 340–46.

69. Loewenstein and Schkade, "Wouldn't It Be Nice?"

70. A.S. Brett, "Limitations of Listing Specific Medical Interventions in Advance Directives," *JAMA* 266 (1991): 825–28.

71. I.S. Kirsch et al., *Adult Literacy in America: A First Look at the Results of the National Adult Literacy Survey,* U.S. Department of Education; August 1993; NCES 93275.

72. Cox and Sachs, "Advance Directives and the Patient Self-Determination Act"; Miles, Koepp, and Weber, "Advance End-of-Life Treatment Planning"; Silveira et al., "Patient's Knowledge of Options at the End of Life"; Coppola et al., "Perceived Benefits and Burdens of Life-Sustaining Treatments."

73. Pope, "The Maladaptation of Miranda to Advance Directives." pp. 139, 165–66.

74. D.J. Doukas and L.B. McCullough, "The Values History: The Evaluation of the Patient's Values and Advance Directives," *Journal of Family Practice* 32, no. 2 (1991): 145–53.

75. Lochner v. New York N. 198 U.S. 45: Supreme Court of the United States; 1905.

76. H.J. Silverman et al., "Implementation of the Patient Self-Determination Act in a Hospital Setting: An Initial Evaluation," *Archives of Internal Medicine* 155, no. 5 (1995: 502–510.

77. Roe et al., "Durable Power of Attorney for Health Care."

78. R.S. Morrison et al., "The Inaccessibility of Advance Directives on Transfer from Ambulatory to Acute Care Settings," *JAMA* 274 (1995): 478–82.

79. Ibid.

80. M. Danis et al., "A Prospective Study of the Impact of Patient Preferences on Life-Sustaining Treatment and Hospital Cost," *Critical Care Medicine* 24, 11 (1996): 1811–17.

81. J.A. Druley et al., "Physicians' Predictions of Elderly Outpatients' Preferences for Life-Sustaining Treatment," *Journal of Family Practice* 37 (1993): 469–75; J. Hare, C. Pratt, and C. Nelson, "Agreement between Patients and Their Self-Selected Surrogates on Difficult Medical Decisions," *Archives of Internal Medicine* 152, no. 5 (1992): 1049–1054; P.M. Layde et al., "Surrogates' Predictions of Seriously Ill Patients' Resuscitation Preferences," *Archives of Family Medicine* 4, no. 6 (1995): 518–23; J.G. Ouslander, A.J. Tymchuk, and B. Rahbar, "Health Care Decisions among Elderly Long-term Care Residents and Their Potential Proxies," *Archives of Internal Medicine* 149 no. 6 (1989): 1367–72; A.B. Seckler et al., "Substituted Judgment: How Accurate Are Proxy Predictions?" *Annals of Internal Medicine* 115 (1991): 92–98; D.P. Sulmasy et al., "The Accuracy of Substituted Judgments in Patients with Terminal Diagnoses," *Annals of Internal Medicine* 128, no. 8 (1998): 621–29; R.F. Uhlmann, R.A. Pearlman, and K.C. Cain, "Physicians' and Spouses' Predictions of Elderly Patients' Resuscitation Preferences," *Journal of Gerontology* 43, no. 5 (1988): M115–M121; R.F. Uhlmann, R.A. Pearlman, and K.C. Cain, "Understanding of Elderly Patients' Resuscitation Preferences by Physicians and Nurses," *Western Journal of Medicine* 150 (1989): 705–707; N.R. Zweibel and C.K. Cassell, "Treatment Choices at the End of Life: A Comparison of Decisions by Older Patients and Their Physician-Selected Proxies," *Gerontologist* 29, no. 5 (1989): 615–21.

82. L. Emanuel, "The Health Care Directive: Learning How to Draft Advance Care Documents," *Journal of the American Geriatrics Society* 39, no. 12

(1991): 1221–28; P.H. Ditto et al., "Fates Worse than Death: The Role of Valued Life Activities in Health-State Evaluations," *Health Psychology* 15, no. 5 (1996): 332–43.

83. K.M. Coppola et al., "Accuracy of Primary Care and Hospital-based Physicians' Predictions of Elderly Outpatients' Treatment Preferences with and without Advance Directives," *Archives of Internal Medicine* 161, no. 3 (2001): 431–40.

84. Ibid.

85. M.D. Goodman, M. Tarnoff, and G.J. Slotman, "Effect of Advance Directives on the Management of Elderly Critically Ill Patients," *Critical Care Medicine* 26, no. 4 (1998): 701–704.

86. Morrison et al., "The Inaccessibility of Advance Directives."

87. M. Danis and J.M. Garrett, "Advance Directives for Medical Care: Reply," *NEJM* 325 (1991): PP NO?.

88. J. Katz, "Informed Consent—A Fairy Tale? Law's vision," *University of Pittsburgh Law Review* 39, no. 2 (1977): 137–74; C.H. Braddock 3rd et al., "Informed Decision Making in Outpatient Practice: Time to Get Back to Basics," *JAMA* 282, no. 24 (1999): 2313–20.

89. C.E. Schneider, "The Best-Laid Plans," *Hastings Center Report* 30, no. 4 (2000): 24–25; C.E. Schneider, "Gang Aft Agley," *Hastings Center Report* 31, no. 1 (2001): 27–28.

90. Teno et al., "Do Advance Directives Provide Instructions that Direct Care?"

91. W.R. Mower and L.J. Baraff, "Advance Directives: Effect of Type of Directive on Physicians' Therapeutic Decisions," *Archives of Internal Medicine* 153 (1993): 375, 378.

92. J. Lynn, "Learning to Care for People with Chronic Illness Facing the End of Life," *JAMA* 284 (2000): 2508–09.

93. J. Teno et al., "The Illusion of End-of-Life Resource Savings with Advance Directives. SUPPORT Investigators. Study to Understand Prognoses and Preferences for Outcomes and Risks of Treatment," *Journal of the American Geriatrics Society* 45, no. 4 (1997): 513–18.

94. A. Fagerlin et al., "Projection in Surrogate Decisions about Life-Sustaining Medical Treatments," *Health Psychology* 20, no. 3 (2001): 166–75.

95. J. Virmani, L.J. Schneiderman, and R.M. Kaplan, "Relationship of Advance Directives to Physician-Patient Communication," *Archives of Internal Medicine* 154 (1994): 909–913.

96. J.A. Tulsky, M.A. Chesney, B. Lo, "How Do Medical Residents Discuss Resuscitation with Patients?" *Journal of General Internal Medicine* 10 no. 8 (1995): 436–42.

97. Tulsky et al., "Opening the Black Box." pp. 441, 445.

98. P.H. Ditto et al., "Advance Directives as Acts of Communication: A Randomized Controlled Trial, *Archives of Internal Medicine* 161, no. 3 (2001): 421–30.

99. R. Baker et al., "Family Satisfaction with End-of-Life Care in Seriously Ill Hospitalized Adults," *Journal of the American Geriatrics Society* 48, no 5 (suppl) (2000): S61–S69.

100. V.P. Tilden et al., "Family Decisionmaking to Withdraw Life-Sustaining Treatments from Hospitalized Patients," *Nursing Research* 50, no. 2 (2001): 105–115.

101. Miles, Koepp, and Weber, "Advance End-of-Life Treatment Planning."

102. Teno et al., "The Illusion of End-of-Life Resource Savings with Advance Directives"; E.J. Emanuel and L.L. Emanuel, "The Economics of Dying: The Illusion of Cost Savings at the End of Life," *NEJM* 330 (1994): 540–44; L.J. Schneiderman et al., "Effects of Offering Advance Directives on Medical Treatments and Costs," *Annals of Internal Medicine* 117, no. 7 (1992): 599–606.

103. J. Sugarman et al., "The Cost of Ethics Legislation: A Look at the Patient Self-Determination Act," *Kennedy Institute of Ethics Journal* 3, no. 4 (1993): 387–99.

104. Pope, "The Maladaptation of Miranda to Advance Directives." pp. 139, 167.

105. Yates and Glick, "The Failed Patient Self-Determination Act"; Sugarman et al., "The Cost of Ethics Legislation."

Susan E. Hickman et al. 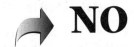 **NO**

Hope for the Future: Achieving the Original Intent of Advance Directives

The development of new, life-prolonging medical technologies in the 1970s aroused concern among Americans about the indiscriminant use of aggressive, life-prolonging treatments. Highly public cases such as those of Karen Ann Quinlan and Nancy Cruzan drew attention to the importance of end of life care planning for healthy adults. Advance directives were developed as a way for people to retain control over their medical care by specifying their treatment values and choices and by naming someone to make medical decisions once they were no longer able to do so. Over the past several decades, it has become clear that statutory advance directives alone have not been as successful as originally hoped in giving patients control over their end of life care. However, the initial goal of advance directives was laudable and is worth preserving. Promising new models have evolved from practice and research that move us closer to achieving the original intent of advance directives.

Most traditional advance directives, such as statutory living wills and surrogate appointments, were created by legislative processes that set specific requirements about content and established rules regarding their use to define the rights of adults to forgo medical treatment, to protect providers who honor these decisions, and to appoint an authorized surrogate decision-maker. Statutory living wills are a tool for patients to express preferences about medical treatments that can be used if a person is no longer able to make his or her own decisions. These documents typically focus on potentially life-prolonging treatments in a very limited set of circumstances, such as when a person is faced with "imminent death regardless of treatment" or is in a "persistent vegetative state." In most states, a person can also designate a surrogate to make decisions in the event the patient loses decisional capacity. Depending on state law, a surrogate may be called a health care proxy or agent, medical power of attorney, or durable power of attorney for health care.

Limitations of Traditional Advance Directives

Despite the hope that traditional advance directives would ensure that patient preferences are honored, numerous studies have found that only a minority (20 to 30 percent) of American adults have an advance directive and that these documents have limited effects on treatment decisions near the end of life, though more recent research suggests use may be higher at the end of life. In addition to a low completion rate, there are many reasons why traditional advance directives are less successful than originally hoped. These reasons include the following:

(1) The focus is often on a patient's legal right to refuse unwanted medical treatments, reflecting the legislative origins of traditional advance directives. Those who complete such documents generally do not receive assistance in understanding or discussing their underlying goals and values.

(2) The instructions given in these documents and the scenarios provided for discussion are generally either too vague to be clear (for example, "If I am close to death") or too medically specific to be helpful in common clinical situations (for example, "If I am in a persistent vegetative state").—five wishes explains this

(3) Vague instructions result in conversations that produce equally vague expressions of wishes such as "Do not keep me alive with machines" or "Let me die if I am a vegetable."

(4) Once advance directives are completed, planning is typically considered finished. A systematic effort to reopen the conversation as a person's health declines is rarely made. The only repeated question that a patient might hear is, "Do you have an advance directive?" as required by the Patient Self-Determination Act.

(5) Traditional advance directives are seen as a right of the patient, with little attention given to routinely integrate planning into the clinical care of patients.

(6) Traditional advance directives are based on the assumption that autonomy is the primary mode of decision-making for most people. However, many people in the United States, particularly those from non-Western cultures, conceptualize the broader social network as the basis of treatment decisions, not the wishes and needs of the individual. Patients may also choose to delegate their autonomy to a family member, religious leader, or others, and defer discussions about prognosis and treatments for cultural or other reasons.

(7) In selecting a surrogate, a patient authorizes someone to speak on his or her behalf; however, advance directives typically do not include directions for the surrogate or health care professionals about treatment preferences unless special instructions are also provided. Additional information about values and goals is important to assist surrogates in decision-making during stressful times.

(8) Some patients may wish for their surrogates' or families' interests to be taken into account in decision-making rather than expecting

the surrogate to base decisions solely on the wishes of the patient using a substituted judgment standard. Research suggests that many patients do not expect surrogates to rigidly follow their traditional advance directives, but rather intend for surrogates to exercise judgment to determine the course of care when there is insufficient information available or for extenuating circumstances.

In response to the difficulties with traditional legalistic advance directives, clinicians and researchers have developed new models that preserve the original goal of advance directives while addressing their shortcomings. One well-known example is "Five Wishes," a document that incorporates a surrogate appointment with a range of wishes about medical, personal, spiritual, and emotional needs (www.agingwithdignity.org). Five Wishes offers advantages over traditional advance directives because it covers a range of issues typically not found in statutory living wills or health care power of attorney documents, such as how comfortable a person wants to be or how he or she wishes to be treated if unable to speak for him or herself. Five Wishes meets the legal requirements for advance directives in thirty-seven states and the District of Columbia. Unfortunately, there are no published research studies to support the efficacy of Five Wishes in guiding surrogates and health care professionals or in ensuring that wishes are honored.

"Let Me Decide" is a recently developed Canadian program with empirical data to support its effectiveness (www.newgrangepress.com). The program was studied in a randomized, controlled trial of 1,292 residents at a group of regional nursing homes and hospitals in Ontario. Residents and their family members had an opportunity to document a range of health care choices regarding levels of care, nutritional support, and cardiopulmonary resuscitation. The program was implemented systematically and nursing home staff received training in how to integrate the advance directive into clinical care. Results indicate that the intervention group had a higher prevalence of planning. Additionally, plans were more specific, residents were less likely to die in the hospital, fewer resources were used, and families were more satisfied with the process than were family members in the control facilities using more traditional advance care planning.[1]

In La Crosse, Wisconsin, "Respecting Choices" began in 1991 as part of a community-wide care planning system (www.gundersenlutheran.com/eolprograms). Local health care systems developed institutional policies to ensure that written advance directives were always available in their medical records when needed. Components of the program include staff education about the program and advance care planning; clearly defined roles and expectations of physicians; training for advanced care planning facilitators; routine public and patient engagement in advanced care planning; clinically relevant advance directives incorporated into clinical care; and written protocols so that emergency personnel can follow physician orders that reflect patient preferences. Quality improvement projects were undertaken to measure outcomes and to improve parts of the system when they did not perform in the way intended.[2]

A study of the Respecting Choices program evaluated La Crosse County deaths over an eleven-month period (524 in all). Eighty-five percent of all decedents had some type of a written advance directive at the time of death; 96 percent of written plans were found in the medical record where the person died; and treatment decisions made in the last weeks of life were consistent with written instructions in 98 percent of the deaths where an advance directive existed. Decedents with written advance directives were also significantly less likely to die in the hospital (31 percent versus 68 percent, p=0.001). Respecting Choices is now being implemented by more than fifty-five communities and organizations in the United States and Canada and is being piloted nationwide in Australia.

One of the most studied systems of advance care planning and documentation is the "Physician Orders for Life-Sustaining Treatment" paradigm, originally developed in Oregon (www.polst.org) and complementary to Respecting Choices (in fact, the Respecting Choices program strongly advocates use of the POLST paradigm to document physician orders in the out-of-hospital setting). The POLST form is designed for patients with serious illness and advanced frailty. The centerpiece of the program is the POLST document, a brightly colored medical order form that converts patient treatment preferences into written medical orders based on a conversation among health care professionals, the patient, and/ or surrogates about treatment goals. The form transfers with patients across care settings to ensure that wishes are honored throughout the health care system. The POLST form is an example of an actionable advance directive that is specific and effective immediately. In a prospective study at eight nursing homes, residents whose POLST forms included a do not resuscitate (DNR) order and an order for comfort measures only were followed for one year. None received unwanted intensive care, ventilator support, or cardiopulmonary resuscitation.[3]

In contrast to the varied out-of-hospital DNR orders used around the country, the POLST paradigm provides patients the opportunity to document treatment goals and preferences for interventions across a range of treatment options, permitting greater individualization.[4] Research suggests that the POLST form accurately represents patient treatment preferences the majority of the time[5] and that treatments at the end of life tend to match orders.[6] A majority of nursing homes and hospices in Oregon use the voluntary POLST Program, and POLST is widely recognized by emergency medical services.[7] At least thirteen states have adapted versions of the POLST program, including Oregon, Washington, West Virginia, Utah, and parts of Wisconsin, New York, Pennsylvania, North Carolina, New Hampshire, Tennessee, and Michigan, reflecting a high degree of acceptance by health care professionals. Each state has made minor alterations to the document to accommodate local regulations and statutes. A National POLST Paradigm Task Force formed in 2004 to support national growth of the program.

Elements of Successful Advance Directive Programs

The newer, more successful, clinically based advance directive programs share key elements: a facilitated process, documentation, proactive but appropriately staged timing, and the development of systems and processes that ensure planning occurs.

First, successful advance directive programs are not limited to the content or rules relating to legal documents. Instead, an individualized plan is developed through a process of interaction with the patient that is specific not only to the patient's values and goals, but also to his or her relationships, culture, and medical condition. Advance care planning should focus on defining "good" care for each patient, rather than on simply listing the right to refuse treatment or promoting individual autonomy. A skilled facilitator can enhance advance care planning by engaging those who are close to the patient so that they understand, support, and follow the plans that are made. The process permits shared or delegated decision-making depending on the beliefs and preferences of the patient. Facilitators should encourage patients and surrogates to discuss how much leeway a surrogate has in decision-making.

Second, for advance directive programs to be implemented successfully as a patient moves between different treatment settings, documentation of wishes, goals, and plans is essential. This documentation should include the identity of a designated surrogate. Ideally, this documentation would be in the form of actionable advance directives that direct treatment with specific medical orders reflecting a patient's current treatment preferences—in contrast to traditional advance directives that address preferences in hypothetical future scenarios. To be truly effective, the actionable advance directive form must be standardized and recognized throughout the broader health care system, and it must provide clear, specific language that is actionable in all settings to which a patient might be transferred. The power of actionable advance directives is most completely realized in a system in which all institutional entities that interact with the patient (health care personnel in emergency medical services, emergency departments, hospitals, nursing homes, hospices, home health care, and others) recognize the actionable advance directive form and are authorized to follow its written orders.

Third, successful advance directive programs also require proactive but appropriately staged timing: some discussion should anticipate health care decisions, but much of it must be revisited as the patient's prognosis becomes known. For an otherwise healthy patient, the presumption is that the treatment goal is to return to his or her prior state of health. Individuals who fit this description do not need an advance directive to guide initial treatment. However, healthy adults can benefit from the process of advance care planning to prepare for sudden, severe illness or injury. Healthy adults should appoint a trusted family member or friend to serve as a health care surrogate who can act as a strong advocate in the event that they are unable to speak for themselves. Healthy adults should also discuss with their surrogates whether and when a permanent loss of neurological function would be so bad that the goals of medical care would change from prolonging life to providing comfort, and they should address the degree of leeway that they grant to the surrogate.

In people with advanced chronic disease and frailty, planning should expand to include discussion of changing treatment goals. Success rates for interventions decline as disease and frailty progress, and patients' evaluations of the desirability of interventions often change in the face of this new reality. Patients and families look to health care professionals to initiate conversations about end of life care planning, and it seems most relevant to broach the topic in the context of a limited prognosis. Once the prognosis has been discussed, health care professionals (but not necessarily physicians) trained to facilitate advance care planning discussions can help guide patients so that plans are specific not only to the patient's experiences, values, and goals, but also to the patient's health condition, culture, and personal relationships. This planning should focus on treatment goals in scenarios likely to occur in the course of that person's chronic disease. Completion of an actionable advance directive may be particularly helpful at this time.

Finally, perhaps the most crucial elements of more successful advance directive programs are policies, procedures, and teamwork within each part of the health care system that ensures advance care planning and implementation occurs. Plans need to be clear and should reflect the individual's values and goals. Plans should be updated over time and available when needed; whenever possible, plans should be honored. A successful model requires the establishment of systems at many levels to achieve these goals. Health care organizations can create policies and procedures to assure that any written plan is available when needed. The roles and responsibilities of different health professionals must be clearly defined so that each person knows his or her part and can perform it. Furthermore, optimal performance of each player's role benefits from periodic assessment, which requires that health organizations conduct quality improvement initiatives to ensure that the implemented system achieves the desired outcomes. Organizations should be prepared to gather the necessary information to improve the system when and where it falls short.

For advance directives to be effective, they need to be integrated into each part of the system of care, including emergency medical service protocols and regulations. State statutes vary regarding traditional advance directives, surrogate appointment, and other relevant factors, such as emergency medical technicians' scope of practice. Therefore, state end of life coalitions consisting of key stakeholders (emergency medicine, long-term care, hospice, nurses, physicians, and health lawyers, among others) may need to identify and overcome state-specific regulatory, legal, and cultural barriers to the implementation of optimal advance care planning.

The original intent of advance directives to enable patients to retain control over their terminal care once they lose decision-making capacity was not fully achieved through the use of the traditional advance directives. New, more successful models address the limitations of the traditional models yet remain true to the concept's original intent. The key elements of these new models are advance care planning in a system with specially trained personnel; highly visible, standardized order forms that are immediately actionable; proactive, appropriately staged timing; ongoing evaluation and quality improvement.

For these new models to be used more broadly, systems to implement them will need to be established in each state and within every health organization. These systems need to ensure that traditional and actionable advance directives are written at the appropriate time, that they are recognized, and that they are honored. Given the initial success of these models, it is reasonable to believe that the original goal of advance directives—to ensure respect for patients' treatment wishes at the end of life—can and will be more completely realized in the future.

References

1. D.W. Molloy et al., "Systematic Implementation of an Advance Directive Program in Nursing Homes: A Randomized Controlled Trial," *Journal of the American Medical Association* 283, no. 11 (2000): 1437–44.

2. B.J. Hammes and B.L. Rooney, "Death and End-of-Life Planning in One Midwestern Community," *Archives of Internal Medicine* 158 (1998): 383–90.

3. S.W. Tolle et al., "A Prospective Study of the Efficacy of the Physician Orders for Life Sustaining Treatment," *Journal of the American Geriatrics Society* 46, no. 9 (1998): 1097–1102.

4. S.E. Hickman et al., "Use of the POLST (Physician Orders for Life-Sustaining Treatment) Program in Oregon: Beyond Resuscitation Status," *Journal of the American Geriatrics Society* 52 (2004): 1424–29.

5. J.L. Meyers et al., "Use of the Physician Orders for Life-Sustaining Treatment (POLST) Form to Honor the Wishes of Nursing Home Residents for End of Life Care: Preliminary Results of a Washington State Pilot Project," *Journal of Gerontological Nursing* 30, no. 9 (2004): 37–46.

6. M.A. Lee et al., "Physician Orders for Life-Sustaining Treatment (POLST): Outcomes in a PACE Program," *Journal of the American Geriatrics Society* 48 (2002): 1219–25.

7. T.A. Schmidt et al., "The Physician Orders for Life-Sustaining Treatment (POLST) Program: Oregon Emergency Medical Technicians' Practical Experiences and Attitudes," *Journal of the American Geriatrics Society* 52 (2004): 1430–34.

EXPLORING THE ISSUE

Have Advance Directives Failed?

Critical Thinking and Reflection

1. How important is it to be able to control or guide in advance the decisions that will eventually be made about your health care at the end of your life? Would you trust family, friends, and physicians to make decisions on your behalf, or with whatever help you are able to offer yourself at the time?
2. How relevant is cost in making public policy to promote or protect a patient's ability to control decisions about end-of-life health care?
3. In what ways does the POLST approach differ from the living wills that Fagerlin and Schneider discuss?
4. What kind of processes might lead to better communication between physicians, families, and patients?

Is There Common Ground?

Many commentators hold that the best approach to end-of-life decision making is all of the above. Attorneys often encourage people both to fill out a living will and to appoint a health care durable power of attorney—in effect, both to try to establish their own preferences and to identify someone who can make decisions that will have to be made by others. If, as Fagerlin and Schneider write is likely, the living will does not anticipate the medical scenarios that a person eventually confronts, then it at least provides the HCDPA, acting as a surrogate decision maker, some indication of the patient's preferences. Many states actually combine the living will and HCDPA appointment into one document.

Similarly, the AARP Web site encourages visitors to look at the Aging with Dignity, which has produced a document titled "Five Wishes" that allows a person both to name someone who can make health care decisions for that person and to identify the kinds of treatments he or she wants or doesn't want.

The POLST approach also continues to gain adherents. Most states either have endorsed or are developing POLST programs, according to the POLST Web site at Oregon Science & Health University (www.ohsu.edu/polst/).

Additional Resources

For information about state policies on advance directives and the different limits they place on the substitute decision maker's power to refuse life-sustaining treatment, specifically artificial nutrition and hydration, see Muriel T. Gillick, "Advance Care Planning," *The New England Journal of Medicine* (February 11, 2005) for a review.

An extensive discussion of end-of-life decision making is available in Nancy Berlinger, Bruce Jennings, and Susan M. Wolf, *The Hastings Center Guidelines for Decisions on Life-Sustaining Treatment and Care Near the End of Life: Revised and Expanded Second Edition* (Oxford University Press, 2013).

The President's Council on Bioethics' 2006 report Taking Care: Ethical Caregiving in an Aging Society argues that advance directives do not account for the possibility that a person might change his or her mind, and that surrogate decision makers should not be bound by patients' prior declarations. The report is available at http://bioethics.georgetown.edu/pcbe /reports/taking_care/taking_care.pdf.

Nancy M.P. King argues in favor of advance directives in *Making Sense of Advance Directives,* rev. ed. (Georgetown University Press, 1996). Among her central points is that advance directives provide only one procedural mechanism for implementing an individual's constitutional right to make decisions concerning his or her own body. See also Robert S. Olick, *Taking Advance Directives Seriously: Prospective Autonomy and Decisions Near the End of Life* (Georgetown University Press, 2001) and Lawrence P. Ulrich and Mark J. Hanson, eds., *The Patient Self-Determination Act: Meeting the Challenge in Patient Care* (Georgetown University Press, 2001). In "What I Learned from Schiavo," Hastings Center Report (November–December 2007), estate law attorney Gerald W. Witherspoon offers advice about advance directives, including the importance of selecting a trusted person as the proxy or surrogate decision maker and making clear this person's authority to prevent challenges.

For further discussion of the POLST approach, see Diane E. Meier and Larry Beresford, "POLST Offers Next Stage in Honoring Patient Preferences," *Journal of Palliative Medicine* (vol. 12, no. 4, 2009).

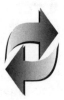

ISSUE 5

Is "Palliative Sedation" Ethically Different from Active Euthanasia?

YES: **American Medical Association**, from "Sedation to Unconsciousness in End-of-Life Care," *Report of the Council on Ethical and Judicial Affairs* (June 2008)

NO: **Margaret P. Battin**, from "Terminal Sedation: Pulling the Sheet Over Our Eyes," *Hastings Center Report* (September–October 2008)

Learning Outcomes

After reading this issue, you should be able to:

- Describe the special challenges of caring for terminally ill patients in the late stages of their illness.
- Describe the concepts of euthanasia, palliative care, and the doctrine of double effect.

ISSUE SUMMARY

YES: The American Medical Association affirms that in cases of extreme suffering the physician's duty to relieve pain and suffering includes palliative sedation—using drugs that result in unconsciousness and may hasten death.

NO: Philosopher Margaret P. Battin believes that palliative or terminal sedation is an unsatisfying compromise that offers no greater protection against abuse than do institutional safeguards established for direct physician aid in dying.

One persistent theme in bioethics is appropriate care and decision making at the end of life. Beginning with the case of Karen Ann Quinlan (see Introduction) and continuing through many highly publicized cases, philosophers, theologians, physicians, policymakers, and patients and family members have struggled with questions about what ethical standards should be used in determining how to use modern medical technology humanely and who should make those decisions. The most publicized cases have concerned young women—Karen Ann Quinlan, Nancy Cruzan, and Terry Schiavo. All suffered traumatic events that put them into long-term, nonresponsive states. But these situations arise even more frequently when individuals with chronic conditions, often frail and elderly, undergo a long period of debilitation before they reach the end of life.

Euthanasia—physician participation in administration of drugs that will result in death—is banned in all states. Only Oregon and Washington have laws that allow physicians under certain circumstances to prescribe but not administer lethal drugs to people at the end of life (see issue 6).

To respect individual autonomy—the right to choose what medical interventions one would or would not accept—many attempts have been made to encourage people to express their wishes through advance directives. As the selections in issue 4 demonstrate, most people do not sign advance directives or in any way indicate their preferences for care at the end of life. Family members are often left to make these decisions based on what they think the patient would have wanted.

Beginning in the 1970s, hospices became an option for people who did not want aggressive medical care. The hospice movement started in Great Britain and emphasized comfort and spiritual care. Today there are over 5,000 hospices in the United States. Contrary to popular perception, which sees hospice as a place where people go to die, most hospice care is provided at home. There are, in addition, some freestanding hospices and hospice units in acute care hospitals and nursing homes. Medicare (the federal health insurance program for people over 65) has a special hospice benefit for people whose life expectancy is 6 months or less. Most people, however, come to hospice very late in the course of their disease, with a median length of stay of 26 days. They and their families fail to obtain the full benefit of the multidisciplinary hospice approach to care.

For many people, one of the drawbacks to hospice is the requirement to give up treatments that are intended to cure the disease. (Medications that ease pain and symptoms are permitted.) Palliative care has become an option in these situations. Palliative care has many of the same goals as hospice—relief of symptoms, multidisciplinary care of the whole person, family involvement—but also allows curative treatments. Importantly, it is available to individuals at any stage of disease. Most palliative care today is provided in hospitals, and there is no special insurance benefit for palliative care at home.

What then is "palliative" or "terminal" sedation and where does it fit in this array of options? Sedation—administering drugs that are to relieve pain or symptoms without causing loss of consciousness—is part of ordinary medical care (unless the patient objects). Depending on the severity of the patient's pain or symptoms, palliative care may include higher levels of medications, which may result in loss of consciousness but is not the intended result. The major controversy concerns the use of drugs in levels that are intended to cause loss of consciousness and are maintained at that level until the patient dies.

In the YES and NO selections, the American Medical Association's Council on Judicial and Ethical Affairs maintains that palliative sedation, within guidelines, is an acceptable extension of the physician's duty to relieve pain and suffering. Philosopher Margaret P. Battin does not object to palliative sedation itself but declares that it is not ethically different from more direct means of ending a patient's life.

YES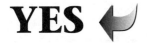

Sedation to Unconsciousness in End-of-Life Care

Introduction

The duty to relieve pain and suffering is central to the physician's role as healer and is an obligation physicians have to their patients. Palliative care is universally accepted as a multidisciplinary approach to prevent and relieve suffering of patients with life-limiting illnesses. In this setting, palliative sedation is an important technique for combating extreme suffering; however, there is much debate over the use of palliative sedation to unconsciousness because of its potential to be misconstrued as active euthanasia. Even when done properly, it may still provoke moral objection due to the mistaken perception of a risk of hastening death. . . .

This report examines the ethics of the palliative use of sedation to unconsciousness as an intervention of last resort for a terminally ill patient to reduce severe, refractory pain or other distressing clinical symptoms that have not been relieved by aggressive symptom-specific palliation. This report will not dwell on the specific ethics of withholding or withdrawing life-sustaining medical treatment, euthanasia, or physician-assisted suicide, all of which are addressed in the AMA's *Code of Medical Ethics,* but may differentiate palliative sedation to unconsciousness from such interventions for the purposes of clarification.

Background

. . . Palliative care is an integral part of the treatment regimen of terminally ill patients. However, even with the highest standards of care and attempts at palliation, it is estimated that between 5% and 35% of patients receiving palliative care in hospice programs experience severe pain and other intractable symptoms in the last week of life.[1] . . .

Clinical Issues

Palliative sedation to unconsciousness is only appropriate for terminally ill patients "as an intervention of last resort to reduce severe, refractory pain or other distressing clinical symptoms that have not been relieved by aggressive symptom-specific palliation." Specifically, such clinical symptoms include pain, nausea and vomiting, shortness of breath, agitated delirium, and dyspnea. Additionally, palliative sedation to unconsciousness has been indicated for patients who exhibit urinary retention due to clot formation, gastrointestinal pain, uncontrolled bleeding, and myoclonus.[2] Severe psychological distress may also warrant palliative sedation to unconsciousness when potentially treatable mental health conditions have been excluded.[2] Purely existential suffering may be defined as the experience of agony and distress that results from living in an unbearable state of existence including, for example, death anxiety, isolation, and loss of control. Some have proposed that such suffering in and of itself should also be recognized as an appropriate indication for palliative sedation to unconsciousness, but this remains controversial.[3] However, the Council concurs with those who argue that existential suffering, distinct from previously listed clinical symptoms, is not an appropriate indication for treatment with palliative sedation to unconsciousness, because the causes of this type of suffering are better addressed by other interventions.[4] For example, palliative sedation to unconsciousness is not the way to address suffering created by social isolation and loneliness; rather such suffering should be addressed by providing the patient with needed social support. For patients whose suffering is existential, it is necessary to show compassion and enlist the support of the patient's broader social and spiritual network in order to address issues which are beyond the scope of clinical care.[5]

Ethical Considerations

As described above, a wide spectrum of actions can be taken to relieve the various forms of suffering a terminally ill patient may experience at the end of life. When the usual armamentarium of medical interventions has been exhausted, choices still remain; these range from letting the terminal illness take its course without further intervention to unacceptable choices, such as euthanasia. Actions that are solely intended to hasten the death of patients, such as physician-assisted suicide or euthanasia, are ethically and medically unacceptable (both are "fundamentally incompatible with the physician's role as healer"). In contrast, the withholding and withdrawing of life-sustaining treatment, when done based on the patient's autonomous refusal of unwanted care, and allowing the natural course of disease to take place, are ethically and medically appropriate. Palliative sedation to unconsciousness is intended to relieve patient suffering and, like withholding or withdrawing life support, may also allow the natural process of terminal disease to take place. A recent review of studies of opiate and sedative use in palliative care concluded that there is no evidence to support shortened survival of terminally ill patients who were sedated.[6,7]

Though evidence suggests that opiate and sedative use in the palliative care setting rarely if ever hastens patient death, ethical issues of "intention" and "proportionality" remain of concern. When exploring the ethics of palliative sedation and differentiating it from those of physician-assisted suicide and euthanasia, it is paramount to consider the primary intention of the measure being utilized. Although intended to relieve suffering, physician-assisted suicide and euthanasia achieve this by bringing about death, where palliative sedation is intended to relieve suffering by providing proportionate sedation. Death due to the course of a terminal illness is anticipated in a patient who receives palliative sedation to unconsciousness. However, bringing about the patient's death is not the intent of the sedation.[8] Although intent cannot be observed directly, it can be gauged in part by examining the medical record. Repeated doses or continuous infusions are indicators of proportionate palliative sedation, whereas one large dose or rapidly accelerating doses out of proportion to the level of immediate patient suffering may signify lack of knowledge or an inappropriate intention to hasten death.[3] These questions about intent demonstrate the importance of careful documentation in the medical record of purpose and strategy for patients receiving any palliative care including palliative sedation to unconsciousness.

The doctrine of double effect illuminates how intent makes some forms of end-of-life care morally permissible and others unacceptable. The principle of double effect is applied to situations where it is impossible to avoid all harmful actions. It requires that the good effect (relieving severe suffering) must outweigh the bad effect (potential to unintentionally hasten death), and that the bad effect (ending the patient's life) cannot be the means of achieving the good effect (relieving suffering).[9] Proportionality is also a central tenant of the principle of double effect; the level of sedation sought (and the associated risk of hastening death) must be in direct relationship with, and justified by,[10,11] the level of unacceptable suffering the patient is experiencing. The greater the patient's pain or suffering, the more a physician must be willing to sedate a patient in order to reduce and hopefully eliminate the unacceptable symptoms. The combination and amount of sedative must be just sufficient, but not more so, to relieve distressing clinical symptoms.[3] Furthermore, the concepts of proportionality and justification help to differentiate palliative sedation from physician-assisted suicide and euthanasia since in the case of palliative sedation the physician aims only to sedate to a level of unconsciousness and no further.[12]

It is also important to consider palliative sedation to unconsciousness from the perspectives of autonomy, beneficence, and non-maleficence. Similar to the ethical argument made for withholding or withdrawing life-sustaining medical treatment where the principle of patient autonomy requires that physicians respect the decision of a patient who possesses decision-making capacity to forgo life-sustaining treatment, autonomous decision-making dictates that a fully informed patient should also be able to choose palliative sedation. A designated surrogate decision-maker would also be able to choose palliative sedation for a patient who lacks decision-making capacity and meets the criteria for receiving sedation at the end of life. Requests for palliative sedation to unconsciousness (by patients or their surrogates) that do not fit within acceptable clinical parameters identified by the definition of palliative sedation are inappropriate. The principle of beneficence dictates taking necessary steps to relieve pain and suffering. When discussing the possibility of palliative sedation, it is necessary to fully inform the patient or surrogate about the various levels of sedation and whether intermittent sedation or continuous sedation to unconsciousness is an appropriate option. Patients and their surrogate decision-makers, with guidance from their physicians, should separately decide whether they will continue to receive any life-sustaining treatments and whether they want to maintain, withhold or withdraw life-sustaining interventions (including nutrition and hydration). . . .

Recommendation

The Council on Ethical and Judicial Affairs recommends that the following be adopted. . . .

The duty to relieve pain and suffering is central to the physician's role as healer and is an obligation physicians have to their patients. Palliative sedation to unconsciousness is the administration of sedative medication to the point of unconsciousness in a terminally ill patient. It is an intervention of last resort to reduce severe, refractory pain or other distressing clinical symptoms that do not respond to aggressive symptom-specific palliation. It is an accepted and appropriate component of end-of-life care under specific, relatively rare circumstances. When symptoms cannot be diminished through all other means of palliation, including symptom-specific treatments, it is the ethical obligation of a physician to offer palliative sedation to unconsciousness as an option for the relief of intractable symptoms. When considering the use of palliative sedation, the following ethical guidelines are recommended:

1. Patients may be offered palliative sedation when they are in the final stages of terminal illness. The rationale for all palliative care measures should be documented in the medical record.
2. Palliative sedation to unconsciousness may be considered for those terminally ill patients whose clinical symptoms have been unresponsive to aggressive, symptom-specific treatments.
3. Physicians should ensure that the patient and/or the patient's surrogate have given informed consent for palliative sedation to unconsciousness.
4. Physicians should consult with a multidisciplinary team, including an expert in the field of palliative care, to ensure that symptom-specific treatments have been sufficiently employed and that palliative sedation to unconsciousness is now the most appropriate course of treatment.
5. Physicians should discuss with their patients considering palliative sedation the care plan relative to degree and length (intermittent or constant) of sedation, and the specific expectations for continuing, withdrawing or withholding future life-sustaining treatments.
6. Once palliative sedation is begun, a process must be implemented to monitor for appropriate care.
7. Palliative sedation is not an appropriate response to suffering that is primarily existential, defined as the experience of agony and distress that may arise from such issues as death anxiety, isolation and loss of control. Existential suffering is better addressed by other

interventions. For example, palliative sedation is not the way to address suffering created by social isolation and loneliness; such suffering should be addressed by providing the patient with needed social support.

8. Palliative sedation must never be used to intentionally cause a patient's death.

References

1. Quill, T. E., Byock, I. R., for the ACP-ASIM End-of-Life Care Consensus Panel. Responding to intractable terminal suffering: the role of terminal sedation and voluntary refusal of food and fluids. *Ann Intern Med.* 2000;132:408–414.

2. National Ethics Committee, Veterans Health Administration. The Ethics of palliative sedation as a therapy of last resort. *Am J Hosp Palliat Med.* 2007;23(6):483–491.

3. de Graeff A, Dean M. Palliative sedation therapy in the last weeks of life: a literature review and recommendations for standards. *J Palliat Med.* 2007 Feb;10(1):67–85.

4. Taylor BR, McCann RM. Controlled sedation for physical and existential suffering? *J of Palliat Med.* 2005;8(1):144–147.

5. Snyder L, Sulmasy DP, for the Etchis and Human Rights Committee, ACP-ASIM. Physician-assisted suicide—Position paper. *Ann Intern Med.* 2001;135:208–216.

6. Charter S, Viola R, Paterson J. Sedation for intractable distress in dying—A survey of experts. *Palliat Med.* 1998;12:255–296.

7. Morita T, Chinone Y, Ikenaga M, Miyoshi M, Nakaho T, Nishitateno K et al. Efficacy and safety of palliative sedation therapy: A multicenter, prospective, observational study conducted on specialized palliative care units in Japan. *J Pain Symptom Manage.* 2005;30(4):320–8.

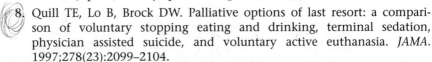

8. Quill TE, Lo B, Brock DW. Palliative options of last resort: a comparison of voluntary stopping eating and drinking, terminal sedation, physician assisted suicide, and voluntary active euthanasia. *JAMA.* 1997;278(23):2099–2104.

9. Quill TE, Dresser R, Brock DW. The rule of double effect—a critique of its role in end-of-life decision making. *N Eng J Med.* 1997;337:1768–1771.

10. Cantor NL, Thomas GC. The legal bounds of physician conduct hastening death. *Buffalo L Rev.* 2000;48(1):83–173.

11. Kollas CD, Boyer-Kollas B, Kollas JW. Criminal prosecutions of physicians providing palliative or end-of-life care. *J Palliat Med.* 2008;11(3):233–241.

12. Emanuel E. Ethics in pain management: an introductory overview. *Pain Med.* 2001:2(2)112–6.

Margaret P. Battin 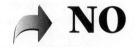 **NO**

Terminal Sedation: Pulling the Sheet Over Our Eyes

$\mathbf{T}$erminal sedation—also called "palliative sedation," "continuous deep sedation," or "primary deep continuous sedation"—has become a new favorite in end-of-life care, a seeming compromise in the debate over physician-assisted dying. Like all compromises, it offers something to each side of a dispute. But it is not a real down-the-middle compromise. It sells out on most of the things that may be important—to both sides. To corrupt an already awkward metaphor, terminal sedation pulls the sheet over our eyes. Terminal sedation may still be an important option in end-of-life care, but we should not present it as the only option in difficult deaths.

Proponents of assisted dying point to autonomy and mercy. The principle of autonomy holds that people are entitled to be the architects, as much as possible, of how they die. (Of course, autonomy has limits—one cannot inflict harm on others—and when one is no longer competent, values and interests may be expressed only indirectly; advance directives or surrogate decision-makers must be brought into play. But the principle itself is clear enough.) The principle of mercy requires that pain and suffering be relieved to the extent possible. These two principles operate in tandem to underwrite physician-assisted dying: physician assistance in bringing about death is to be provided just when the person voluntarily seeks it and just when it serves to avoid pain and suffering or the prospect of them. *Both* requirements must be met.

Opponents base their objections to physician-assisted dying on two other concerns. One is the sanctity of life, a religious or secular absolute respect for life that is held to entail the wrongness of killing, suicide, and murder. This principled objection holds regardless of whether a patient seeks assistance in dying in the face of pain and suffering. The second objection is that physician-assisted dying might lead to abuse. This concern is often spelled out in two ways: physician-assisted dying risks undercutting the integrity of the medical profession, and institutional or social pressures might make people victims of assisted dying they did not want.

These latter objections operate independently. One could be opposed to aid in dying on sanctity-of-life grounds even without fearing the slippery slope, and one could worry about the slippery slope without accepting the sanctity-of-life concerns. Often, however, these two concerns are fused in a

From *Hastings Center Report*, September/October 2008, pp. 27–30. Copyright © 2008 by The Hastings Center. Reprinted by permission of the publisher and Margaret P. Battin.

general objection—a joint claim that it is wrong for doctors to kill and that if doctors *do* kill, even in sympathetic cases like that of the seriously suffering and already dying patient who begs for help, then they might start killing in other, more worrisome cases as well. In short, it's autonomy *and* mercy on the one side, sanctity of life *and/or* the possibility of abuse on the other. That's the standoff over physician-assisted dying, argued in a kaleidoscope of ways over the past several decades.

Terminal sedation is often proffered as an alternative last resort measure that can overcome these practical and ideological disputes. In the 1997 cases *Washington v. Glucksberg* and *Vacco v. Quill,* the Supreme Court recognized the legality of providing pain relief in palliative care even if doing so might shorten life, provided the intention was to relieve pain. But careful scrutiny of terminal sedation—particularly sedation to unconsciousness, in which nutrition and hydration are withheld—suggests that it is not much of a compromise after all.

An Inadequate Compromise

Consider how terminal sedation fails to meet the concerns that underlie the dispute.

Autonomy

Consent of the person affected is central to the concept of autonomy, but it is not and—as a consequence of some political interpretations—*cannot* be honored in decisions to use terminal sedation. First, terminal sedation is often used for patients suffering from severe pain, for whom pain management has failed, but if pain is severe enough, reflective, unimpaired consent may no longer be possible. Decision-making must be deflected to a second party. (Of course, voluntary, informed consent is often challenged by pain: consider women in the throes of labor consenting to an epidural or a caesarean, or trauma victims consenting to surgery.)

More importantly, even when the decision is made in advance of the onset of intense pain, the focus of consent is obscured. Terminal sedation may end pain, but it also ends life. It does so in two ways: it immediately ends sentient life and the possibility for social interaction, and then, because artificial nutrition and hydration are usually withheld, it also ends biological life. But because the assumption is that sedation is used just to end pain, without the *intention* of ending life, the patient cannot be asked for consent to end his or her life, but only to relieve his or her pain. Of course, the consent process could include some mention of the possibility that relieving pain might inadvertently shorten life, but if the acknowledgment that life will be ended is stronger than that, the question of what is intended will arise. Thus, the focus of consent is on avoiding pain, but it should be on causing death.

The new euphemism, "palliative sedation," now often used instead of the more distressing "terminal sedation," only reinforces this problem. By avoiding the word "terminal" and hence any suggestion that death may be coming, the most important feature of this practice is obscured and terminal sedation is confused with "palliative care." Thus, the patient cannot consent to the really significant decision—whether his or her life shall be ended now. Autonomy is therefore undercut whether the patient's capacity for reflection is impaired by severe pain or not.

Mercy

Terminal sedation is typically used only at the very end of the downhill course, and only when the patient's pain has become extreme and other palliative measures are not effective. A broad study of pooled data over the last forty years on pain in cancer found that 59 percent of patients on anticancer treatment and 64 percent of patients with advanced metastatic disease experience pain.[1] Agitation, delirium, dyspnea, seizures, urinary and fecal retention, and nausea and protracted vomiting are also problems. Bernard Lo and Gordon Rubenfeld, writing in the *Journal of the American Medical Association,* discuss a forty-nine-year-old cancer patient given very high doses of morphine who developed myoclonus: seizures in the extremities and eventually in the whole body, producing intense pain.[2] As they say of palliative sedation for her and other dying patients: "We turn to it when everything else hasn't worked."

Terminal sedation to unconsciousness can certainly provide relief from such suffering, but some patients wish to avoid this long downhill course— especially the last stages of it. The use of terminal sedation "to relieve pain" presupposes that the patient is *already* experiencing pain. It provides no rationale for sedating a patient who is not currently in pain. Thus, the rationale for the use of terminal sedation in effect *requires* that the patient suffer.

The Sanctity of Life

The dispute over the principle of the wrongness of killing, or the sanctity of life, has focused mainly on ending a person's life before it would "naturally" end. Terminal sedation does not honor this principle. Rather, it unarguably causes death, and it does so in a way that is not "natural."

It is important to be perfectly clear about the process. Terminal sedation commonly involves two components: (1) inducing sedation, and (2) withholding the administration of fluids and nutrition. The first is not intrinsically lethal,[3] but the second is, if pursued long enough. Patients who are sedated to the degree involved in terminal sedation cannot eat or drink, and without "artificial" nutrition and hydration will necessarily die, virtually always before they would have died otherwise. Patients are sometimes sedated to unconsciousness with food and fluids continued—a practice that extends the dying period (and the cost), but this is not the usual form.

The death itself is not "natural," either. The airy, rather romantic notion of "natural" death usually refers to death that results from an underlying disease, but in terminal sedation death typically results from or is accelerated by dehydration. This is not "natural" dehydration; it is induced by a physician. If respect for the sanctity of life means that a patient's life should not be caused to end, but rather that death must occur only as the result of the underlying disease process, then terminal sedation does not honor this principle.

The Possibility of Abuse

This concern takes two general forms: (1) concern that the integrity of the medical profession will be undercut, and (2) concern that various familial, institutional, or social pressures will maneuver the patient into death when that would have been neither her choice nor in accord with her interests. Yet there is nothing in the practice of terminal sedation that offers greater protection against the possibility of abuse in either of these forms than does direct physician-assisted dying. Is the integrity of the medical profession likely to be undercut? There are many vivid forms of this charge leveled against direct physician-assisted dying—that physicians are overworked, anxious to cover their mistakes, unwilling to work with patients they dislike, biased against patients of certain class or racial backgrounds, beholden to cost pressures from their HMOs, and so on—but there is no reason to assume that terminal sedation would be less subject to these abuses than direct aid in dying. Indeed, direct aid in dying, at least as it is legally practiced in Oregon, requires a series of safeguards—confirmation of a terminal diagnosis, oral and written consent, a waiting period, and more—that do not come into play in terminal sedation. Terminal sedation has no institutional safeguards built in.

What about the sorts of familial, institutional, or social pressures that opponents claim would maneuver a patient into choosing death when that would not have been his choice? In terminal sedation, the choice a patient faces is already obscured: it is not framed as a choice of death versus life, but only as pain versus the relief of pain—a seemingly far easier choice to make, and hence one presumably far more easily shaped by external pressures from greedy family members, overworked or intolerant physicians, or the agents of cost-conscious institutions. *You don't need to suffer like this* is all they need to say.

In short, terminal sedation offers no greater protection against abuse than do the institutional safeguards established for (direct) physician aid in dying.

The Case in Favor of Terminal Sedation

Several writers in the field have argued, as I have, that terminal sedation fails to satisfy fully any of the major principles on either side of the aid in dying disputes. Timothy Quill, describing in close detail the "ambiguity of clinical intentions," has pointed out that it is virtually impossible for the clinician administering terminal sedation to intend palliation but not intend that death occur.[4] David Orentlicher lambasted the 1997 Supreme Court decision in *Washington v. Glucksberg* and *Vacco v. Quill* for "rejecting physician-assisted suicide, embracing euthanasia."[5] Tim Quill, Rebecca Dresser, and Dan Brock have skewered the Court's tortuous use of double-effect reasoning in supporting the practice of terminal sedation while rejecting voluntary, patient-requested physician-assisted suicide.[6]

Just the same, a case may be made for terminal sedation. It offers a definitive response to uncontrollable suffering. The gradual induction of death over the several days or more that terminal sedation takes may appeal to some patients and their families, especially if this slow process is perceived as gentler and easier for the patient, and as permitting the family more time to absorb the reality of their loss. It may also be perceived as less final than physician-assisted death: some forms of palliative sedation involve lightening up on the level of sedation periodically—for example, once a day—to see if the patient is still suffering.

The argument in favor of terminal sedation is one of perceptions: it may *feel* natural (even if it is not), it may *feel* safer (even if it offers less protection from abuse), it may *feel* like something the patient can openly choose (even if the choice is constructed in a way that obscures its real nature), and it may *feel* to the physician as if it is more in keeping with medical codes that prohibit killing (even if it still brings about death). We live in a society that tolerates many obfuscations and hypocrisies, and this may be another one we ought to embrace.

The Need for Guidelines

But we should do so with caution, and with a measure of skepticism about efforts to promote it. Some months before the November ballot that would include the state of Washington's measure I-1000, which is modeled on Oregon's Death with Dignity Act, the American Medical Association Council on Ethical and Judicial Affairs issued a report on "Sedation to Unconsciousness in End-of-Life Care."[7] This report makes an earnest effort to try to preclude many of the practical and ethical difficulties with palliative sedation. For example, the report acknowledges the importance of patient or surrogate consent. It insists that the patient's symptoms really warrant this measure. It emphasizes the importance of interdisciplinary consultation and careful monitoring. And it distinguishes between physical and existential suffering, insisting that palliative sedation may be appropriate in the former but that measures like social supports are to be used for the latter.

However, in its effort to distinguish palliative sedation (it avoids the expression "terminal sedation") from euthanasia, the report undercuts its own courage in addressing these difficult issues by trying to argue that palliative sedation (the permissible strategy) has nothing in common with euthanasia (the impermissible strategy). It does not distinguish between voluntary euthanasia (legal in the Netherlands and Belgium), nonvoluntary euthanasia (of a patient no longer capable of expressing his wishes or of giving legal consent), and involuntary euthanasia (against the patient's wishes). It fails to notice that the Dutch and the Nazi senses of "euthanasia" are entirely different, and that one could welcome the former while reviling the latter.

The AMA report distinguishes palliative sedation from euthanasia (or physician-assisted suicide or aid in dying) on the basis of intention—an application of the well-worn principle of double effect—and then attempts to infer intent from the pattern of practice. "One large dose" or "rapidly accelerating doses" of morphine may signify a bad intention—seeking to cause death—whereas "repeated doses or continuous infusions" are benign. This is naive in the extreme. It's the slyest courtier who poisons the emperor gradually; what could equally well be inferred from repeated doses and continuous infusions is a clever attempt to cover one's tracks. Nor is it clear what counts as "large doses" or other treatment measures in this simplistic dichotomy.

Is a fentanyl patch in a fentanyl-naive patient "rapidly accelerating" or "continuously infusing" when opioid tolerance may be in question? If a hydromorphone infusion for a patient with myoclonus is increased overnight from forty milligrams per hour to one hundred, does the increase count as "rapidly accelerating"? Are one hundred milligram boluses of hydromorphone given every fifteen to thirty minutes on top of a one hundred milligram/hour infusion considered to be "large doses," or are they merely "repeated" doses? What about the doses involved in initiating palliative sedation for this patient: a loading dose of phenobarbital and maintenance on a continuous phenobarbital infusion, together with intravenous dantrolene to lessen the myoclonus? In the case of the forty-nine-year-old cancer patient discussed by Lo and Rubenfeld, the patient died within approximately four hours of the initiation of palliative sedation. Indeed, the average survival in terminal sedation cases is just 1.5 to 3.1 days.[8]

What is astonishing is the AMA's attempt to try to differentiate between different sorts of clinical intentions on the basis of observed practice, when it is simply not possible—nor morally defensible—to draw this false bright line between them. These unworkable distinctions can only exacerbate the unease and legal dread in physicians who work to ease their patients' dying.

It's not that palliative sedation/sedation to unconsciousness/terminal sedation is wrong. It's that it can be practiced hypocritically, as the AMA report seems to ensure. Because there is so much anxiety that it might be confused with euthanasia, the features that it shares with euthanasia are obscured or sanitized. This is where the sheet is pulled over our eyes. The implausible effort to draw a completely bright line between continuous terminal sedation and euthanasia makes the practice of terminal sedation both more dangerous and more dishonest than it should be—and makes what can be a decent and humane practice morally problematic.

Another factor that hasn't been adequately explored is where terminal sedation ought to fit on a spectrum of end-of-life options: much of the "compromise" discussion seems to suggest that terminal sedation is the one and only way to deal with difficult deaths. But there are many last resort options, including patient-elected cessation of eating and drinking and direct physician-assisted dying. Terminal sedation is not an acceptable "compromise" if it overshadows these alternatives.

There is no reason why everyone facing a predictable, potentially difficult death should die in the same way. Knowing that pain is likely in some diseases and that even with the best palliative care not all pain can be relieved, some patients will prefer to avoid the worst, so to speak, and choose an earlier, gentler way out. Some will want to hang on as long as possible, in spite of everything. There is no reason that terminal sedation should not be recognized as an option, but there are excellent reasons why it should not be seen as the *only* option—or even the best option—for easing a bad death.

References

1. M.H. van den Beuken-van Everdingen et al., "Prevalence of Pain in Patients with Cancer: A Systematic Review of the Last 40 Years," *Annals of Oncology* 18, no. 9 (2007): 1437–49.

2. B. Lo and G. Rubenfeld, "Palliative Sedation in Dying Patients: 'We Turn to It When Everything Else Hasn't Worked,'" *Journal of the American Medical Association* 294 (2005): 1810–16.

3. For an analysis of data from the National Hospice Outcomes Project concerning whether opioids used in terminal illness cause death, see R.K. Portenoy et al., "Opioid Use and Survival at the End of Life: A Survey of a Hospice Population," *Journal of Pain and Symptom Management* 32, no. 6 (2006): 532–40.

4. T.E. Quill, "The Ambiguity of Clinical Intentions," *New England Journal of Medicine* 329 (1993): 1039–40.

5. D. Orentlicher, "The Supreme Court and Terminal Sedation: Rejecting Assisted Suicide, Embracing Euthanasia," *Hastings Constitutional Law Quarterly* 24, no. 4 (1997): 947–68.

6. T.E. Quill, R. Dresser, and D.W. Brock, "The Rule of Double Effect: A Critique of Its Role in End-of-Life Decision Making," *New England Journal of Medicine* 227 (1997): 1768–71.

7. American Medical Association Council on Ethical and Judicial Affairs, CEJA Report 5-A-08, "Sedation to Unconsciousness in End-of-Life Care."

8. C. Vena, K. Kuebler, and S.E. Schrader, "The Dying Process," in K. Kuebler, M.P. David, and C.C. Moore, eds., *Palliative Practices* (St. Louis, Mo.: Elsevier Mosby, 2005), 346, citing data from 1998 and 2000. See also Veterans Affairs National Ethics Teleconference, Terminal Sedation, August 27, 2002, online at http://www.ethics.va.gov/ETHICS/docs/net/NET_Topic_20020827_Terminal_Sedation.doc.

EXPLORING THE ISSUE

Is "Palliative Sedation" Ethically Different from Active Euthanasia?

Critical Thinking and Reflection

1. Do you agree with Battin that palliative sedation is tantamount to killing a terminally ill person, and why? If palliative sedation hastens death, is that, in your view, morally wrong? How compelling do you find Battin's thoughts about mercy?
2. Do you accept the "doctrine of double effect" as an explanation for why it might hasten death yet be acceptable? Or do you think that if it hastens death, then whether hastening death is acceptable must be confronted head on?
3. The AMA's Council on Ethical and Judicial Affairs offers a number of recommendations intended to ensure that palliative sedation at the end of life is not misused. Do those recommendations seem adequate to you? Too restrictive?

Is There Common Ground?

Everyone agrees that patients in the last throes of a terminal illness should be made as comfortable as possible. There is also broad agreement among ethicists and palliative care specialists that this justifies palliation strong enough to make the patient unconscious.

How far to go with palliative sedation seems to depend, as Battin notes, on how much value one attaches to biological life as opposed to freedom from suffering and the ability to live out one's life in the manner one wishes. The debate about the value of biological life is often cast as a sharp contrast: Either we believe that life is sacred, or we reject that idea altogether. If we uphold it, then we think it should be preserved even at the cost of suffering and turmoil, and even if the person's life story has essentially ended. Some years ago, however, the legal theorist Ronald Dworkin argued in the book *Life's Dominion: An Argument about Abortion, Euthanasia, and Individual Freedom* that many people actually accept both sides of this contrast to some degree: They think that biological life has value in and of itself, and that suffering should be curtailed and the person's wishes honored. They just differ on exactly where they strike the balance.

Additional Resources

Several Web sites carry posts opposing palliative sedation, some equating it to abortion or euthanasia. See, for example, www.hospicepatients.org, sponsored by the Hospice Patients Alliance, a "watchdog" organization.

For a set of professional recommendations of the use of palliative sedation on patients very near death, see Timothy W. Kirk and Margaret M. Mahon, "National Hospice and Palliative Care Organization (NHPCO) Position Statement and Commentary on the Use of Palliative Sedation in Imminently Dying Terminally Ill Patients," *Journal of Pain and Symptom Management* (vol. 39, no. 5, 2010); www.nhpco.org/i4a/pages/index.cfm?pageid=4673. Also, see National Ethics Committee, Veterans Health Administration, "The Ethics of Palliative Sedation as a Therapy of Last Resort," *American Journal of Hospice and Palliative Care* (vol. 23, no. 6, 2007).

Palliative care is also discussed in Nancy Berlinger, Bruce Jennings, and Susan M. Wolf, *The Hastings Center Guidelines for Decisions on Life-Sustaining Treatment and Care Near the End of Life: Revised and Expanded Second Edition* (Oxford University Press, 2013).

In "Last-Resort Options for Palliative Sedation," Timothy E. Quill, Bernard Lo, Dan W. Brock, and Alan Meisel recommend that palliative care and hospice programs develop clear policies about various levels of palliative sedation, including mechanisms for training and ensuring clinician competency (*Annals of Internal Medicine*, September 15, 2009).

After reviewing organizational guidelines around palliative sedation, Jeffrey Berger concluded that "current guidelines treat palliative sedation to unconsciousness as an effective medical treatment for terminally ill patients who need relief from severe symptoms, yet also restrict its use in ways that are extraordinary for medical treatments." He proposes loosening the guidelines that require imminent death and the failure of other aggressive measures ("Rethinking Guidelines for the Use of Palliative Sedation," *Hastings Center Report*, May–June 2010).

In "Responding to Intractable Terminal Suffering: The Role of Terminal Sedation and Voluntary Refusal of Food and Fluids," Timothy E. Quill and Ira Byock, writing for the American College of Physicians–American Society of Internal Medicine End-of-Life Consensus Panel, assert that terminal sedation and voluntary refusal of hydration and nutrition are options that substantially increase patients' choices (*Annals of Internal Medicine*, March 7, 2000).

Erich H. Loewy, a physician, offers a personal commentary in "Terminal Sedation, Self-Starvation, and Orchestrating the End of Life," *Archives of Internal Medicine* (February 12, 2001). He believes that when end-of-life care is skillfully orchestrated by a well-trained and practiced team, "few persons will want to take refuge in these options of last resort." He says that there is an enormous difference between allowing people to end their lives in this way and encouraging it.

ISSUE 6

Should Physicians Be Allowed to Assist in Patient Suicide?

YES: **Marcia Angell**, from "The Supreme Court and Physician-Assisted Suicide—The Ultimate Right," *The New England Journal of Medicine* (January 2, 1997)

NO: **Kathleen M. Foley**, from "Competent Care for the Dying Instead of Physician-Assisted Suicide," *The New England Journal of Medicine* (January 2, 1997)

Learning Outcomes

After reading this issue, you should be able to:

- Discuss the ethical dilemma posed by physician-assisted suicide.
- Explain the differences between active and passive euthanasia and between voluntary and involuntary euthanasia.

ISSUE SUMMARY

YES: Physician Marcia Angell asserts that a physician's main duties are to respect patient autonomy and to relieve suffering, even if that sometimes means assisting in a patient's death.

NO: Physician Kathleen M. Foley counters that if physician-assisted suicide becomes legal, it will begin to substitute for interventions that otherwise might enhance the quality of life for dying patients.

Since the early 1980s, physicians, lawyers, philosophers, and judges have examined questions about withholding life-sustaining treatment. Their deliberations have resulted in a broad consensus that competent adults have the right to make decisions about their medical care, even if those decisions seem unjustifiable to others and even if they result in death. Furthermore, the right of individuals to name others to carry out their prior wishes or to make decisions if they should become incompetent is now well established. Thirty-eight states now have legislation allowing advance directives (commonly known as "living wills").

The debate in specific cases continues (see, e.g., issue 5 on palliative seda-tion), but on the whole, patients' rights to self-determination have been bol-stered by 80 or more legal cases, dozens of reports, and statements made by medical societies and other organizations.

As often occurs in bioethical debate, the resolution of one issue only highlights the lack of resolution about another. There is clearly no consensus about either euthanasia or physician-assisted suicide.

Like truth telling, euthanasia is an old problem given new dimensions by the ability of modern medical technology to prolong life. The word itself is Greek (literally, *happy death*) and the Greeks wrestled with the question of whether, in some cases, people would be better off dead. But the Hippocratic Oath in this instance was clear: "I will neither give a deadly drug to anybody if asked for it, nor will I make a suggestion to that effect." On the other hand, if the goal of medicine is not simply to prolong life but to reduce suffering, at some point the question of what measures should be taken or withdrawn will inevitably arise. The problem is: When death is inevitable, how far should one go in hastening it?

The majority of cases in which euthanasia is raised as a possibility are among the most difficult ethical issues to resolve, for they involve the con-flict between a physician's duty to preserve life and the burden on the patient and the family that is created by fulfilling that duty. One common distinction is between *active* euthanasia (i.e., some positive act such as administering a lethal injection) and *passive* euthanasia (i.e., an inaction such as deciding not to administer antibiotics when the patient has a severe infection). Another common distinction is between *voluntary* euthanasia (i.e., the patient wishes to die and consents to the action that will make it happen) and *involuntary—or better, nonvoluntary*—euthanasia (i.e., the patient is unable to consent, perhaps because he or she is in a coma).

The YES and NO selections address a particularly controversial aspect of this issue. Is it ethical for a physician to assist in a hopelessly ill patient's suicide? Marcia Angell argues that sometimes hastening death should be an option for physicians although "reluctantly as a last resort." Angell states that a physician must consider patient autonomy and suffering when deciding upon care. Kathleen M. Foley contends that the medical profession should take the lead in developing guidelines for the end of life. This means that one must not confuse compassion for a patient's suffering with competence in care.

YES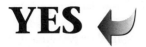

Marcia Angell

The Supreme Court and Physician-Assisted Suicide—The Ultimate Right

The importance and contentious issue of physician-assisted suicide, now being argued before the U.S. Supreme Court, is the subject of the following two editorials. Writing in favor of permitting assisted suicide under certain circumstances is the Journal's executive editor, Dr. Marcia Angell. Arguing against it is Dr. Kathleen Foley, co-chief of the Pain and Palliative Care Service of Memorial Sloan-Kettering Cancer Center in New York. We hope these two editorials, which have in common the authors' view that care of the dying is too often inadequate, will help our readers in making their own judgments.

—Jerome P. Kassirer, M.D.

The U.S. Supreme Court will decide later this year whether to let stand decisions by two appeals courts permitting doctors to help terminally ill patients commit suicide.[1] The Ninth and Second Circuit Courts of Appeals last spring held that state laws in Washington and New York that ban assistance in suicide were unconstitutional as applied to doctors and their dying patients.[2, 3] If the Supreme Court lets the decisions stand, physicians in 12 states, which include about half the population of the United States, would be allowed to provide the means for terminally ill patients to take their own lives, and the remaining states would rapidly follow suit. Not since *Roe* v. *Wade* has a Supreme Court decision been so fateful.

The decision will culminate several years of intense national debate, fueled by a number of highly publicized events. Perhaps most important among them is Dr. Jack Kevorkian's defiant assistance in some 44 suicides since 1990, to the dismay of many in the medical and legal establishments, but with substantial public support, as evidenced by the fact that three juries refused to convict him even in the face of a Michigan statute enacted for that purpose. Also since 1990, voters in three states have considered ballot initiatives that would legalize some form of physician-assisted dying, and in 1994 Oregon became the first state to approve such a measure.[4] (The Oregon law was stayed pending a court challenge.) Several surveys indicate that roughly two thirds of the American public now support physician-assisted suicide,[5, 6] as do more than half the doctors in the United States,[6, 7] despite the fact that influential physicians' organizations are opposed. It seems clear that many Americans are now so concerned about

From *The New England Journal of Medicine*, January 2, 1997, pp. 50–53. Copyright © 1997 by Massachusetts Medical Society. All rights reserved. Reprinted by permission.

the possibility of a lingering, high-technology death that they are receptive to the idea of doctors' being allowed to help them die.

In this editorial I will explain why I believe the appeals courts were right and why I hope the Supreme Court will uphold their decisions. I am aware that this is a highly contentious issue, with good people and strong arguments on both sides. The American Medical Association (AMA) filed an amicus brief opposing the legalization of physician-assisted suicide,[8] and the Massachusetts Medical Society, which owns the *Journal,* was a signatory to it. But here I speak for myself, not the *Journal* or the Massachusetts Medical Society. The legal aspects of the case have been well discussed elsewhere, to me most compellingly in Ronald Dworkin's essay in the *New York Review of Books.*[9] I will focus primarily on the medical and ethical aspects.

I begin with the generally accepted premise that one of the most important ethical principles in medicine is respect for each patient's autonomy, and that when this principle conflicts with others, it should almost always take precedence. This premise is incorporated into our laws governing medical practice and research, including the requirement of informed consent to any treatment. In medicine, patients exercise their self-determination most dramatically when they ask that life-sustaining treatment be withdrawn. Although others may sometimes consider the request ill-founded, we are bound to honor it if the patient is mentally competent—that is, if the patient can understand the nature of the decision and its consequences.

A second starting point is the recognition that death is not fair and is often cruel. Some people die quickly, and others die slowly but peacefully. Some find personal or religious meaning in the process, as well as an opportunity for a final reconciliation with loved ones. But others, especially those with cancer, AIDS, or progressive neurologic disorders, may die by inches and in great anguish, despite every effort of their doctors and nurses. Although nearly all pain can be relieved, some cannot, and other symptoms, such as dyspnea, nausea, and weakness, are even more difficult to control. In addition, dying sometimes holds great indignities and existential suffering. Patients who happen to require some treatment to sustain their lives, such as assisted ventilation or dialysis, can hasten death by having the life-sustaining treatment withdrawn, but those who are not receiving life-sustaining treatment may desperately need help they cannot now get.

If the decisions of the appeals courts are upheld, states will not be able to prohibit doctors from helping such patients to die by prescribing a lethal dose of a drug and advising them on its use for suicide. State laws barring euthanasia (the administration of a lethal drug by a doctor) and assisted suicide for patients who are not terminally ill would not be affected. Furthermore, doctors would not be *required* to assist in suicide; they would simply have that option. Both appeals courts based their decisions on constitutional questions. This is important, because it shifted the focus of the debate from what the majority would approve through the political process, as exemplified by the Oregon initiative, to a matter of fundamental rights, which are largely immune from the political process. Indeed, the Ninth Circuit Court drew an explicit analogy between suicide and abortion, saying that both were personal choices protected by the

Constitution and that forbidding doctors to assist would in effect nullify these rights. Although states could regulate assisted suicide, as they do abortion, they would not be permitted to regulate it out of existence.

It is hard to quarrel with the desire of a greatly suffering, dying patient for a quicker, more humane death or to disagree that it may be merciful to help bring that about. In those circumstances, loved ones are often relieved when death finally comes, as are the attending doctors and nurses. As the Second Circuit Court said (in the case of *Quill v. Vacco*), the state has no interest in prolonging such a life. Why, then, do so many people oppose legalizing physician-assisted suicide in these cases? There are a number of arguments against it, some stronger than others, but I believe none of them can offset the overriding duties of doctors to relieve suffering and to respect their patients' autonomy. Below I list several of the more important arguments against physician-assisted suicide and discuss why I believe they are in the last analysis unpersuasive.

Assisted suicide is a form of killing, which is always wrong. In contrast, withdrawing life-sustaining treatment simply allows the disease to take its course. There are three methods of hastening the death of a dying patient: withdrawing life-sustaining treatment, assisting suicide, and euthanasia. The right to stop treatment has been recognized repeatedly since the 1976 case of Karen Ann Quinlan[10] and was affirmed by the U.S. Supreme Court in the 1990 Cruzan decision[11] and the U.S. Congress in its 1990 Patient Self-Determination Act.[12] Although the legal underpinning is the right to be free of unwanted bodily invasion, the purpose of hastening death was explicitly acknowledged. In contrast, assisted suicide and euthanasia have not been accepted; euthanasia is illegal in all states, and assisted suicide is illegal in most of them.

Why the distinctions? Most would say they turn on the doctor's role: whether it is passive or active. When life-sustaining treatment is withdrawn, the doctor's role is considered passive and the cause of death is the underlying disease, despite the fact that switching off the ventilator of a patient dependent on it looks anything but passive and would be considered homicide if done without the consent of the patient or a proxy. In contrast, euthanasia by the injection of a lethal drug is active and directly causes the patient's death. Assisting suicide by supplying the necessary drugs is considered somewhere in between, more active than switching off a ventilator but less active than injecting drugs, hence morally and legally more ambiguous.

I believe, however, that these distinctions are too doctor-centered and not sufficiently patient-centered. We should ask ourselves not so much whether the doctor's role is passive or active but whether the *patient's* role is passive or active. From that perspective, the three methods of hastening death line up quite differently. When life-sustaining treatment is withdrawn from an incompetent patient at the request of a proxy or when euthanasia is performed, the patient may be utterly passive. Indeed, either act can be performed even if the patient is unaware of the decision. In sharp contrast, assisted suicide, by definition, cannot occur without the patient's knowledge and participation. Therefore, it must be active—that is to say, voluntary. That is a crucial distinction, because it provides an inherent safeguard against abuse that is not present with the other two methods of hastening death. If the loaded term "kill" is to be used, it is not the doctor who kills, but the patient. Primarily because euthanasia can be performed without the patient's participation, I oppose its legalization in this country.

Assisted suicide is not necessary. All suffering can be relieved if care givers are sufficiently skillful and compassionate, as illustrated by the hospice movement. I have no doubt that if expert palliative care were available to everyone who needed it, there would be few requests for assisted suicide. Even under the best of circumstances, however, there will always be a few patients whose suffering simply cannot be adequately alleviated. And there will be some who would prefer suicide to any other measures available, including the withdrawal of life-sustaining treatment or the use of heavy sedation. Surely, every effort should be made to improve palliative care, as I argued 15 years ago,[13] but when those efforts are unavailing and suffering patients desperately long to end their lives, physician-assisted suicide should be allowed. The argument that permitting it would divert us from redoubling our commitment to comfort care asks these patients to pay the penalty for our failings. It is also illogical. Good comfort care and the availability of physician-assisted suicide are no more mutually exclusive than good cardiologic care and the availability of heart transplantation.

Permitting assisted suicide would put us on a moral "slippery slope." Although in itself assisted suicide might be acceptable, it would lead inexorably to involuntary euthanasia. It is impossible to avoid slippery slopes in medicine (or in any aspect of life). The issue is how and where to find a purchase. For example, we accept the right of proxies to terminate life-sustaining treatment, despite the obvious potential for abuse, because the reasons for doing so outweigh the risks. We hope our procedures will safeguard patients. In the case of assisted suicide, its voluntary nature is the best protection against sliding down a slippery slope, but we also need to ensure that the request is thoughtful and freely made. Although it is possible that we may someday decide to legalize voluntary euthanasia under certain circumstances or assisted suicide for patients who are not terminally ill, legalizing assisted suicide for the dying does not in itself make these other decisions inevitable. Interestingly, recent reports from the Netherlands, where both euthanasia and physician-assisted suicide are permitted, indicate that fears about a slippery slope there have not been borne out.[14, 15, 16]

Assisted suicide would be a threat to the economically and socially vulnerable. The poor, disabled, and elderly might be coerced to request it. Admittedly, overburdened families or cost-conscious doctors might pressure vulnerable patients to request suicide, but similar wrongdoing is at least as likely in the case of withdrawing life-sustaining treatment, since that decision can be made by proxy. Yet, there is no evidence of widespread abuse. The Ninth Circuit Court recalled that it was feared *Roe v. Wade* would lead to coercion of poor and uneducated women to request abortions, but that did not happen. The concern that coercion is more likely in this era of managed care, although understandable, would hold suffering patients hostage to the deficiencies of our health care system. Unfortunately, no human endeavor is immune to abuses. The question is not whether a perfect system can be devised, but whether abuses are likely to be sufficiently rare to be offset by the benefits to patients who otherwise would be condemned to face the end of their lives in protracted agony.

Depressed patients would seek physician-assisted suicide rather than help for their depression. Even in the terminally ill, a request for assisted suicide might signify treatable depression, not irreversible suffering. Patients suffering greatly at the end of life may also be depressed, but the depression does not necessarily explain their decision to commit suicide or make it irrational. Nor is it simple to diagnose depression in terminally ill patients. Sadness is to be expected, and some of the vegetative symptoms of depression are similar to the symptoms of terminal illness. The success of antidepressant treatment in these circumstances is also not ensured. Although there are anecdotes about patients who changed their minds about suicide after treatment,[17] we do not have good studies of how often that happens or the relation to antidepressant treatment. Dying patients who request assisted suicide and seem depressed should certainly be strongly encouraged to accept psychiatric treatment, but I do not believe that competent patients should be *required* to accept it as a condition of receiving assistance with suicide. On the other hand, doctors would not be required to comply with all requests; they would be expected to use their judgment, just as they do in so many other types of life-and-death decisions in medical practice.

Doctors should never participate in taking life. If there is to be assisted suicide, doctors must not be involved. Although most doctors favor permitting assisted suicide under certain circumstances, many who favor it believe that doctors should not provide the assistance.[6, 7] To them, doctors should be unambiguously committed to life (although most doctors who hold this view would readily honor a patient's decision to have life-sustaining treatment withdrawn). The AMA, too, seems to object to physician-assisted suicide primarily because it violates the profession's mission. Like others, I find that position too abstract.[18] The highest ethical imperative of doctors should be to provide care in whatever way best serves patients' interests, in accord with each patient's wishes, not with a theoretical commitment to preserve life no matter what the cost in suffering.[19] If a patient requests help with suicide and the doctor believes the request is appropriate, requiring someone else to provide the assistance would be a form of abandonment. Doctors who are opposed in principle need not assist, but they should make their patients aware of their position early in the relationship so that a patient who chooses to select another doctor can do so. The greatest harm we can do is to consign a desperate patient to unbearable suffering—or force the patient to seek out a stranger like Dr. Kevorkian. Contrary to the frequent assertion that permitting physician-assisted suicide would lead patients to distrust their doctors, I believe distrust is more likely to arise from uncertainty about whether a doctor will honor a patient's wishes.

Physician-assisted suicide may occasionally be warranted, but it should remain illegal. If doctors risk prosecution, they will think twice before assisting with suicide.   This argument wrongly shifts the focus from the patient to the doctor. Instead of reflecting the condition and wishes of patients, assisted suicide would reflect the courage and compassion of their doctors. Thus, patients with doctors like Timothy Quill, who described in a 1991 *Journal* article how he helped a patient take her life,[20] would get the help they need and want, but similar patients with less steadfast doctors would not. That makes no sense.

People do not need assistance to commit suicide. With enough determination, they can do it themselves.   This is perhaps the cruelest of the arguments against physician-assisted suicide. Many patients at the end of life are, in fact, physically unable to commit suicide on their own. Others lack the resources to do so. It has sometimes been suggested that they can simply stop eating and drinking and kill themselves that way. Although this method has been described as peaceful under certain conditions,[21] no one should count on that. The fact is that this argument leaves most patients to their suffering. Some, usually men, manage to commit suicide using violent methods. Percy Bridgman, a Nobel laureate in physics who in 1961 shot himself rather than die of metastatic cancer, said in his suicide note, "It is not decent for Society to make a man do this to himself."[22]

My father, who knew nothing of Percy Bridgman, committed suicide under similar circumstances. He was 81 and had metastatic prostate cancer. The night before he was scheduled to be admitted to the hospital, he shot himself. Like Bridgman, he thought it might be his last chance. At the time, he was not in extreme pain, nor was he close to death (his life expectancy was probably longer than six months). But he was suffering nonetheless—from nausea and the side effects of antiemetic agents, weakness, incontinence, and hopelessness. Was he depressed? He would probably have freely admitted that he was, but he would have thought it beside the point. In any case, he was an intensely private man who would have refused psychiatric care. Was he overly concerned with maintaining control of the circumstances of his life and death? Many people would say so, but that was the way he was. It is the job of medicine to deal with patients as they are, not as we would like them to be.

I tell my father's story here because it makes an abstract issue very concrete. If physician-assisted suicide had been available, I have no doubt my father would have chosen it. He was protective of his family, and if he had felt he had the choice, he would have spared my mother the shock of finding his body. He did not tell her what he planned to do, because he knew she would stop him. I also believe my father would have waited if physician-assisted suicide had been available. If patients have access to drugs they can take when they choose, they will not feel they must commit suicide early, while they are still able to do it on their own. They would probably live longer and certainly more peacefully, and they might not even use the drugs.

Long before my father's death, I believed that physician-assisted suicide ought to be permissible under some circumstances, but his death strengthened my conviction that it is simply a part of good medical care—something to be done reluctantly and sadly, as a last resort, but done nonetheless. There should be safeguards to ensure that the decision is well considered and consistent, but they should not be so daunting or violative of privacy that they become obstacles instead of protections. In particular, they should be directed not toward reviewing the reasons for an autonomous decision, but only toward ensuring that the decision is indeed autonomous. If the Supreme Court upholds the decisions of the appeals courts, assisted suicide will not be forced on either patients or doctors, but it will be a choice for those patients who need it and those doctors willing to help. If, on the other hand, the Supreme Court overturns the lower courts' decisions, the issue will continue to be grappled with state by state, through the political process. But sooner or later, given the need and the widespread public support, physician-assisted suicide will be demanded of a compassionate profession.

References

1. Greenhouse L. High court to say if the dying have a right to suicide help. New York Times. October 2, 1996:A1.
2. Compassion in Dying v. Washington, 79 F.3d 790 (9th Cir. 1996).
3. Quill v. Vacco, 80 F.3d 716 (2d Cir. 1996).
4. Annas GJ. Death by prescription—the Oregon initiative. N Engl J Med 1994;331:1240–3.
5. Blendon RJ, Szalay US, Knox RA. Should physicians aid their patients in dying? The public perspective. JAMA 1992;267:2658–62.
6. Bachman JG, Alcser KH, Doukas DJ, Lichtenstein RL, Corning AD, Brody H. Attitudes of Michigan physicians and the public toward legalizing physician-assisted suicide and voluntary euthanasia. N Engl J Med 1996;334:303–9.
7. Lee MA, Nelson HD, Tilden VP, Ganzini L, Schmidt TA, Tolle SW. Legalizing assisted suicide—views of physicians in Oregon. N Engl J Med 1996;334:310–5.
8. Gianelli DM. AMA to court: no suicide aid. American Medical News. November 25, 1996:1, 27, 28.
9. Dworkin R. Sex, death, and the courts. New York Review of Books. August 8, 1996.
10. In re: Quinlan, 70 N.J. 10, 355 A.2d 647 (1976).
11. Cruzan v. Director, Missouri Department of Health, 497 U.S. 261, 110 S.Ct. 2841 (1990).
12. Omnibus Budget Reconciliation Act of 1990, P.L. 101–508, sec. 4206 and 4751, 104 Stat. 1388, 1388–115, and 1388–204 (classified respectively at 42 U.S.C. 1395cc(f) (Medicare) and 1396a(w) (Medicaid) (1994)).
13. Angell M. The quality of mercy. N Engl J Med 1982;306:98–9.
14. van der Maas PJ, van der Wal G, Haverkate I, et al. Euthanasia, physician-assisted suicide, and other medical practices involving the end of life in the Netherlands, 1990–1995. N Engl J Med 1996;335:1699–705.

15. van der Wal G, van der Maas PJ, Bosma JM, et al. Evaluation of the notification procedure for physician-assisted death in the Netherlands. N Engl J Med 1996;335:1706–11.

16. Angell M. Euthanasia in the Netherlands—good news or bad? N Engl J Med 1996;335:1676–8.

17. Chochinov HM, Wilson KG, Enns M, et al. Desire for death in the terminally ill. Am J Psychiatry 1995;152:1185–91.

18. Cassel CK, Meier DE. Morals and moralism in the debate over euthanasia and assisted suicide. N Engl J Med 1990;323:750–2.

19. Angell M. Doctors and assisted suicide. Ann R Coll Physicians Surg Can 1991;24:493–4.

20. Quill TE. Death and dignity—a case of individualized decision making. N Engl J Med 1991;324:691–4.

21. Lynn J, Childress JF. Must patients always be given food and water? Hastings Cent Rep 1983;13(5):17–21.

22. Nuland SB. How we die. New York: Alfred A. Knopf, 1994:152.

Kathleen M. Foley

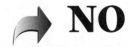 **NO**

Competent Care for the Dying Instead of Physician-Assisted Suicide

While the Supreme Court is reviewing the decisions by the Second and Ninth Circuit Courts of Appeals to reverse state bans on assisted suicide, there is a unique opportunity to engage the public, health care professionals, and the government in a national discussion of how American medicine and society should address the needs of dying patients and their families. Such a discussion is critical if we are to understand the process of dying from the point of view of patients and their families and to identify existing barriers to appropriate, humane, compassionate care at the end of life. Rational discourse must replace the polarized debate over physician-assisted suicide and euthanasia. Facts, not anecdotes, are necessary to establish a common ground and frame a system of health care for the terminally ill that provides the best possible quality of living while dying.

The biased language of the appeals courts evinces little respect for the vulnerability and dependency of the dying. Judge Stephen Reinhardt, writing for the Ninth Circuit Court, applied the liberty-interest clause of the Fourteenth Amendment, advocating a constitutional right to assisted suicide. He stated, "The competent terminally ill adult, having lived nearly the full measure of his life, has a strong interest in choosing a dignified and humane death, rather than being reduced to a state of helplessness, diapered, sedated, incompetent."[1] Judge Roger J. Miner, writing for the Second Circuit Court of Appeals, applied the equal-rights clause of the Fourteenth Amendment and went on to emphasize that the state "has no interest in prolonging a life that is ending."[2] This statement is more than legal jargon. It serves as a chilling reminder of the low priority given to the dying when it comes to state resources and protection.

The appeals courts' assertion of a constitutional right to assisted suicide is narrowly restricted to the terminally ill. The courts have decided that it is the patient's condition that justifies killing and that the terminally ill are special—so special that they deserve assistance in dying. This group alone can receive such assistance. The courts' response to the New York and Washington cases they reviewed is the dangerous form of affirmative action in the name of compassion. It runs the risk of further devaluing the lives of terminally ill patients and may provide the excuse for society to abrogate its responsibility for their care.

Both circuit courts went even further in asserting that physicians are already assisting in patients' deaths when they withdraw life-sustaining

From *The New England Journal of Medicine*, January 2, 1997, pp. 54–58. Copyright © 1997 by Massachusetts Medical Society. All rights reserved. Reprinted by permission.

treatments such as respirators or administer high doses of pain medication that hasten death. The appeals courts argued that providing a lethal prescription to allow a terminally ill patient to commit suicide is essentially the same as withdrawing life-sustaining treatment or aggressively treating pain. Judicial reasoning that eliminates the distinction between letting a person die and killing runs counter to physicians' standards of palliative care.[3] The courts' purported goal in blurring these distinctions was to bring society's legal rules more closely in line with the moral value it places on the relief of suffering.[4]

In the real world in which physicians care for dying patients, withdrawing treatment and aggressively treating pain are acts that respect patients' autonomous decisions not to be battered by medical technology and to be relieved of their suffering. The physician's intent is to provide care, not death. Physicians do struggle with doubts about their own intentions.[5] The courts' arguments fuel their ambivalence about withdrawing life-sustaining treatments or using opioid or sedative infusions to treat intractable symptoms in dying patients. Physicians are trained and socialized to preserve life. Yet saying that physicians struggle with doubts about their intentions in performing these acts is not the same as saying that their intention is to kill. In palliative care, the goal is to relieve suffering, and the quality of life, not the quantity, is of utmost importance.

Whatever the courts say, specialists in palliative care do not think that they practice physician-assisted suicide or euthanasia.[6] Palliative medicine has developed guidelines for aggressive pharmacologic management of intractable symptoms in dying patients, including sedation for those near death.[3, 7, 8] The World Health Organization has endorsed palliative care as an integral component of a national health care policy and has strongly recommended to its member countries that they not consider legalizing physician-assisted suicide and euthanasia until they have addressed the needs of their citizens for pain relief and palliative care.[9] The courts have disregarded this formidable recommendation and, in fact, are indirectly suggesting that the World Health Organization supports assisted suicide.

Yet the courts' support of assisted suicide reflects the requests of the physicians who initiated the suits and parallels the numerous surveys demonstrating that a large proportion of physicians support the legalization of physician-assisted suicide.[10, 11, 12, 13, 14, 15] A smaller proportion of physicians are willing to provide such assistance, and an even smaller proportion are willing to inject a lethal dose of medication with the intent of killing a patient (active voluntary euthanasia). These survey data reveal a gap between the attitudes and behavior of physicians; 20 to 70 percent of physicians favor the legalization of physician-assisted suicide, but only 2 to 4 percent favor active voluntary euthanasia, and only approximately 2 to 13 percent have actually aided patients in dying, by either providing a prescription or administering a lethal injection. The limitations of these surveys, which are legion, include inconsistent definitions of physician-assisted suicide and euthanasia, lack of information about nonrespondents, and provisions for maintaining confidentiality that have led to inaccurate reporting.[13, 16] Since physicians' attitudes toward alternatives to assisted suicide have not been studied, there is a void in our knowledge about the priority that physicians place on physician-assisted suicide.

The willingness of physicians to assist patients in dying appears to be determined by numerous complex factors, including religious beliefs, personal values, medical specialty, age, practice setting, and perspective on the use of financial resources.[13, 16, 17, 18, 19] Studies of patients' preferences for care at the end of life demonstrate that physicians' preferences strongly influence those of their patients.[13] Making physician-assisted suicide a medical treatment when it is so strongly dependent on these physician-related variables would result in a regulatory impossibility.[19] Physicians would have to disclose their values and attitudes to patients to avoid potential conflict.[13] A survey by Ganzini et al. demonstrated that psychiatrists' responses to requests to evaluate patients were highly determined by their attitudes.[13] In a study by Emanuel et al., depressed patients with cancer said they would view positively those physicians who acknowledged their willingness to assist in suicide. In contrast, patients with cancer who were suffering from pain would be suspicious of such physicians.[11]

In this controversy, physicians fall into one of three groups. Those who support physician-assisted suicide see it as a compassionate response to a medical need, a symbol of nonabandonment, and a means to reestablish patients' trust in doctors who have used technology excessively.[20] They argue that regulation of physician-assisted suicide is possible and, in fact, necessary to control the actions of physicians who are currently providing assistance surreptitiously.[21] The two remaining groups of physicians oppose legalization.[19, 22, 23, 24] One group is morally opposed to physician-assisted suicide and emphasizes the need to preserve the professionalism of medicine and the commitment to "do no harm." These physicians view aiding a patient in dying as a form of abandonment, because a physician needs to walk the last mile with the patient, as a witness, not as an executioner. Legalization would endorse justified killing, according to these physicians, and guidelines would not be followed, even if they could be developed. Furthermore, these physicians are concerned that the conflation of assisted suicide with the withdrawal of life support or adequate treatment of pain would make it even harder for dying patients, because there would be a backlash against existing policies. The other group is not ethically opposed to physician-assisted suicide and, in fact, sees it as acceptable in exceptional cases, but these physicians believe that one cannot regulate the unregulatable.[19] On this basis, the New York State Task Force on Life and the Law, a 24-member committee with broad public and professional representation, voted unanimously against the legalization of physician-assisted suicide.[24] All three groups of physicians agree that a national effort is needed to improve the care of the dying. Yet it does seem that those in favor of legalizing physician-assisted suicide are disingenuous in their use of this issue as a wedge. If this form of assistance with dying is legalized, the courts will be forced to broaden the assistance to include active voluntary euthanasia and, eventually, assistance in response to requests from proxies.

One cannot easily categorize the patients who request physician-assisted suicide or euthanasia. Some surveys of physicians have attempted to determine retrospectively the prevalence and nature of these requests.[10] Pain, AIDS, and neurodegenerative disorders are the most common conditions in patients requesting assistance in dying. There is a wide range in the age of such patients, but many are younger persons with AIDS.[10] From the limited data available, the factors most commonly involved in requests for assistance are concern about future loss of control, being or becoming a burden to others, or being unable to care for oneself and fear of severe pain.[10] A small number of recent studies have directly asked terminally ill patients with cancer or AIDS about their desire for death.[25, 26, 27] All these studies show that the desire for death is closely associated with depression and that pain and lack of social support are contributing factors.

Do we know enough, on the basis of several legal cases, to develop a public policy that will profoundly change medicine's role in society?[1, 2] Approximately 2.4 million Americans die each year. We have almost no information on how they die and only general information on where they die. Sixty-one percent die in hospitals, 17 percent in nursing homes, and the remainder at home, with approximately 10 to 14 percent of those at home receiving hospice care.

The available data suggest that physicians are inadequately trained to assess and manage the multifactorial symptoms commonly associated with patients' requests for physician-assisted suicide. According to the American Medical Association's report on medical education, only 5 of 126 medical schools in the United States require a separate course in the care of the dying.[28] Of 7048 residency programs, only 26 percent offer a course on the medical and legal aspects of care at the end of life as a regular part of the curriculum. According to a survey of 1068 accredited residency programs in family medicine, internal medicine, and pediatrics and fellowship programs in geriatrics, each resident or fellow coordinates the care of 10 or fewer dying patients annually.[28] Almost 15 percent of the programs offer no formal training in terminal care. Despite the availability of hospice programs, only 17 percent of the training programs offer a hospice rotation, and the rotation is required in only half of those programs; 9 percent of the programs have residents or fellows serving as members of hospice teams. In a recent survey of 55 residency programs and over 1400 residents, conducted by the American Board of Internal Medicine, the residents were asked to rate their perception of adequate training in care at the end of life. Seventy-two percent reported that they had received adequate training in managing pain and other symptoms; 62 percent, that they had received adequate training in telling patients that they are dying; 38 percent, in describing what the process will be like; and 32 percent, in talking to patients who request assistance in dying or a hastened death (Blank L: personal communication).

The lack of training in the care of the dying is evident in practice. Several studies have concluded that poor communication between physicians and patients, physicians' lack of knowledge about national guidelines for such care, and their lack of knowledge about the control of symptoms are barriers to the provision of good care at the end of life.[23, 29, 30]

Yet there is now a large body of data on the components of suffering in patients with advanced terminal disease, and these data provide the basis for treatment algorithms.[3] There are three major factors in suffering: pain and other physical symptoms, psychological distress, and existential distress (described as the experience of life without meaning). It is not only the patients who suffer but also their families and the health care professionals attending them. These experiences of suffering are often closely and inextricably related. Perceived distress in any one of the three groups amplifies distress in the others.[31, 32]

Pain is the most common symptom in dying patients, and according to recent data from U.S. studies, 56 percent of outpatients with cancer, 82 percent of outpatients with AIDS, 50 percent of hospitalized patients with various diagnoses, and 36 percent of nursing home residents have inadequate management of pain during the course of their terminal illness.[33, 34, 35, 36] Members of minority groups and women, both those with cancer and those with AIDS, as well as the elderly, receive less pain treatment than other groups of patients. In a survey of 1177 physicians who had treated a total of more than 70,000 patients with cancer in the previous six months, 76 percent of the respondents cited lack of knowledge as a barrier to their ability to control pain.[37] Severe pain that is not adequately controlled interferes with the quality of life, including the activities of daily living, sleep, and social interactions.[33, 38]

Other physical symptoms are also prevalent among the dying. Studies of patients with advanced cancer and of the elderly in the year before death show that they have numerous symptoms that worsen the quality of life, such as fatigue, dyspnea, delirium, nausea, and vomiting.[36, 38]

Along with these physical symptoms, dying patients have a variety of well-described psychological symptoms, with a high prevalence of anxiety and depression in patients with cancer or AIDS and the elderly.[27, 39] For example, more than 60 percent of patients with advanced cancer have psychiatric problems, with adjustment disorders, depression, anxiety, and delirium reported most frequently. Various factors that contribute to the prevalence and severity of psychological distress in the terminally ill have been identified.[39] The diagnosis of depression is difficult to make in medically ill patients[3, 26, 40]; 94 percent of the Oregon psychiatrists surveyed by Ganzini et al. were not confident that they could determine, in a single evaluation, whether a psychiatric disorder was impairing the judgment of a patient who requested assistance with suicide.[13]

Attention has recently been focused on the interaction between uncontrolled symptoms and vulnerability to suicide in patients with cancer or AIDS.[41] Data from studies of both groups of patients suggest that uncontrolled pain contributes to depression and that persistent pain interferes with patients' ability to receive support from their families and others. Patients with AIDS have a high risk of suicide that is independent of physical symptoms. Among New York City residents with AIDS, the relative risk of suicide in men between the ages of 20 and 59 years was 36 times higher than the risk among men without AIDS in the same age group and 66 times higher than the risk in the general population.[41] Patients with AIDS who committed suicide generally did so within nine months after receiving the diagnosis; 25 percent had made a previous suicide attempt, 50 percent had reported severe depression, and 40 percent had seen a psychiatrist within four days before committing suicide. As previously noted, the desire to die is most closely associated with the diagnosis of depression.[26, 27] Suicide is the eighth leading cause of death in the United States, and the incidence of suicide is higher in patients with cancer or AIDS and in elderly men than in the general population. Conwell and Caine reported that depression was underdiagnosed by primary care physicians in a cohort of elderly patients who subsequently committed suicide; 75 percent of the patients had seen a primary care physician during the last month of life but had not received a diagnosis of depression.[22]

The relation between depression and the desire to hasten death may vary among subgroups of dying patients. We have no data, except for studies of a small number of patients with cancer or AIDS. The effect of treatment for depression on the desire to hasten death and on requests for assistance in doing so has not been examined in the medically ill population, except for a small study in which four of six patients who initially wished to hasten death changed their minds within two weeks.[26]

There is also the concern that certain patients, particularly members of minority groups that are estranged from the health care system, may be reluctant to receive treatment for their physical or psychological symptoms because of the fear that their physicians will, in fact, hasten death. There is now some evidence that the legalization of assisted suicide in the Northern Territory of Australia has undermined the Aborigines' trust in the medical care system[42]; this experience may serve as an example for the United States, with its multicultural population.

The multiple physical and psychological symptoms in the terminally ill and elderly are compounded by a substantial degree of existential distress. Reporting on their interviews with Washington State physicians whose patients had requested assistance in dying, Back et al. noted the physicians' lack of sophistication in assessing such nonphysical suffering.[10]

In summary, there are fundamental physician-related barriers to appropriate, humane, and compassionate care for the dying. These range from attitudinal and behavioral barriers to educational and economic barriers. Physicians do not know enough about their patients, themselves, or suffering to provide assistance with dying as a medical treatment for the relief of suffering. Physicians need to explore their own perspectives on the meaning of suffering in order to develop their own approaches to the care of the dying. They need insight into how the nature of the doctor-patient relationship influences their own decision making. If legalized, physician-assisted suicide will be a substitute for rational therapeutic, psychological, and social interventions that might otherwise enhance the quality of life for patients who are dying. The medical profession needs to take the lead in developing guidelines for good care of dying patients. Identifying the factors related to physicians, patients, and the health care system that pose barriers to appropriate care at the end of life should be the first step in a national dialogue to educate health care professionals and the public on the topic of death and dying. Death is an issue that society as a whole faces, and it requires a compassionate response. But we should not confuse compassion with competence in the care of terminally ill patients.

References

1. Reinhardt, Compassion in Dying v. State of Washington, 79 F. 3d 790 9th Cir. 1996.
2. Miner, Quill v. Vacco 80 F. 3d 716 2nd Cir. 1996.
3. Doyle D, Hanks GWC, MacDonald N. The Oxford textbook of palliative medicine. New York: Oxford University Press, 1993.
4. Orentlicher D. The legalization of physician-assisted suicide. N Engl J Med 1996;335:663–7.
5. Wilson WC, Smedira NG, Fink C, McDowell JA, Luce JM. Ordering and administration of sedatives and analgesics during the withholding and withdrawal of life support from critically ill patients. JAMA 1992; 267:949–53.
6. Foley KM. The relationship of pain and symptom management to patient requests for physician-assisted suicide. J Pain Symptom Manage 1991;6:289–97.
7. Cherny NI, Coyle N, Foley KM. Guidelines in the care of the dying patient. Hematol Oncol Clin North Am 1996;10:261–86.
8. Cherny NI, Portenoy RK. Sedation in the management of refractory symptoms: guidelines for evaluation and treatment. J Palliat Care 1994;10(2): 31–8.
9. Cancer pain relief and palliative care. Geneva: World Health Organization, 1989.
10. Back AL, Wallace JI, Starks HE, Pearlman RA. Physician-assisted suicide and euthanasia in Washington State: patient requests and physician responses. JAMA 1996;275:919–25.
11. Emanuel EJ, Fairclough DL, Daniels ER, Clarridge BR. Euthanasia and physician-assisted suicide: attitudes and experiences of oncology patients, oncologists, and the public. Lancet 1996;347:1805–10.
12. Lee MA, Nelson HD, Tilden VP, Ganzini L, Schmidt TA, Tolle SW. Legalizing assisted suicide—views of physicians in Oregon. N Engl J Med 1996;334: 310–5.
13. Ganzini L, Fenn DS, Lee MA, Heintz RT, Bloom JD. Attitudes of Oregon psychiatrists toward physician-assisted suicide. Am J Psychiatry 1996; 153:1469–75.
14. Cohen JS, Fihn SD, Boyko EJ, Jonsen AR, Wood RW. Attitudes toward assisted suicide and euthanasia among physicians in Washington State. N Engl J Med 1994;331:89–94.
15. Doukas DJ, Waterhouse D, Gorenflo DW, Seid J. Attitudes and behaviors on physician-assisted death: a study of Michigan oncologists. J Clin Oncol 1995;13:1055–61.
16. Morrison S, Meier D. Physician-assisted dying: fashioning public policy with an absence of data. Generations. Winter 1994:48–53.
17. Portenoy RK, Coyle N, Kash K, et al. Determinants of the willingness to endorse assisted suicide: a survey of physicians, nurses, and social workers. Psychosomatics (in press).

18. Fins J. Physician-assisted suicide and the right to care. Cancer Control 1996;3:272–8.

19. Callahan D, White M. The legalization of physician-assisted suicide: creating a regulatory Potemkin Village. U Richmond Law Rev 1996;30:1–83.

20. Quill TE. Death and dignity—a case of individualized decision making. N Engl J Med 1991;324:691–4.

21. Quill TE, Cassel CK, Meier DE. Care of the hopelessly ill—proposed clinical criteria for physician-assisted suicide. N Engl J Med 1992;327:1380–4.

22. Conwell Y, Caine ED. Rational suicide and the right to die—reality and myth. N Engl J Med 1991;325:1100–3.

23. Foley KM. Pain, physician assisted suicide and euthanasia. Pain Forum 1995;4:163–78.

24. When death is sought: assisted suicide and euthanasia in the medical context. New York: New York State Task Force on Life and the Law, May 1994.

25. Brown JH, Henteleff P, Barakat S, Rowe CJ. Is it normal for terminally ill patients to desire death? Am J Psychiatry 1986;143:208–11.

26. Chochinov HM, Wilson KG, Enns M, et al. Desire for death in the terminally ill. Am J Psychiatry 1995;152:1185–91.

27. Breitbart W, Rosenfeld BD, Passik SD. Interest in physician-assisted suicide among ambulatory HIV-infected patients. Am J Psychiatry 1996;153:238–42.

28. Hill TP. Treating the dying patient: the challenge for medical education. Arch Intern Med 1995;155:1265–9.

29. Callahan D. Once again reality: now where do we go? Hastings Cent Rep 1995;25(6):Suppl:S33–S36.

30. Solomon MZ, O'Donnell L, Jennings B, et al. Decisions near the end of life: professional views on life-sustaining treatments. Am J Public Health 1993;83:14–23.

31. Cherny NI, Coyle N, Foley KM. Suffering in the advanced cancer patient: definition and taxonomy. J Palliat Care 1994;10(2):57–70.

32. Cassel EJ. The nature of suffering and the goals of medicine. N Engl J Med 1982;306:639–45.

33. Cleeland CS, Gonin R, Hatfield AK, et al. Pain and its treatment in outpatients with metastatic cancer. N Engl J Med 1994;330:592–6.

34. Breitbart W, Rosenfeld BD, Passik SD, McDonald MV, Thaler H, Portenoy RK. The undertreatment of pain in ambulatory AIDS patients. Pain 1996;65:243–9.

35. The SUPPORT Principal Investigators. A controlled trial to improve care for seriously ill hospitalized patients. JAMA 1995;274:1591–8.

36. Seale C, Cartwright A. The year before death. Hants, England: Avebury, 1994.

37. Von Roenn JH, Cleeland CS, Gonin R, Hatfield AK, Pandya KJ. Physician attitudes and practice in cancer pain management: a survey from the Eastern Cooperative Oncology Group. Ann Intern Med 1993;119:121–6.

38. Portenoy RK. Pain and quality of life: clinical issues and implications for research. Oncology 1990;4:172–8.

39. Breitbart W. Suicide risk and pain in cancer and AIDS patients. In: Chapman CR, Foley KM, eds. Current and emerging issues in cancer pain. New York: Raven Press, 1993.

40. Chochinov H, Wilson KG, Enns M, Lander S. Prevalence of depression in the terminally ill: effects of diagnostic criteria and symptom threshold judgments. Am J Psychiatry 1994;151:537–40.

41. Passik S, McDonald M, Rosenfeld B, Breitbart W. End of life issues in patients with AIDS: clinical and research considerations. J Pharm Care Pain Symptom Control 1995;3:91–111.

42. NT "success" in easing rural fear of euthanasia. The Age. August 31, 1996:A7.

EXPLORING THE ISSUE

Should Physicians Be Allowed to Assist in Patient Suicide?

Critical Thinking and Reflection

1. In your view, does a person's autonomy ever encompass a right to end one's own life? If so, under what circumstances and with what safeguards?
2. What is the most compelling kind of reason for permitting physician-assisted suicide—the curtailment of the patient's suffering, or the completion of the patient's life plans?
3. If a patient who expresses a desire to die is diagnosed with depression, should the depression be treated before agreeing to help the patient die?
4. If physician-assisted death is permitted, would physicians' role as caregivers be undermined? Do you see physician-assisted death more as a case of commitment to patients or abandonment of patients? Why?

Is There Common Ground?

In 1997, Oregon became the first state to implement a law legalizing physician-assisted suicide. The Death with Dignity Act was originally passed in 1994, but its implementation was delayed until 1997, when it was upheld by a large majority of voters. Under this law, a person who is mentally competent and suffering from a terminal illness (likely to die within 6 months) may receive lethal drugs from a physician. The person has to consult two doctors and wait 15 days before obtaining the drugs. A similar law was enacted in Washington in 2008, and the Montana Supreme Court decision in the 2010 case *Baxter v. Montana* has made physician-assisted suicide permissible in Montana. Efforts to make physician-assisted suicide legal in other states have so far failed but have not stopped. The Death with Dignity Act was offered as a ballot measure in Massachusetts in 2012.

Very few patients in Oregon actually use the option of requesting physician-assisted suicide, and the number has remained stable since 2002. Fewer than 1,000 people have obtained prescriptions for drugs to end their lives, and about 600 have actually used the drugs, according to Oregon's Public Health Division. Those most likely to request drugs were married, white, more highly educated, and had cancer as a primary diagnosis. Physicians who wrote prescriptions have reported that patient requests stemmed from concerns related to loss of autonomy, decreasing ability to participate in enjoyable activities, and loss of dignity, rather than unbearable pain. Nearly all patients were enrolled in hospice and had health insurance. Washington's experience with physician-assisted suicide has been similar so far to Oregon's.

In the Netherlands, euthanasia—defined as "the intentional termination of the life of a patient at his or her request by a physician"—was legalized in 2002. The practice had occurred before 2002 without repercussions for the physician. About 9,700 requests are made each year. Those who oppose the practice claim that not all requests are voluntary.

Additional Resources

Information about the experience in Oregon is available from the Oregon Department of Human Services and is available at http://public.health.oregon .gov/ProviderPartnerResources/EvaluationResearch/DeathwithDignityAct/Pages /index.aspx.

Susan Tolle and colleagues have published research on how many people in Oregon consider physician-assisted suicide as compared to the number who follow through with it, and on the barriers to fulfilling their intentions (Susan W. Tolle et al., "Characteristics and Proportion of Dying Oregonians Who Personally Consider Physician-Assisted Suicide," *Journal of Clinical Ethics* [Summer 2004]).

In "Legal Regulation of Physician-Assisted Death—The Latest Report Cards," *The New England Journal of Medicine* (May 10, 2007), Timothy E. Quill concludes that legalization has resulted in more open conversation and careful evaluation of end-of-life options.

In November 2008, voters in the state of Washington approved a measure similar to Oregon's law. In 1991, voters rejected a bill that would allow doctors to administer the lethal medications; the 2008 version requires patients to take the medications on their own.

A review of the impact in Oregon and the Netherlands of physician-assisted suicide on "vulnerable" groups such as the elderly, women, people with low educational status, racial and ethnic minorities, and people with psychiatric illness found no evidence that these groups were disproportionately involved. The only people with a heightened risk were people with AIDS. Those who received physician-assisted suicide were more likely to be better educated, have more economic and social resources, and professional status (Margaret P. Battin et al., "Legal Physician-Assisted Dying in Oregon and the Netherlands: Evidence Concerning the Impact on Patients in 'Vulnerable' Groups," *Journal of Medical Ethics* [2007]).

Physician-Assisted Dying: The Case for Palliative Care and Patient Choice, edited by Timothy E. Quill and Margaret P. Battin, is a collection of articles that presents the case for the legalization of physician-assisted dying (Johns Hopkins University Press, 2004). Opposing the practice are the authors in *The Case Against Assisted Suicide*, edited by Kathleen E. Foley and Herbert Hendin (Johns Hopkins University Press, 2002). See also Arthur L. Caplan, Lois Snyder, and Kathy Feber-Langendoen, "The Role of Guidelines in the Practice of Physician-Assisted Suicide," *Annals of Internal Medicine* (March 21, 2000). The entire issue is devoted to this subject.

Internet References . . .

NARAL Online

This is the home page of the National Abortion and Reproductive Rights Action League (NARAL), an organization that works to promote reproductive freedom and dignity for women and their families.

www.naral.org

Students for Life

This organization, run by students at Simon Fraser University in Vancouver, Canada, lists Web sites representing the diversity of pro-life views.

www.studentsforlife.org

National Advocates for Pregnant Women

This organization participates in and provides resources on the debate over punishing women who expose their fetuses to drugs.

www.advocatesforpregnantwomen.org/

Centers for Disease Control

The CDC provides information about assisted reproductive technologies and clinics that offer ART.

www.cdc.gov/art/

Choices in Reproduction

*F*ew bioethical issues could be of greater personal and social significance than questions concerning reproduction. Advances in medical technology, such as in vitro fertilization and egg donation, have opened new possibilities for infertile couples, while challenging traditional notions of family. How to responsibly use these technologies to help people have families presents special challenges. Another type of technological advance, the ability to see images of the developing fetus, has enhanced our understanding of both normal growth and birth defects. This technology has provided evidence of the impact of the mother's behavior on fetal development. While many behaviors of pregnant women expose fetuses to risk, and while fathers' exposure to chemicals and other toxic substances also affects fetuses, attention has focused mainly on the mothers' use of illegal drugs. Preventing risk to fetuses raises troubling questions concerning the role of police and the courts in medical matters and the best way to assist drug-addicted women. The most polarized question remains the morality of abortion, where common ground is elusive. The issues in this unit come to grips with some of the most perplexing and fundamental questions that confront medical practitioners, individual women and their partners, and society in general.

- Is Abortion Immoral?
- Should There Be Legal Limits on How Many Embryos Can Be Transferred into a Woman Who Wants to Be Pregnant?
- Should a Pregnant Woman Be Punished for Exposing Her Fetus to Risk?

ISSUE 7

Is Abortion Immoral?

YES: Patrick Lee and Robert P. George, from "The Wrong of Abortion," in Andrew Cohen and Christopher Heath Wellman, eds., *Contemporary Debates in Applied Ethics* (Blackwell, 2004)

NO: Margaret Olivia Little, from "The Morality of Abortion," in Bonnie Steinbock, John D. Arras, and Alex John London, eds., *Ethical Issues in Modern Medicine* (McGraw-Hill, 2002)

Learning Outcomes

After reading this issue, you should be able to:

- Discuss the ethical dilemma posed by abortion.
- Describe the concepts of personhood and parenthood and some of the different accounts that may be given of them.

ISSUE SUMMARY

YES: Philosopher Patrick Lee and professor of jurisprudence Robert P. George assert that human embryos and fetuses are complete (though immature) human beings and that intentional abortion is unjust and objectively immoral.

NO: Philosopher Margaret Olivia Little believes that the moral status of the fetus is only one aspect of the morality of abortion. She points to gestation as an intimacy, motherhood as a relationship, and creation as a process to advance a more nuanced approach.

$\mathbf{A}$bortion is the most divisive bioethical issue of our time. The issue has been a persistent one in history, but in the past 30 years or so the debate has polarized. One view—known as "pro-life"—sees abortion as the wanton slaughter of innocent life. The other view—"pro-choice"—considers abortion as an option that must be available to women if they are to control their own reproductive lives. According to the pro-life view, women who have access to "abortion on demand" put their own selfish whims ahead of an unborn child's right to life. According to the pro-choice view, women have the right to choose to have an abortion—especially if there is an overriding reason, such as preventing the birth of a child with a severe genetic defect or one conceived as a result of rape or incest.

Behind these strongly held convictions, as political scientist Mary Segers has pointed out, are widely differing views of what determines value (i.e., whether value is inherent in a thing or ascribed to it by human beings), the relation between law and morality, and the use of limits of political solutions to social problems, as well as the value of scientific progress. Those who condemn abortion as immoral generally follow a classical tradition in which abortion is a public matter because it involves our conception of how we should live together in an ideal society. Those who accept the idea of abortion, on the other hand, generally share the liberal, individualistic ethos of contemporary society. They believe that abortion is a private choice, and that public policy should reflect how citizens actually behave, not some unattainable ideal.

This is what we know about abortion practices in America today: Abortion has been legal since the 1973 Supreme Court decision of *Roe v. Wade* declared that a woman has a constitutional right to privacy, which includes an abortion. According to the National Center on Health Statistics, abortion at 8 weeks or less gestation is seven times safer than childbirth, although there are some unknown risks—primarily the effect of repeated abortions on subsequent pregnancies.

In the past few decades, the demographic profile of women who have abortions has changed significantly, according to data collected by the Guttmacher Institute, a private research organization. Relatively fewer white childless teenagers are choosing abortion, while more low-income women of color in their 20s and 30s who already have children are having abortions. Non-Hispanic white women account for 36 percent of abortions, non-Hispanic black women for 30 percent, Hispanic women for 25 percent, and women of other races for 9 percent.

Overall the abortion rate dropped by about one-third from 1978 to 2008, from a high of around 28 abortions for every thousand women aged 15–44 to about 20 per thousand in 2008. Some of the reasons are the use of long-acting hormonal contraceptives, a lower pregnancy rate among teenagers, and growing use of emergency contraception. According to 2011 data available from the Guttmacher Institute, the typical woman having an abortion is between the ages of 20 and 30, has never married, lives in a metropolitan area, and is a Christian (37 percent identify as Protestant and 28 percent as Catholic). Most women who have an abortion already have a child, and 44 percent have incomes below the federal poverty level.

The YES and NO selections offer thoughtful and reasoned but opposing views on abortion. Patrick Lee and Robert P. George conclude that being a mother generates a special responsibility and that the sacrifice morally required of the mother is less burdensome than the harm that would be done by expelling the child, causing his or her death, to escape that responsibility. They see abortion as objectively immoral. Margaret Olivia Little believes that if we acknowledge gestation as an intimacy, motherhood as a relationship, and creation as a process, we will be better able to appreciate the moral textures of abortion.

YES ↵   Patrick Lee and
           Robert P. George

The Wrong of Abortion

Much of the public debate about abortion concerns the question whether deliberate feticide ought to be unlawful, at least in most circumstances. We will lay that question aside here in order to focus first on the question: is the choice to have, to perform, or to help procure an abortion morally wrong?

We shall argue that the choice of abortion is objectively immoral. By "objectively" we indicate that we are discussing the choice itself, not the (subjective) guilt or innocence of someone who carries out the choice: someone may act from an erroneous conscience, and if he is not at fault for his error, then he remains subjectively innocent, even if his choice is objectively wrongful.

The first important question to consider is: what is killed in an abortion? It is obvious that some living entity is killed in an abortion. And no one doubts that the moral status of the entity killed is a central (though not the only) question in the abortion debate. We shall approach the issue step by step, first setting forth some (though not all) of the evidence that demonstrates that what is killed in abortion—a human embryo—is indeed a human being, then examining the ethical significance of that point.

Human Embryos and Fetuses Are Complete (though Immature) Human Beings

It will be useful to begin by considering some of the facts of sexual reproduction. The standard embryology texts indicate that in the case of ordinary sexual reproduction the life of an individual human being begins with complete fertilization, which yields a genetically and functionally distinct organism, possessing the resources and active disposition for internally directed development toward human maturity.[1] In normal conception, a sex cell of the father, a sperm, unites with a sex cell of the mother, an ovum. Within the chromosomes of these sex cells are the DNA molecules which constitute the information that guides the development of the new individual brought into being when the sperm and ovum fuse. When fertilization occurs, the 23 chromosomes of the sperm unite with the 23 chromosomes of the ovum. At the end of this process

From *Contemporary Debates in Applied Ethics* by Andrew Cohen and Christopher Heath Weelman, eds., 2004, pp. 13–15, 20–25. Copyright © 2004 by Blackwell Publishing, Ltd. Reprinted by permission.

there is produced an entirely new and distinct organism, originally a single cell. This organism, the human embryo, begins to grow by the normal process of cell division—it divides into 2 cells, then 4, 8, 16, and so on (the divisions are not simultaneous, so there is a 3-cell stage, and so on). This embryo gradually develops all of the organs and organ systems necessary for the full functioning of a mature human being. His or her development (sex is determined from the beginning) is very rapid in the first few weeks. For example, as early as eight or ten weeks of gestation, the fetus has a fully formed, beating heart, a complete brain (although not all of its synaptic connections are complete—nor will they be until sometime *after* the child is born), a recognizably human form, and the fetus feels pain, cries, and even sucks his or her thumb.

There are three important points we wish to make about this human embryo. First, it is from the start *distinct* from any cell of the mother or of the father. This is clear because it is growing in its own distinct direction. Its growth is internally directed to its own survival and maturation. Second, the embryo is *human:* it has the genetic makeup characteristic of human beings. Third, and most importantly, the embryo is a *complete* or *whole* organism, though immature. The human embryo, from conception onward, is fully programmed actively to develop himself or herself to the mature stage of a human being, and, *unless prevented by disease or violence, will actually do so, despite possibly significant variation in environment* (in the mother's womb). None of the changes that occur to the embryo after fertilization, for as long as he or she survives, generates a new direction of growth. Rather, *all* of the changes (for example, those involving nutrition and environment) either facilitate or retard the internally directed growth of this persisting individual.

Sometimes it is objected that if we say human embryos are human beings, on the grounds that they have the potential to become mature humans, the same will have to be said of sperm and ova. This objection is untenable. The human embryo is radically unlike the sperm and ova, the sex cells. The sex cells are manifestly not *whole* or *complete* organisms. They are not only genetically but also functionally identifiable as parts of the male or female potential parents. They clearly are destined either to combine with an ovum or sperm or die. Even when they succeed in causing fertilization, they do not survive; rather, their genetic material enters into the composition of a distinct, new organism.

Nor are human embryos comparable to somatic cells (such as skin cells or muscle cells), though some have tried to argue that they are. Like sex cells, a somatic cell is functionally only a part of a larger organism. The human embryo, by contrast, possesses from the beginning the internal resources and active disposition to develop himself or herself to full maturity; all he or she needs is a suitable environment and nutrition. The direction of his or her growth *is not extrinsically determined,* but the embryo is internally directing his or her growth toward full maturity.

So, a human embryo (or fetus) is not something distinct from a human being; he or she is not an individual of any non-human or intermediate species. Rather, an embryo (and fetus) is a human being at a certain (early) stage of development—the embryonic (or fetal) stage. In abortion, what is killed is a human being, a whole living member of the species *homo sapiens*, the same *kind* of entity as you or I, only at an earlier stage of development. . . .

The Argument That Abortion Is Justified as Non-Intentional Killing

Some "pro-choice" philosophers have attempted to justify abortion by denying that all abortions are intentional killing. They have granted (at least for the sake of argument) that an unborn human being has a right to life but have then argued that this right does not entail that the child *in utero* is morally entitled to the use of the mother's body for life support. In effect, their argument is that, at least in many cases, abortion is not a case of intentionally killing the child, but a choice not to provide the child with assistance, that is, a choice to expel (or "evict") the child from the womb, despite the likelihood or certainty that expulsion (or "eviction") will result in his or her death (Little, 1999; McDonagh, 1996; Thomson, 1971).

Various analogies have been proposed by people making this argument. The mother's gestating a child has been compared to allowing someone the use of one's kidneys or even to donating an organ. We are not *required* (morally or as a matter of law) to allow someone to use our kidneys, or to donate organs to others, even when they would die without this assistance (and we could survive in good health despite rendering it). Analogously, the argument continues, a woman is not morally required to allow the fetus the use of her body. We shall call this "the bodily rights argument."

It may be objected that a woman has a special responsibility to the child she is carrying, whereas in the cases of withholding assistance to which abortion is compared there is no such special responsibility. Proponents of the bodily rights argument have replied, however, that the mother has not voluntarily assumed responsibility for the child, or a personal relationship with the child, and we have strong responsibilities to others only if we have voluntarily assumed such responsibilities (Thomson, 1971) or have consented to a personal relationship which generates such responsibilities (Little, 1999). True, the mother may have voluntarily performed an act which she knew may result in a child's conception, but that is distinct from consenting to gestate the child if a child is conceived. And so (according to this position) it is not until the woman consents to pregnancy, or perhaps not until the parents consent to care for the child by taking the baby home from the hospital or birthing center, that the full duties of parenthood accrue to the mother (and perhaps the father).

In reply to this argument we wish to make several points. We grant that in some few cases abortion is not intentional killing, but a choice to expel the child, the child's death being an unintended, albeit foreseen and (rightly or wrongly) accepted, side effect. However, these constitute a small minority of abortions. In the vast majority of cases, the death of the child *in utero* is precisely the object of the abortion. In most cases the end sought is to avoid being a parent; but abortion brings that about only by bringing it about that the child dies. Indeed, the attempted abortion would be considered by the woman requesting it and the abortionist performing it to have been *unsuccessful* if the child survives. In most cases abortion *is* intentional killing. Thus, even if the bodily rights argument succeeded, it would justify only a small percentage of abortions.

Still, in some few cases abortion is chosen as a means precisely toward ending the condition of pregnancy, and the woman requesting the termination of her pregnancy would not object if somehow the child survived. A pregnant woman may have less or more serious reasons for seeking the termination of this condition, but if that is her objective, then the child's death resulting from his or her expulsion will be a side effect, rather than the means chosen. For example, an actress may wish not to be pregnant because the pregnancy will change her figure during a time in which she is filming scenes in which having a slender appearance is important; or a woman may dread the discomforts, pains, and difficulties involved in pregnancy. (Of course, in many abortions there may be mixed motives: the parties making the choice may intend both ending the condition of pregnancy and the death of the child.)

Nevertheless, while it is true that in some cases abortion is not intentional killing, it remains misleading to describe it simply as choosing not to provide bodily life support. Rather, it is actively expelling the human embryo or fetus from the womb. There is a significant moral difference between *not doing* something that would assist someone, and *doing* something that causes someone harm, even if that harm is an unintended (but foreseen) side effect. It is more difficult morally to justify the latter than it is the former. Abortion is the *act* of extracting the unborn human being from the womb—an extraction that usually rips him or her to pieces or does him or her violence in some other way.

It is true that in some cases causing death as a side effect is morally permissible. For example, in some cases it is morally right to use force to stop a potentially lethal attack on one's family or country, even if one foresees that the force used will also result in the assailant's death. Similarly, there are instances in which it is permissible to perform an act that one knows or believes will, as a side effect, cause the death of a child *in utero*. For example, if a pregnant woman is discovered to have a cancerous uterus, and this is a proximate danger to the mother's life, it can be morally right to remove the cancerous uterus with the baby in it, even if the child will die as a result. A similar situation can occur in ectopic pregnancies. But in such cases, not only is the child's death a side effect, but the mother's life is in proximate danger. It is worth noting also that in these cases *what is done* (the means) is the correction of a pathology (such as a cancerous uterus, or a ruptured uterine tube). Thus, in such cases, not only the child's death, but also the ending of the pregnancy, are side effects. So, such acts are what traditional casuistry referred to as *indirect* or *non-intentional,* abortions.

But it is also clear that not every case of causing death as a side effect is morally right. For example, if a man's daughter has a serious respiratory disease and the father is told that his continued smoking in her presence will cause her death, it would obviously be immoral for him to continue the smoking. Similarly, if a man works for a steel company in a city with significant levels of air pollution, and his child has a serious respiratory problem making the air pollution a danger to her life, certainly he should move to another city. He should move, we would say, even if that meant he had to resign a prestigious position or make a significant career change.

In both examples, (a) the parent has a special responsibility to his child, but (b) the act that would cause the child's death would avoid a harm to the parent but cause a significantly worse harm to his child. And so, although the harm done would be a side effect, in both cases the act that caused the death would be an *unjust* act, and morally wrongful *as such*. The special responsibility of parents to their children requires that they *at least* refrain from performing acts that cause terrible harms to their children in order to avoid significantly lesser harms to themselves.

But (a) and (b) also obtain in intentional abortions (that is, those in which the removal of the child is directly sought, rather than the correction of a life-threatening pathology) even though they are not, strictly speaking, intentional killing. First, the mother has a special responsibility to her child, in virtue of being her biological mother (as does the father in virtue of his paternal relationship). The parental relationship itself—not just the voluntary acceptance of that relationship—gives rise to a special responsibility to a child.

Proponents of the bodily rights argument deny this point. Many claim that one has full parental responsibilities only if one has voluntarily assumed them. And so the child, on this view, has a right to care from his or her mother (including gestation) only if the mother has accepted her pregnancy, or perhaps only if the mother (and/or the father?) has in some way voluntarily begun a deep personal relationship with the child (Little, 1999).

But suppose a mother takes her baby home after giving birth, but the only reason she did not get an abortion was that she could not afford one. Or suppose she lives in a society where abortion is not available (perhaps very few physicians are willing to do the grisly deed). She and her husband take the child home only because they had no alternative. Moreover, suppose that in their society people are not waiting in line to adopt a newborn baby. And so the baby is several days old before anything can be done. If they abandon the baby and the baby is found, she will simply be returned to them. In such a case the parents have not voluntarily assumed responsibility; nor have they consented to a personal relationship with the child. But it would surely be wrong for these parents to abandon their baby in the woods (perhaps the only feasible way of ensuring she is not returned), even though the baby's death would be only a side effect. Clearly, we recognize that parents do have a responsibility to make sacrifices for their children, even if they have not voluntarily assumed such responsibilities, or given their consent to the personal relationship with the child.

The bodily rights argument implicitly supposes that we have a primordial right to construct a life simply as we please, and that others have claims on us only very minimally or through our (at least tacit) consent to a certain sort of relationship with them. On the contrary, we are by nature members of communities. Our moral goodness or character consists to a large extent (though not solely) in contributing to the communities of which we are members. We ought to act for our genuine good or flourishing (we take that as a basic ethical principle), but our flourishing involves being in communion with others. And communion with others of itself—even if we find ourselves united with others because of a physical or social relationship which precedes our consent—entails duties or responsibilities. Moreover, the contribution we are morally required to make to others will likely bring each of us some discomfort and pain. This is not to say that we should simply ignore our own good, for the sake of others. Rather, since what (and who) I am is in part constituted by various relationships with others, not all of which are initiated by my will, my genuine good includes the contributions I make to the relationships in which I participate. Thus, the life we constitute by our free choices should be in large part a life of mutual reciprocity with others.

For example, I may wish to cultivate my talent to write and so I may want to spend hours each day reading and writing. Or I may wish to develop my athletic abilities and so I may want to spend hours every day on the baseball field. But if I am a father of minor children, and have an adequate paying job working (say) in a coal mine, then my clear duty is to keep that job. Similarly, if one's girlfriend finds she is pregnant and one is the father, then one might also be morally required to continue one's work in the mine (or mill, factory, warehouse, etc.).

In other words, I have a duty to do something with my life that contributes to the good of the human community, but that general duty becomes specified by my particular situation. It becomes specified by the connection or closeness to me of those who are in need. We acquire special responsibilities toward people, not only by *consenting* to contracts or relationships with them, but also by having various types of union with them. So, we have special responsibilities to those people with whom we are closely united. For example, we have special responsibilities to our parents, and brothers and sisters, even though we did not choose them.

The physical unity or continuity of children to their parents is unique. The child is brought into being out of the bodily unity and bodies of the mother and the father. The mother and the father are in a certain sense prolonged or continued in their offspring. So, there is a natural unity of the mother with her child, and a natural unity of the father with his child. Since we have special responsibilities to those with whom we are closely united, it follows that we in fact do have a special responsibility to our children anterior to our having voluntarily assumed such responsibility or consented to the relationship.[2]

The second point is this: in the types of case we are considering, the harm caused (death) is much worse than the harms avoided (the difficulties in pregnancy). Pregnancy can involve severe impositions, but it is not nearly as bad as death—which is total and irreversible. One needn't make light of the burdens of pregnancy to acknowledge that the harm that is death is in a different category altogether.

The burdens of pregnancy include physical difficulties and the pain of labor, and can include significant financial costs, psychological burdens, and interference with autonomy and the pursuit of other important goals (McDonagh, 1996: ch. 5). These costs are not inconsiderable. Partly for that reason, we owe our mothers gratitude for carrying and giving birth to us. However, where pregnancy does not place a woman's life in jeopardy or threaten grave and lasting damage to her physical health, the harm done to other goods is not total. Moreover, most of the harms involved in pregnancy are not irreversible: pregnancy is a nine-month task—if the woman and man are not in a good position to raise the child, adoption is a possibility. So the difficulties of pregnancy, considered together, are in a different and lesser category than death. Death is not just worse in degree than the difficulties involved in pregnancy; it is worse in kind.

It has been argued, however, that pregnancy can involve a unique type of burden. It has been argued that the *intimacy* involved in pregnancy is such that if the woman must remain pregnant without her consent then there is inflicted on her a unique and serious harm. Just as sex with consent can be a desired experience but sex without consent is a violation of bodily integrity, so (the argument continues) pregnancy involves such a close physical intertwinement with the fetus that not to allow abortion is analogous to rape—it involves an enforced intimacy (Boonin, 2003: 84; Little, 1999: 300–3).

However, this argument is based on a false analogy. Where the pregnancy is unwanted, the baby's "occupying" the mother's womb may involve a harm; but the child is committing no injustice against her. The baby is not forcing himself or herself on the woman, but is simply growing and developing in a way quite natural to him or her. The baby is not performing any action that could in any way be construed as aimed at violating the mother.[3]

It is true that the fulfillment of the duty of a mother to her child (during gestation) is unique and in many cases does involve a great sacrifice. The argument we have presented, however, is that being a mother *does* generate a special responsibility, and that the sacrifice morally required of the mother is less burdensome than the harm that would be done to the child by expelling the child, causing his or her death, to escape that responsibility. Our argument equally entails responsibilities for the father of the child. His duty does not involve as direct a bodily relationship with the child as the mother's, but it may be equally or even more burdensome. In certain circumstances, his obligation to care for the child (and the child's mother), and especially his obligation to provide financial support, may severely limit his freedom and even require months or, indeed, years, of extremely burdensome physical labor. Historically, many men have rightly seen that their basic responsibility to their family (and country) has entailed risking, and in many cases, losing, their lives. Different people in different circumstances, with different talents, will have different responsibilities. It is no argument against any of these responsibilities to point out their distinctness.

So, the burden of carrying the baby, for all its distinctness, is significantly less than the harm the baby would suffer by being killed; the mother and father have a special responsibility to the child; it follows that intentional abortion (even in the few cases where the baby's death is an unintended but foreseen side effect) is unjust and therefore objectively immoral.

Notes

1. See, for example: Carlson (1994: chs. 2–4); Gilbert (2003: 183–220, 363–90); Larson (2001: chs. 1–2); Moore and Persaud (2003: chs. 1–6); Muller (1997: chs. 1–2); O'Rahilly and Mueller (2000: chs. 3–4).

2. David Boonin claims, in reply to this argument—in an earlier and less developed form, presented by Lee (1996: 122)—that it is not clear that it is impermissible for a woman to destroy what is a part of, or a continuation of, herself. He then says that to the extent the unborn human being is united to her in that way, "it would if anything seem that her act is *easier* to justify than if this claim were not true" (2003: 230). But Boonin fails to grasp the point of the argument (perhaps understandably since it was not expressed very clearly in the earlier work he is discussing). The unity of the child to the mother is the basis for this child being related to the woman in a different way from how other children are. We ought to pursue our own good *and the good of others with whom we are united in various ways.* If that is so, then the closer someone is united to us, the deeper and more extensive our responsibility to the person will be.

3. In some sense being bodily "occupied" when one does not wish to be *is* a harm; however, just as the child does not (as explained in the text), neither does the state inflict this harm on the woman, in circumstances in which the state prohibits abortion. By prohibiting abortion the state would only prevent the woman from performing an act (forcibly detaching the child from her) that would unjustly kill this developing child, who is an innocent party.

References

Boonin, David (2003). *A Defense of Abortion.* New York: Cambridge University Press.

Carlson, Bruce (1994). *Human Embryology and Developmental Biology.* St. Louis, MO: Mosby.

Gilbert, Scott (2003). *Developmental Biology,* 7th edn. Sunderland, MA: Sinnauer Associates.

Larson, William J. (2001). *Human Embryology,* 3rd edn. New York: Churchill Livingstone.

Lee, Patrick (1996). *Abortion and Unborn Human Life.* Washington, DC: Catholic University of America Press.

Little, Margaret Olivia (1999). "Abortion, intimacy, and the duty to gestate." *Ethical Theory and Moral Practice,* 2: 295–312.

McDonagh, Eileen (1996). *Breaking the Abortion Deadlock: From Choice to Consent.* New York: Oxford University Press.

Moore, Keith, and Persaud, T. V. N. (2003). *The Developing Human, Clinically Oriented Embryology,* 7th edn. New York: W. B. Saunders.

Muller, Werner A. (1997). *Developmental Biology.* New York: Springer Verlag.

O'Rahilly, Ronan, and Mueller, Fabiola (2000). *Human Embryology and Teratology,* 3rd edn. New York: John Wiley & Sons.

Thomson, Judith Jarvis (1971). "A defense of abortion." *Philosophy and Public Affairs,* 1: 47–66; reprinted, among other places, in Feinberg (1984, pp. 173–87).

Margaret Olivia Little 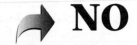 **NO**

The Morality of Abortion

Introduction

It is often noted that the public discussion of abortion's moral status is disappointingly crude. The positions staked out and the reasoning proffered seem to reflect little of the subtlety and nuance—not to mention ambivalence—that mark more private reflections on the subject. Despite attempts by various parties to find middle ground, the debate remains largely polarized—at its most dramatic, with extreme conservatives claiming abortion the moral equivalent of murder even as extreme liberals think it devoid of moral import.

To some extent, this polarization is due to the legal battle that continues to shadow moral discussions: admission of ethical nuance, it is feared, will play as concession on the deeply contested question of whether abortion should be a legally protected option for women. But to some extent, blame for the continued crudeness can be laid at the doorstep of moral theory itself.

For one thing, the ethical literature on abortion has focused its attention almost exclusively on the thinnest moral assessment—on whether and when abortion is "morally permissible." That question is, of course, a crucial one, its answer often desperately sought. But many of our deepest struggles with the morality of abortion concern much more textured questions about its placement on the scales of *decency, respectfulness,* and *responsibility.* It is one thing to decide that an abortion was permissible, quite another to decide that it was *honorable;* one thing to decide that an abortion was impermissible, quite another to decide that it was *monstrous.* It is these latter categories that determine what we might call the thick moral interpretation of the act—and, with it, the meaning the woman must live with, and the reactive attitudes such as disgust, forbearance, or admiration that she and others think the act deserves. A moral theory that moves too quickly or focuses too exclusively on moral permissibility won't address these crucial issues. . . .

To make progress on abortion's moral status, it thus turns out, requires us not just to arbitrate already familiar controversies in metaphysics and ethics, but to attend to the distinctive aspects of pregnancy that often stand at their margins. In the following, I want to argue that if we acknowledge gestation as an *intimacy,* motherhood as a *relationship,* and creation as a *process,* we will be in a far better position to appreciate the moral textures of abortion. I explore these textures, in the first half on stipulation that the fetus is a person, in the second half under supposition that early human life has an important value worthy of respect.

Fetal Personhood: From Wrongful Interference to Positive Responsibilities

If fetuses are persons, then abortion is surely an enormously serious matter: What is at stake is nothing less than the life of a creature with full moral standing. To say that the stakes are high, though, is not to say that moral analysis is obvious (which is why elsewhere in moral theory, conversation usually starts, not stops, once we realize people's lives are at issue). I think the most widely held objection to abortion is badly misguided; more importantly, it obscures the deeper ethical question at issue.

On the usual view, it is perfectly obvious what to say about abortion on supposition of fetal personhood: if fetuses are persons, then abortion is murder. Persons, after all, have a fundamental right to life, and abortion, it would seem, counts as its gross violation. On this view, we can assess the status of abortion quite cleanly. In particular, we needn't delve too deeply into the burdens that continued gestation might present for women—not because their lives don't matter or because we don't sympathize with their plight, but because we don't take hardship as justification for murder.

In fact, though, abortion's assimilation to murder will seem clear-cut only if we have already ignored key features of gestation. While certain metaphors depict gestation as passive carriage—as though the fetus were simply occupying a room until it is born—the truth is of course far different. One who is gestating is providing the fetus with sustenance—donating nourishment, creating blood, delivering oxygen, providing hormonal triggers for development—without which it could not live. For a fetus, to live *is* to be receiving aid. And whether the assistance is delivered by way of intentional activity (as when the woman eats or takes her prenatal vitamins) or by way of biological mechanism, assistance it plainly is. But this has crucial implications for abortion's alleged status as murder. To put it simply, the right to life, as Judith Thomson famously put it, does not include the right to have all assistance needed to maintain that life (Thomson, 1971). Ending gestation will, at early stages at least, certainly lead to the fetus's demise, but that does not mean that doing so would constitute murder. . . .

Even if the fetus is a person, then, abortion would not be murder. More broadly put, abortion, whatever its rights and wrongs, isn't a species of *wrongful interference*.

None of this, though, is to say that abortion under such supposition is therefore unproblematic. It is to argue, instead, that the crucial moral issue needs to be re-located. Wrongful interference is a central concern in morality, but it isn't the only one. We are also concerned with notions of *neglect, abandonment* and *disregard*. These are issues that involve abrogations of positive responsibilities to help others, not injunctions against interfering with them.

If fetuses are persons, the question we really need to decide is what positive responsibilities, if any, do pregnant women have to continue gestational assistance? This is a question that takes us into far richer, and far more interesting, territory than that occupied by discussions of murder.

One issue it raises is: what do pregnant women owe to the fetuses they carry as a matter of *general beneficence?* Philosophers, of course, familiarly divide over the ambitions of beneficence, generically construed; but abortion raises distinct difficulties of its own. On the one hand, the beneficence called for here is of a particularly urgent kind: the stakes are life and death, and the pregnant woman is the *only* one who can render the assistance needed. It's a rare (and, many of us will think, dreadful) moral theory that will think she faces no responsibilities to assist here: passing a drowning person for mere convenience when no one else is within shouting distance is a very good example of moral indecency. On the other hand, gestation is not just any activity. It involves sharing one's very body. It brings with it an emotional intertwinement that can reshape one's entire life. It brings another person into one's family. Being asked to gestate another person, that is, isn't like being asked to write a check to support an impoverished child; it's like being asked to adopt the child. Doing so is a caring, compassionate act; it is also an enormous undertaking that has reverberations for an entire lifetime. Deciding whether, and if so when, such action is obligatory rather than admirable is no light matter.

I don't think moral theory has begun to address the rich questions at issue here. When are intimate actions owed to generic others? How do we weigh the sacrifice morality requires of us when it is measured, not in terms of risk, but of intertwinement? What should we think of such obligations if the required acts would be performed under conditions of profound self-alienation? The *type* of issue paradigmatically represented by gestation—an assistance that combines life and death stakes with deep intimacy—is virtually nowhere discussed in ethical theory. (We aren't called upon in the usual course of events to save people's lives by, say, having sexual intercourse with them.) By ignoring these issues, mainstream moral theory has ended up deeply underselling the moral complexity of abortion.

Difficult as these questions are, though, it is actually a second issue, I suspect, that is responsible for much of the passion that surrounds abortion on supposition of fetal personhood. On reflection, many will say, the issues confronting the pregnant woman aren't about generic beneficence at all. The considerations she faces are not just those that would face someone uniquely well placed to serve as Good Samaritan to some stranger—as when one passes the drowning person: for the pregnant woman and fetus, crucially, aren't strangers. If the fetus is a person, many will say, it is *her child;* and for this reason she has special responsibilities to meet its needs. In the end, I believe, much of the animating concern with abortion is not about what we owe to generic others; it's about what parents owe their children.

But if it's parenthood that is carrying normative weight, then we need an ethics of parenthood—a theory of what makes someone a parent in this thickly normative sense and what the contours of its responsibilities really are. This should raise something of a warning flag. Philosophers, it must be said, have by and large done a rather poor job when it comes to parenthood—variously avoiding it, romanticizing it, or assimilating it to categories, like contractual relations, to which it stands in paradigmatic contrast. This general shortcoming is evident in discussions of abortion, where two remarkably unhelpful models dominate.

One position, advocated by Judith Thomson and some of the most recent treatments of abortion, is a classically liberal one. It agrees that special responsibilities attach to parenthood but argues that parenthood is thereby a status that is entered into only by consent. That consent is usually tacit, to be sure—taking the baby home from the hospital qualifies; nonetheless, special responsibilities to a child accrue only when one voluntarily assumes them.

Such a model is surely an odd one. The model yields the plausible view that the rape victim does not face the very same set of duties as many other pregnant women, but it does so by implying that a man who fathers a child during a one-night stand has no special responsibilities toward that child unless he decides he does. Perhaps most strikingly, such a view has no resources for acknowledging that there may be moral reasons why one *should* consent to the status. Those who sustain a biological connection may have a tendency to enter the role of parent, but on this scheme it's a mere psychological proclivity that rides atop nothing normative.

Another position is classically conservative. According to this view, the special responsibilities of parenthood are grounded in biological progenitorship. It is blood ties, to use the old-fashioned vernacular—"passing on one's genes," in more current translation—that makes one a parent and grounds heightened responsibilities. This view has its own blind spot. It has the resources for agreeing that a man who fathers a child from a one-night stand faces special responsibilities for the child whether he likes it or not, but none for distinguishing between the responsibilities of someone who has served as the special steward for a child—who has engaged for years in the *activity* of parenting—and the responsibilities of someone who bears literally no connection beyond a genetic or causal contribution to existence. On this view, a sperm donor faces all the responsibilities of a social father.

What both positions have in common is the supposition that parenthood is an all or nothing affair. Applied to pregnancy, the gestating woman either owes everything we imagine we owe to the children we love and rear or she owes nothing beyond general beneficence unless she decides she does. But parenthood—like all familial relations—is surely a more complicated moral notion than this. Parenthood, and its attendant responsibilities, admit of *layers*. It has a crucial existence as a social *role*—something with institutionally defined entrances, exits, and expectations that can attach to us quite independently of what our self-conceptions might say. It also has a crucial existence as a *relationship*—an emotional connection, a shared history, an intertwinement of lives. It is because of that intertwinement that parents' motivation to sacrifice is so often immediate. But it is also because of that relationship that even especially ambitious sacrifices are legitimately expected, and why failure to undertake them would be so problematic: absent unusual circumstances, it becomes a betrayal of the relationship itself. In short, parenthood is not monolithic: some of the responsibilities we paradigmatically associate as parental attach, not to the role, but to the relationship that so often accompanies it.

These layers matter especially when we get to gestation, for the pregnant woman stands precisely at their intersection. If a fetus is a person, then there is surely an important sense in which she is its mother: to regard her as just a passing stranger uniquely able to help it would grossly distort the situation. But she is not yet a mother most thickly described—a mother in standing relationship with a child, with the responsibilities born of shared history and the enterprise of caretaking.

These demarcations are integral, I think, to understanding the distinctive sorts of conflicts that pregnancy can represent—including, most notably, the conflicts it can bring *within* the mantle of motherhood. Women sometimes decide to abort even though they regard the fetus they carry as their child, because they realize, grimly, that bringing this child into the world will leave too little room to care adequately for the children they are already raising. This is a conflict we cannot even name, much less arbitrate, on standard views—if the fetus is her child, how could she possibly choose to sacrifice its life unless the stakes are literally equivalent for the others? But this is to ignore the layers of parenthood. She occupies the *role* of mother to the fetus, but with the other children, she is, by dint of time, interaction, and intertwinement, in a *relationship* of motherhood. The fetus is her baby, then—not just some passing stranger she alone can help—which is why this conflict brings the kind of agony it does. But if it is her child in the role sense only, she does not yet owe all that she owes to her other children. Depending on the circumstances, other family members with whom she is already in relationship may, tragically, come first.

None of this is to make light to the responsibilities pregnant women face on supposition of fetal personhood. If fetuses are persons, such responsibilities are surely profound. It is, rather, to insist that they admit of layer and degree, and that these distinctions, while delicate, are crucial to capturing the *types* of tragedy—and the types of moral compromise—abortion can here represent.

The Sanctity of Life: Respect Revisited

. . . For many women who contemplate abortion, the desire to end pregnancy is not, or not centrally, a desire to avoid the nine months of pregnancy; it is to avoid what lies on the far side of those months—namely, motherhood. If gestation were simply a matter of rendering, say, somewhat risky assistance to help a burgeoning human life they've come across—if they could somehow render that assistance without thereby adding a member to their family—the decision faced would be a far different one. But gestation doesn't just allow cells to become a person; it turns one into a mother.

One of the most common reasons women give for wanting to abort is that they do not want to become a mother—now, ever, again, with this partner, or no reliable partner, with these few resources, or these many that are now, after so many years of mothering, slated finally to another cause. Nor does adoption represent a universal solution. To give up a child would be for some a life-long trauma; others occupy fortunate circumstances that would, by their own lights, make it unjustified to give over a child for others to rear. Or again—and most frequently—she doesn't want to raise a child just now but knows that if she *does* carry the pregnancy to term, she won't *want* to give up the child for adoption. Gestation, she knows, is likely to reshape her heart and soul, transforming her into a mother emotionally, not just officially; and it is precisely that transformation she does not want to undergo. It is because continuing pregnancy brings with it this new identity and, likely, relationship, then, that many feel it legitimate to decline.

But pregnancy's connection to motherhood also enters the phenomenology of abortion in just the opposite direction. For some women, that it would be her child is precisely why she feels she must continue the pregnancy—even if motherhood is not what she desired. To be pregnant is to have one's potential child knocking at one's door; to abort is to turn one's back on it, a decision, many women say, that would haunt them forever. On this view, the desire to avoid motherhood, so compelling as a reason to contracept, is uneasy grounds to abort: for once an embryo is on the scene, it isn't about rejecting motherhood, it's about rejecting one's *child.* Not literally, of course, since there is no child yet extant to stand as the object of rejection. But the stance one should take to pregnancy, sought or not, is one of *acceptance:* when a potential family member is knocking at the door, one should move over, make room, and welcome her in.

These two intuitive stances represent just profoundly different ways of gestalting the situation of ending pregnancy. On the first view, abortion is closer to contraception—hardly equivalent, because it means the demise of something of value. But the desire to avoid the enterprise and identity of motherhood is an understandable and honorable basis for deciding to end a pregnancy. Given that there is no child yet on the scene, one does not owe special openness to the relationship that stands at the end of pregnancy's trajectory. On the second view, abortion is closer to exiting a parental relationship—hardly equivalent, for one of the key relata is not yet fully present. But one's decision about whether to continue the pregnancy already feels specially constrained: that one would be related to the resulting person exerts now some moral force. It would take especially grave reasons to refuse assistance here, for the norms of parenthood already have a toehold. Assessing the moral status of abortion, it turns out, then, is not just about assessing the contours of generic respect owed to burgeoning human life, it's about assessing the salience of *impending relationship.* And this is an issue that functions in different ways for different women—and, sometimes, in one and the same woman.

In my own view, until the fetus is a person, we should recognize a moral prerogative to decline parenthood and end the pregnancy. Not because motherhood is necessarily a burden (though it can be); but because it so thoroughly changes what we might call one's fundamental practical identity. The enterprise of mothering restructures the self—changing the shape of one's heart, the primary commitments by which one lives one's life, the terms by which one judges one's life a success or a failure. If the enterprise is eschewed and one decides to give the child over to another, the identity of mother still changes the normative facts that are true of one, as there is now someone by whom one does well or poorly. And either way—whether one rears the child or lets it go—to continue a pregnancy means that a piece of one's heart, as the saying goes, will forever walk outside one's body. As profound as the respect we should have for burgeoning human life, we should acknowledge moral prerogatives over identity-constituting commitments and enterprises as profound as motherhood.

But I also don't think this is the whole of the moral story. If women find themselves with different ways of gestalting the prospective relationship involved in pregnancy, it is in part because they have different identities, commitments, and ideals that such a prospect intersects with—commitments which, while permissibly idiosyncratic, are morally authoritative for *them*. If a woman feels already duty-bound by the norms of parenthood to nurture this creature, it may be for the very good reason that, in an important personal sense, she already *is* its mother. She finds herself—perhaps to her surprise, happy or otherwise—with a maternal commitment to this creature. As philosophers forget but women and men have long known, something can be your child even if it is not yet a person. But taking on the identity of mother towards something just *is* to take on certain imperatives about its well-being as categorical. Her job is thus clear—it's to help this creature reach its fullest potential. For other women, the identity is still something that can be assessed—tried on, perhaps accepted, but perhaps declined: in which case respect is owed, but is saved, or confirmed, for others—other relationships, other projects, other passions.

And again, if a woman feels she owes a stance of welcome to burgeoning human life that comes her way, it may be, not because she thinks such a stance authoritative for all, but because of the virtues around which her practical identity is now oriented: receptivity to life's agenda, for instance, or responsiveness to that which is most vulnerable. For another woman, the executive virtues to be exercised tug in just the other direction: loyalty to treasured life plans, a commitment that it be she, not the chances of biology, that should determine her life's course, bolstering self-direction after a life too long ruled by serendipity and fate.

Deciding when it is morally decent to end a pregnancy, it turns out, is an admixture of settling impersonally or universally authoritative moral requirements, and of discovering and arbitrating—sometimes after agonizing deliberation, sometimes in a decision no less deep for its immediacy—one's own commitments, identity, and defining virtues.

A similarly complex story appears when we turn to the second theme. Another thread that appears in many women's stories in the face of unsought pregnancy is respect for the weighty responsibility involved in creating human life. Once again, it is a theme that pulls and tugs in different directions.

In its most familiar direction, it shows up in many stories of why an unsought pregnancy is continued. Many people believe that one's responsibility to nurture new life is importantly amplified if one is responsible for bringing about its existence in the first place. Just what it takes to count as responsible here is a point on which individuals diverge (whether voluntary but contracepted intercourse is different from intercourse without use of birth control, and again from intentionally deciding to become pregnant at the IVF clinic). But triggering the relevant standard of responsibility for creation, it is felt, brings with it a heightened responsibility to nurture: it is disrespectful to create human life only to allow it to wither. Put more rigorously, one who is responsible for bringing about a creature that has intrinsic value in virtue of its potential to become a person has a special responsibility to enable it to reach that end state.

But the idea of respect for creation is also, if less frequently acknowledged, sometimes the reason why women are moved to *end* pregnancies. As Barbara Katz Rothman (1985) puts it, decisions to abort often represent, not a decision to destroy, but a refusal to create. Many people have deeply felt convictions about the circumstances under which they feel it right for them to bring a child into the world—can it be brought into a decent world, an intact family, a society that can minimally respect its agency? These considerations may persist even after conception has taken place; for while the *embryo* has already been created, a person has not. Some women decide to abort, that is, not because they do not *want* the resulting child—indeed, they may yearn for nothing more, and desperately wish that their circumstances were otherwise—but because they do not think bringing a child into the world the right thing for them to do.

These are abortions marked by moral language. A woman wants to abort because she knows she couldn't give up a child for adoption but feels she couldn't give the child the sort of life, or be the sort of parent, she thinks a child *deserves;* a woman who would have to give up the child thinks it would be *unfair* to bring a child into existence already burdened by rejection, however well grounded its reasons; a woman living in a country marked by poverty and gender apartheid wants to abort because she decides it would be *wrong* for her to bear a daughter whose life, like hers, would be filled with so much injustice and hardship.

Some have thought that such decisions betray a simple fallacy: unless the child's life were literally going to be worse than non-existence, how can one abort out of concern for the future child? But the worry here isn't that one would be imposing a *harm* on the child by bringing it into existence (as though children who are in the situations mentioned have lives that aren't worth living). The claim is that bringing about a person's life in these circumstances would do violence to her ideals of creating and parenthood. She does not want to bring into existence a daughter she cannot love and care for, she does not want to bring into existence a person whose life will be marked by disrespect or rejection.

Nor does the claim imply judgment on women who *do* continue pregnancies in similar circumstances—as though there were here an obligation to abort. For the norms in question, once again, need not be impersonally authoritative moral chums. Like ideals of good parenting, they mark out considerations all should be sensitive to, perhaps, but equally reasonable people may adhere to different variations and weightings. Still, they are normative for those who do have them; far from expressing mere matters of taste, the ideals one does accept carry an important kind of categoricity, issuing imperatives whose authority is not reducible to mere desire. These are, at root, issues about *integrity,* and the importance of maintaining integrity over one's participation in this enterprise precisely because it is so normatively weighty.

What is usually emphasized in the morality of abortion is the ethics of destruction; but there is a balancing ethics of creation. And for many people, conflict about abortion is a conflict *within* that ethics. On the one had, we now have on hand an entity that has a measure of sanctity: that it has begun is reason to help it continue—perhaps especially if one had a role in its procreation—which is why even early abortion is not normatively equivalent to contraception. On the other hand, not to end a pregnancy *is* to do something else, namely, to continue creating a person, and for some women, pregnancy strikes in circumstances in which they cannot countenance that enterprise. For some, the sanctity of developing human life will be strong enough to tip the balance towards continuing the pregnancy; for others, their norms of respectful creation will hold sway. For those who believe that the norms governing creation of a person are mild relative to the normative telos of embryonic life, being a responsible creator means continuing to gestate, and doing the best one can to bring about the conditions under which that creation will be more respectful. For others, though, the normativity of fetal telos is mild and their standards of respectful creation high, and the lesson goes in just the other direction: it is a sign of respect not to continue creating when certain background conditions, such as a loving family or adequate resources, are not in place.

However one thinks these issues settle out, they will not be resolved by austere contemplation of the value of human life. They require wrestling with the rich meanings of creation, responsibility, and kinship. And these issues, I have suggested, are just as much issues about one's integrity as they are about what is impersonally obligatory. On many treatments of abortion, considerations about whether or not to continue a pregnancy are exhausted by preferences, on the one hand, and universally authoritative moral demands, on the other; but some of the most important terrain lies in between.

References

Rothman, B. K. (1989). *Recreating motherhood: ideology and technology in a patriarchal society.* New York: Norton.

Thomson, J. J. (1971). A defense of abortion. *Philosophy and Public Affairs,* 1, 47–66.

EXPLORING THE ISSUE

Is Abortion Immoral?

Critical Thinking and Reflection

1. What different meanings can be given to the concepts of "human" and "person"? What do Lee and George mean when they describe the human embryo as a "whole" or "complete" organism?
2. Commentators who defend a pro-choice position sometimes argue that an early embryo has a value greater than the value of an ordinary tissue sample but less than the value of a person; how does that idea square with your views?
3. What different views of maternal commitment to a child or potential child are found in the YES and NO selections? What are the different views of parenthood?
4. Judith Thomson, whose earlier and very influential discussion of abortion is discussed in both of these selections, argued that abortion is permissible even if the fetus is a person. Explain her argument and whether or not you agree with it.

Is There Common Ground?

Surely the central issue in abortion is simply what "person" actually means. Political opposition to abortion has therefore centered in recent years on other topics in reproduction that raise the question of fetal personhood. See issue 9.

A common view about fetal personhood is that it somehow progresses slowly, that there is no one moment at which a person suddenly comes into existence. The embryo or early fetus is therefore less likely to be considered a person than the late-term fetus. In line with this, the Centers for Disease Control and Prevention reports that more than half of all abortions in the United States are performed during the first 8 weeks of pregnancy, and 88 percent before the 12th week. Although uncommon, abortions performed in the second trimester of pregnancy are very controversial. Most often the reasons are fetal abnormalities, illness in the mother, or late diagnosis of pregnancy in a teenager. The procedure, which involves delivering a dead but intact fetus, is particularly troubling. The technical term is "intact dilatation and extraction," but the more commonly used (and emotionally loaded) term is "partial-birth abortion."

In June 2000, the U.S. Supreme Court struck down a Nebraska law making it a crime to perform a partial-birth abortion. The five-to-four vote was the first abortion rights ruling in 8 years. Congress twice passed a bill banning partial-birth abortions, and President Bill Clinton twice vetoed it. President

George W. Bush, however, signed the Partial-Birth Abortion Ban Act of 2003. In June 2004, a federal judge in San Francisco struck down the bill, ruling that the law jeopardizes other legal forms of abortion and threatens the health of women. The U.S. federal government appealed, and the case of *Gonzales v. Carhart* went to the U.S. Supreme Court in 2006. In April 2007, by a five-to-four majority, the U.S. Supreme Court upheld the federal ban, which is limited to a particular, rarely used procedure.

In October 2008, the Court declined to review a New Jersey court's decision in *Acuna v. Turkish* that state law did not require a physician to inform a woman considering a first-trimester abortion that it would result in killing an "existing human being."

Additional Resources

Lawrence O. Gostin criticizes the Supreme Court ruling in *Gonzales* on grounds of its interference with clinical freedom, trust in the judiciary, and the autonomy of women ("Abortion Politics," *Journal of the American Medical Association* [October 3, 2007]). For the Court opinion, with concurrence and dissents, see www.law.cornell.edu/supct/html/05-380.ZO.html.

While most attention focuses on federal challenges to *Roe v. Wade*, state legislatures have been very active in this arena. See www.stateline.org for information on abortion regulations in specific states.

For a history of the political and ethical issues surrounding abortion in the United States, see Eva R. Rubin, *The Abortion Controversy: A Documentary History* (Greenwood, 1994). See also Robert M. Baird and Stuart E. Rosenbaum, *The Ethics of Abortion: Pro-Life vs. Pro-Choice*, 3rd ed. (Prometheus Books, 2001).

ISSUE 8

Should There Be Legal Limits on How Many Embryos Can Be Transferred into a Woman Who Wants to Be Pregnant?

YES: David Orentlicher, from "Multiple Embryo Transfers: Time for Policy," *Hastings Center Report* (May/June 2010)

NO: John A. Robertson, from "The Octuplet Case—Why More Regulation Is Not Likely," *Hastings Center Report* (March/April 2009)

Learning Outcomes

After reading this issue, you should be able to:

- Discuss the potential harms and benefits, and the issues of parental rights, associated with multiple birth pregnancies when in vitro fertilization (IVF) is used.
- Discuss the regulation of assisted reproduction technologies in the United States.

ISSUE SUMMARY

YES: Professor of medicine David Orentlicher argues that the practice of transferring multiple embryos to a woman's uterus, which came to public attention with the case of Nadya Suleman in 2009, is dangerous for both children and mothers and should be discouraged by federal policy.

NO: Lawyer John A. Robertson holds that professional guidelines on embryo transfer are enough, and that hard and fast legal limits on embryo transfer would be seen as violating parents' rights.

Louise Brown, born in England in July 1978, was the first baby to have been conceived using IVF. She was known at that time as the first "test tube baby" because fertilization in IVF occurs outside the woman's body ("in vitro" means "in glass" in Latin). Her birth immediately generated a flurry of ethical debate about whether babies born through IVF would be harmed, about the implications for women's health and role in family and society, about the implications for families about whether IVF is an unnatural and therefore unacceptable way of producing children, and about the implications of IVF for families.

Strictly speaking, "test tube baby" is inaccurate, since fertilization in IVF occurs not in a test tube but in a glass dish. A typical IVF procedure goes as follows. First, the woman is injected with hormones that stimulate her ovaries to produce multiple eggs—more eggs than would normally be produced at any one time. When the eggs are released by the ovaries, the physician draws them into a hollow needle inserted into the woman's body, and then places them in glass dishes. Sperm, collected from the woman's partner or from a donor by asking the man to masturbate, are added to the dishes, and the dishes are placed in an incubator that mimics the conditions of the woman's body. If all goes well, a sperm cell combines with the egg in each dish, producing a new cell that begins to divide into multiple cells, forming an embryo. When the embryos reach the four- to sixteen-cell stage, one or more are drawn into a hollow needle and released in the woman's uterus—a process known as "embryo transfer"—where they implant, resulting in pregnancy.

IVF is used to circumvent a variety of fertility problems, including blocked fallopian tubes, ovulation problems, endometriosis, and low sperm counts. However, because it is complicated, sometimes onerous for the woman, and expensive (over $10,000 per cycle, on average), it is not the first medical response to a fertility problem, and the vast majority of couples with fertility problems never use it. Nor are the success rates especially encouraging: According to the Centers for Disease Control, which keeps statistics on the use of assisted reproductive technologies (ARTs) in the United States, about 30 percent of IVF cycles lead to a pregnancy, and a little over 20 percent to a live birth. (The success rates decline with the woman's age.) Nonetheless, IVF is estimated to have led to close to 500,000 births in the United States, according to the American Society for Reproductive Medicine, and about 1 percent of all babies born in the United States are conceived using IVF.

Because fertility clinics compete with each other partly on the basis of their success rates at producing pregnancies, and because prospective parents want to avoid paying for repeat cycles, both clinics and parents have an incentive to transfer multiple embryos at a time in order to increase the odds that at least one will implant. If multiple embryos are transferred, however, they may all implant, which carries a greater risk of medical problems for the mother and especially for the children. Also, of course, the parents may not be prepared financially or psychologically to raise more than one child. When a multifetal pregnancy occurs, "selective reduction" can be used to remove one or more of the fetuses, but reduction carries its own medical risks, and of course it raises the concerns associated with abortion.

The American Society for Reproductive Medicine (ASRM) recommends limits on the number of embryos that can be transplanted, but the recommendations are not strict requirements—a fact that was illuminated in 2009 by the case of Nadya Suleman, dubbed "Octomom" by the media when she gave birth to eight children after having 12 embryos transferred to her uterus simultaneously. Six implanted, but two of those then split into new embryos, raising the total to eight. (Suleman initially claimed that only six embryos had been transferred, but Dr. Kamrava later admitted he had transferred 12.) In general, the development and clinical use of ARTs proceeds with very little coordinated oversight in the United States. By contrast, the United Kingdom has provided oversight through the Human Fertilisation and Embryology Authority, a nongovernmental body that is given responsibility by the government for licensing and monitoring clinics and laboratories that work on ARTs.

The YES and NO selections discuss the regulation of IVF and other ARTs in the United States and reach different conclusions about whether it ought to be changed. David Orentlicher argues that the practice of transferring multiple embryos is dangerous and the current professional guidelines discouraging the practice should be supplemented with federal policy. John Robertson argues that the professional guidelines will prove adequate and that laws to explicitly ban multiple embryo transfers would violate parents' rights.

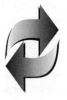

YES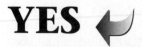

David Orentlicher

Multiple Embryo Transfers: Time for Policy

The birth of eight children to Nadya Suleman led to an outcry over the common practice in assisted reproduction of transferring multiple embryos to a woman's uterus. The practice increases the chances of a live birth, but also raises the likelihood of multiple births, with their risks and costs. It is time for the United States to enact policy that will limit the number of embryos transferred to a woman.

Health Problems

In vitro fertilization in the United States often leads to multiple births. More than 30 percent of deliveries using fresh embryos and nearly 25 percent of those using frozen ones result in multiple births,[1] with 48 percent of all IVF infants born in multiple births.[2]

Any multiple birth raises health risks. Among twins, more than 60 percent are born prematurely; among triplets or other multiples, more than 95 percent are premature.[3] Primarily for this reason, IVF twins, triplets, and other multiples are more likely than singletons to require neonatal intensive care, to develop cognitive and physical disabilities, and to die. Twins have an infant mortality rate four to five times that of singletons; triplets have an eight- to tenfold increase.[4] These infants are also at increased risk for cerebral palsy, deafness, and blindness, and they exhibit delayed language development and lower verbal intelligence.[5] Multiple births pose greater health risks for the mother as well. They increase the risk for maternal hypertension, preeclampsia, hemorrhage, Cesarean section, and death, as well as for postpartum depression and high parenting stress.[6]

These risks drive up the cost of health care. In one study, the delivery-associated hospital costs were twice as high per child for twins as for singletons, and four times higher for triplets.[7] Lifetime medical costs may be two hundred times higher.[8]

IVF patients might be willing to assume the increased risks of multiple births in order to increase their likelihood of having at least one child. Studies indicate, however, that the success rate improves only marginally with multiple transfers, and some studies have found no difference. In one study involving women younger than age thirty-six with good-quality embryos,

From *Hastings Center Report*, May–June 2010, pp. 12–13. Copyright © 2010 by The Hastings Center. Reprinted by permission of Wiley-Blackwell via Rightslink.

double-embryo transfers increased the live birth rate from 39 to 43 percent, but the multiple birth rate increased from 1 to 33 percent.[9] In another study of women with good prospects for successful IVF, those with single-embryo transfers had the higher live birth rate—41 percent versus 36 percent for the double-embryo transfers. Moreover, the multiple birth rate rose from zero for single-embryo transfers to 37 percent for double-embryo transfers.[10] For women who have less favorable prospects, on the other hand, a double-embryo transfer may significantly increase the chances of success. In one study, it doubled the pregnancy rate.[11]

To be sure, there are other tradeoffs between single- and double-embryo transfers. To achieve a comparable overall live birth rate, women using single-embryo transfers may need to undergo two IVF cycles instead of one, doubling their cost of treatment. And older women who want two children may prefer to have twins rather than successive singletons. Because of the decline in fertility with advancing age, a forty-year-old woman may not be able to become pregnant a second time.[12]

The Response

Professional guidelines discourage multiple-embryo transfers, especially for women under age thirty-five. Suleman's physician transferred six embryos for her pregnancy, but Society for Assisted Reproductive Technology and American Society for Reproductive Medicine guidelines indicate that she should have received only one or two. Yet IVF procedures with two or more embryos are still common. Nearly 90 percent of embryo transfers involve at least two embryos, and more than 40 percent involve at least three.[13] To be sure, the percentage of IVF procedures with more than two embryos has recently declined, but the shift has been to double- rather than single-embryo transfers. As a result, triplet or high-order births have declined while twin births have increased.[14]

If professional guidelines have not been effective, what other approaches might make sense? This depends on why physicians transfer multiple embryos. Studies do not generate uniform data, but a few considerations appear important. Several of these reflect patient preference. First, when patients weigh the chances of successful IVF and the risks of multiple births, the desire to have at least one child appears stronger than the desire to avoid multiple births.[15] To the extent that IVF patients believe multiple-embryo transfers are more likely to succeed, they will prefer the multiple-embryo transfer. Second, IVF patients generally bear the full cost of their treatment. If a single-embryo transfer is less successful than a multiple-embryo transfer, then single-embryo transfers will require more IVF cycles (and higher fees) for one child. And patients who want two children may prefer having twins with one IVF cycle than singletons in two cycles. Finally, some patients simply want twins.

Multiple-embryo transfers may also be driven by physician preference. IVF clinics compete for patients, and maximizing overall birth rate is one way to do this, especially since the federal government publishes clinics' success rates on the Internet. However, empirical data suggest that competition among IVF clinics may not have a significant effect on multiple birth rates.[16]

These considerations suggest three changes in law and practice to reduce multiple births from IVF.

Education

Some IVF patients prefer multiple-embryo transfers because they underestimate both the success rate of single-embryo transfers and the health risks for multiple-birth children. Most probably assume they will increase their chances of success with multiple-embryo transfer, and many do not appreciate the extent to which twins and triplets have elevated health risks, especially with television shows like *Jon and Kate Plus Eight*. When IVF patients receive information about the health risks of multiple births, they become more interested in single-embryo transfers.[17]

Funding

Financial considerations may also lead patients to prefer multiple-embryo transfer. IVF can cost as much as $15,000. If a couple wants two children, they may want to have both in one IVF cycle. If insurers covered the cost of IVF, though, then the financial pressure on patients would be eased.

Although studies based on interviews of IVF patients come to different conclusions about the significance of cost on patient preference, one study of U.S. IVF practices indicates that costs are important. The study compared embryo transfers in states that require insurers to cover IVF costs with those in states that do not. In states with mandated coverage, there were more IVF cycles, with fewer embryos transferred per cycle and fewer multiple births.[18]

The funding of IVF services can better align patient incentives with societal interests. While patients face higher costs from multiple, single-embryo IVF cycles, society bears higher costs from multiple-embryo cycles. The higher costs of multiple IVF cycles are more than offset by higher health care costs from more multiple births.[19] Finally, considerations of equity justify funding for IVF services. Infertility can be a serious disability that warrants medical care, just as other disabilities do.

Legal Limits on Transfer

Important though they are, education and funding are probably not enough. Legal limits on transfer may be necessary. Data from Sweden demonstrate that this strategy can be effective. Sweden allows only single-embryo transfers, although double-embryo transfers are permitted for women at low risk of multiple births.[20] After the law was adopted, the birth rate did not change, but the multiple-birth rate dropped from 35 to 5 percent.[21]

A similar U.S. policy would balance a desire to avoid multiple births with the goal of achieving successful pregnancies. Physicians would transfer a single embryo unless a transfer of two was justified by the mother's age, poorer-quality embryos, or no prior success with IVF. To ensure adherence, advance approval of double-embryo transfers would probably be necessary. If the outcomes were similar to those in Sweden, and if transfer restrictions were coupled with insurance coverage of IVF, the restrictions would not limit reproductive rights.

Notes

1. Centers for Disease Control and Prevention, *2006 Assisted Reproductive Technology Success Rates: National Summary and Fertility Clinic Reports* (Atlanta, Ga.: Centers for Disease Control and Prevention, 2008), 22, 55.

2. S. Sunderam et al., "Assisted Reproductive Technology Surveillance—United States, 2006," *MMWR Surveillance Summaries* 58, SS-5 (2009): 1–25, at 8.

3. Centers for Disease Control and Prevention, *2006 Assisted Reproductive Technology Success Rates*, at 23.

4. B. Luke and M.B. Brown, "The Changing Risk of Infant Mortality by Gestation, Plurality, and Race: 1989–1991 versus 1999–2001," *Pediatrics* 118 (2006): 2488–97, at 2492.

5. C.R. Newton et al., "Factors Affecting Patients' Attitudes toward Single- and Multiple-Embryo Transfer," *Fertility and Sterility* 87 (2007): 269–78, at 269.

6. G.L. Ryan et al., "The Desire of Infertile Patients for Multiple Births," *Fertility and Sterility* 81 (2004): 500–504, at 503; B.J. Van Voorhis, "In Vitro Fertilization," *New England Journal of Medicine* 356 (2007): 379–86, at 382.

7. T. Callahan et al., "The Economic Impact of Multiple-Gestation Pregnancies and the Contribution of Assisted-Reproduction Techniques to Their Incidence," *New England Journal of Medicine* 331 (1994): 244–49.

8. FIGO Committee for the Ethical Aspects of Human Reproduction and Women's Health, "Ethical Guidelines in the Prevention of Iatrogenic Multiple Pregnancy," *European Journal of Obstetrics and Gynecology and Reproductive Biology* 96 (2001): 209–210.

9. A. Thurin et al., "Elective Single-Embryo Transfer versus Double-Embryo Transfer in In Vitro Fertilization," *New England Journal of Medicine* 351 (2004): 2392–2402.

10. H.G.M. Lukassen et al., "Two Cycles with Single Embryo Transfer Versus One Cycle with Double Embryo Transfer: A Randomized Controlled Trial," *Human Reproduction* 20 (2005): 702–8.

11. A.P.A. Van Montfoort et al., "In Unselected Patients, Elective Single Embryo Transfer Prevents Multiples, but Results in Significantly Lower Pregnancy Rates Compared with Double Embryo Transfer: A Randomized Controlled Trial," *Human Reproduction* 21 (2006): 338–43.

12. N. Gleicher and D. Barad, "The Relative Myth of Elective Single Embryo Transfer," *Human Reproduction* 21 (2006): 1337–44, at 1340.

13. Centers for Disease Control and Prevention, *2006 Assisted Reproductive Technology Success Rates*, at 44.

14. S.L. Boulet et al., "Perinatal Outcomes of Twin Births Conceived Using Assisted Reproduction Technology: A Population-Based Study," *Human Reproduction* 23 (2008): 1941–48, at 1941.

15. Ryan et al., "The Desire of Infertile Patients," 502.

16. A.Z. Steiner, R.J. Paulson, and K.E. Hartmann, "Effects of Competition among Fertility Centers on Pregnancy and High-Order Multiple Gestation Rates," *Fertility and Sterility* 83 (2005): 1429–34.

17. Newton et al., "Factors Affecting Patients' Attitudes," 274–75.

18. T. Jain, B.L. Harlow, and M.D. Hornstein, "Insurance Coverage and Outcomes of In Vitro Fertilization," *New England of Medicine* 347 (2002): 661–66.

19. Lukassen et al., "Two Cycles with Single Embryo Transfer," 706.

20. P.O. Karlström and C. Bergh, "Reducing the Impact of Embryos Transferred in Sweden—Impact on Delivery and Multiple Birth Rates," *Human Reproduction* 22 (2007): 2202–7, at 2203.

21. Ibid.

John A. Robertson 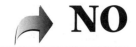 **NO**

The Octuplet Case—Why More Regulation Is Not Likely

In vitro fertilization and assisted reproductive technologies, or ARTs, have always posed a regulatory conundrum. They've been hugely successful (52,000 births from 152,000 IVF cycles in 2005) and are firmly established as the treatment of choice for many kinds of infertility.[1] But over the years there has been a steady drip of ethical lapses, from doctors who oversell their success rates to theft of eggs and embryos. A 1992 federal law arranges for accurate reporting of success rates and encourages accreditation of IVF laboratories, but there is no centralized licensing and control authority to enforce it (as exists, for example, in the United Kingdom) and thus few teeth to it.[2]

The IVF industry argues that there is more regulation in place than meets the eye, citing the many federal and state laws that impinge on IVF practice in some way.[3] It also is active in developing ethical and practice guidelines, though it has little muscle to enforce them. Critics of the industry argue that it's like the wild west—anything goes if patients can pay, often to that patient's detriment. Yet these critics are remarkably silent on what specific form more regulation should take. The Bush-appointed President's Council on Bioethics was concerned enough to spend two years examining the field but found no reason to urge major regulatory intervention.

The octuplet case has peeled back the ART industry's claim that everything is fine and dandy. In the end, however, it is unlikely to bring major changes to how IVF is conducted and regulated. This is in part due to the case being such an outlier. If the situation had not arisen in real life, it would have been hard to imagine it: an unemployed, thirty-three-year-old single mother of six IVF children with some evidence of personal instability has her IVF doctor implant six frozen embryos in her uterus. She then ends up giving birth to eight children and touching off a media firestorm.

The "octomom" has been widely reviled as an example of irresponsible reproductive behavior, not just because the octuplets, born at thirty-one weeks, are at high risk for cerebral palsy and learning disabilities, but because she doesn't have the money to pay for their care, nor a husband or partner to help with it. She is partially estranged from her family and depends on the kindness of strangers and Medicaid to pay the enormous medical and rearing costs of an additional eight premature infants.

From *Hastings Center Report*, March–April 2009, pp. 26–28. Copyright © 2009 by The Hastings Center. Reprinted by permission of Wiley-Blackwell via Rightslink.

Nevertheless, the decision to transfer the embryos initially had some defenders. One noted fertility specialist in Los Angeles, Jeffrey Steinberg, was quoted in the *Philadelphia Inquirer* as saying, "Who am I to say that six is the limit. There are people who love big families." Jamie Grifo, who is paid approximately $2.3 million annually by New York University medical school for his fertility skills, was similarly quoted in the *New York Times:* "I don't think it's our job to tell them how many babies they are allowed to have. I am not a policeman for reproduction in the United States."

However, since the first reports, few other doctors have publicly defended Dr. Michael Kamrava's decision to transfer six embryos. His Web site reportedly proclaimed that he was an "internationally recognized leader in the field of in-vitro fertilization whose work has led to breakthrough technology." Although no law directly regulates who may have IVF procedures or the number of embryos to transfer, Dr. Kamrava appears to have violated the American Society of Reproductive Medicine's guideline to transfer only two embryos for healthy women under thirty-five (one if they have already had an IVF birth) and has offered no justification for doing so.[4] It is noteworthy that his program—one of many in the Los Angeles area—had a very low success rate.

So what, if anything, should be done about this? Since ART, like most medical procedures, relies heavily on professional self-regulation, let us first examine whether professional self-regulation can prevent such situations, and then turn to the possibility of legal change.

The ASRM has two sets of guidelines that pertain to this situation. Its ethics committee statement on "Child-Rearing Ability and the Provision of Fertility Services" discusses situations in which the patient appears unlikely to be able to provide adequate childrearing.[5] The statement says that programs may deny services to patients if they have a substantial basis for thinking that any given patient will not be adequate to the task. The statement is careful to say that this judgment is not easy to make and should be arrived at as a group. It also warns against assuming that having a disability alone is enough to support such a judgment.

Based on this guidance, a doctor should have no doubt that he could have refused to provide any services to a woman in Suleman's position, not just her request to transfer six embryos at once. The statement also says, however, that a doctor is still free to treat, except in cases where clear significant harm to offspring is likely. While that provision might have justified the doctor if he were transferring one or two embryos, the transfer of six crosses that line, since higher-order multifetal gestation clearly poses a threat of harm to offspring.

The second set of ASRM guidelines are those concerning the number of embryos to be transferred that I mentioned above. The ASRM's affiliate group of reproductive endocrinologists, the Society of Assisted Reproductive Technology (SART), developed the practice guidelines. They are quite clear that no more than two embryos should be transferred for women under thirty-five, and only one if the mother has already given birth through IVF. There is no question that transferring six violated the professional guideline.

Critics, however, would argue that even clear professional guidelines are not adequate to deal with such cases. The ethics statement on reproductive services and inadequate childrearing leaves much room for individual judgment and does not explicitly condemn providing services in this kind of case. And like the embryo transfer policy, no sanction exists for violating it beyond expulsion or suspension from those societies and loss of the right to use that affiliation on Web sites and in advertising. Since Dr. Kamrava was a member of SART at the time of the embryo transfer, it will be interesting to see what action, if any, SART takes for violation of its guidelines.

The ASRM guidelines do, however, have some bite if taken as an indicator of the standard of care for doctors practicing reproductive medicine. The California state medical licensing board will probably take them into account in determining whether to renew Dr. Kamrava's license to practice in California, which expires on November 30, 2009. The guidelines could also be used in tort actions against doctors by patients or offspring, though litigation in this case appears unlikely.

What, then, about legislation to curb such incidents in the future? There are some theoretic possibilities here, but all have problems. First is the question of providing IVF to a person who already has six children by IVF. While small families are now in vogue, it wasn't so long ago that large families were both desired and praised. Indeed, the UN Convention Against Elimination of All Forms of Discrimination Against Women gives women the same rights as men "to decide freely and responsibly on the number and spacing of their children." While India and China have had social policies against large families, we in the United States do not. I suspect that the courts would look with deep constitutional suspicion on laws that limit the number of children one may have.[6] Even Supreme Court Justice Antonin Scalia, who has nine children, might agree that there are constitutional problems with number limits on reproduction. The mode of conception of previous or next children—coital or ART—should not change this conclusion.

So what about laws that restrict reproduction when parents lack the means to care for the child? Such a law would penalize the poor and smack of classism. Limiting public assistance is not a good remedy, since it's the children who are penalized. Nor would compulsory reversible contraception fly. At best, one might be able to restrict ART for persons who already have children they are unable to care for by penalizing the doctors who provide the service, but such a law would interfere with the right of such persons to have additional children. In addition, it would require more screening of IVF patients than is now done. Most of these patients would not be in the doctor's office in the first place unless they were able to afford the treatment (which is quite pricey), and most would presumably then be able to pay the costs of rearing the resulting child.

Perhaps the best that the law can do here is to give greater legal effect to ASRM guidelines, as Missouri recently proposed. But this then shifts the focus to the development of those guidelines. Medical guidelines are never ethically neutral: normative choices are always hidden in the factual specifications. If the guidelines are to be the equivalent of law, then how they are arrived at will have to be more closely scrutinized, the process of writing them opened up, and measures taken to assure they do not simply protect the interests of doctors.

I believe that we'll have to stick with professional guidelines to prevent future higher-order multiple cases despite their limited bite because, as Yeats put it, "nothing better can be had." Guidelines do have some effect— professional shame and reputational standing matter, even if coercive sanctions matter more.

More importantly, though, we should put outliers like the Suleman case to the side and focus on the more important question of how best to reduce the continuing high rate of twin and triplet births in ARTs. In 2005, 35 percent of ART births were multiple, the vast majority being twins.[7] The ASRM has been successful in bringing the triplet-plus rate down from 6 percent in 2001 to 2 percent in 2007, and that rate is expected to drop even further.[8] But reducing the number of twins is much harder. Infertile patients view twins as a good outcome, overlooking the higher risks of twin pregnancies to both the mother and offspring. Also, with little insurance coverage for IVF, many parents like the idea of "getting two for the price of one." The rate of twins is lower in Europe but is still around 22 percent, which is considerably higher than the background rate from coital conception of 5 percent.[9] The best solution here would be single embryo transfer in patients under thirty-five, backed by repeated transfer of single frozen embryos if a fresh cycle fails to produce a pregnancy. Reaching such a goal will require a concerted effort comprised of patient education, insurance coverage, and changes in professional practice standards. Like much else in reproductive medicine, the law is usually too blunt an instrument to do the job.

References

1. https://www.sartcorsonline.com/rptCSR_PublicMultYear.aspx?ClinicPKID=0;   see also V.L. Wright et al., "Assisted Reproductive Technology Surveillance— United States, 2005," *Mortality and Morbidity Weekly Report* 57, Surveillance Summary no. 5 (2008): 1–23.

2. Fertility Clinic Success Rate and Certification Act of 1992, Pub. L. No. 102–493, 106 Stat. 3146.

3. D. Adamson, "Regulation of Assisted Reproductive Technologies in the United States," *Fertility and Sterility* 78, no. 5 (2002): 932–42.

4. The Practice Committee of the Society for Assisted Reproductive Technology, The American Society for Reproductive Medicine, "Guidelines on the Number of Embryos Transferred," *Fertility and Sterility* 82, Suppl. 1 (2004): 1–2.

5. The Ethics Committee of the American Society for Reproductive Medicine, "Child-Rearing Ability and the Provision of Fertility Services," *Fertility and Sterility* 82 (2004): 564.

6. See, e.g., *Skinner v. Oklahoma*, 316 U.S. 535 (1942).

7. https://www.sartcorsonline.com/rptCSR_PublicMultYear.aspx?ClinicPKID=0.

8. R.W. Rebar and A.H. DeCherney, "Assisted Reproduction in the United States," *New England Journal of Medicine* 350 (2004): 1603–5.

9. A. Andersen et al., The European IVF-Monitoring (EIM) Consortium, for the European Society of Human Reproduction and Embryology (ESHRE), "Assisted Reproductive Technology in Europe, 2004: Results Generated from European Registers by ESHRE," *Human Reproduction* 23, no. 4 (2008): 756.

EXPLORING THE ISSUE

Should There Be Legal Limits on How Many Embryos Can Be Transferred into a Woman Who Wants to Be Pregnant?

Critical Thinking and Reflection

1. Robertson argues that the regulatory picture is complicated, but that the use of IVF is in fact legally limited. What imposes limits, in his account, and how do they function?
2. How does Robertson think policy should deal with the tension between preventing harm to children and protecting parental rights resolved? How would Orentlicher address that tension, and which approach do you find more effective?
3. How would you decide when a risk of harm to children is severe enough to make a policy limiting that harm advisable?

Is There Common Ground?

Following the birth of the Suleman octuplets, Dr. Michael Kamrava was expelled from the American Society for Reproductive Medicine and lost his license to practice medicine in California. Losing membership in ASRM does not prevent a physician from practicing, but loss of a license does. In November 2009, the ASRM also announced that it had revised its guidelines for embryo transfer, recommending that for women who are under 35 years of age and have a favorable chance of becoming pregnant, "consideration should be given to transferring only a single embryo," and that no more than two embryos should be transferred simultaneously.

Some U.S. commentators have called for the formation in the United States of a body similar to the U.K. Human Fertilisation and Embryology Authority, but there has been no movement toward that goal outside academia.

Additional Resources

For information about ART generally and about the success rates of clinics that offer ART, see the Centers for Disease Control Web site, www.cdc.gov/art/.

The American Society for Reproductive Medicine offers information about IVF and other assisted reproduction technologies at www.reproductivefacts.org/. See also the Web site of the Society for Assisted Reproductive Technology, www.sart.org/.

For a broad discussion of U.S. regulation of assisted reproduction technologies, and recommendations for creation of a U.S. version of the HFEA, see Erik Parens and Lori P. Knowles, "Reprogenetics and Public Policy: Reflections and Recommendations," *Hastings Center Report* (July–August 2003, supplement).

Camille M. Davidson argues that federal law should require insurers to cover IVF services because covering cost of IVF would greatly reduce patients' and physicians' incentive to transfer multiple embryos. See "Octomom and Multi-Fetal Pregnancies: Why Federal Legislation Should Require Insurers to Cover in Vitro Fertilization," *William and Mary Journal of Women and the Law* (vol. 17, 2010).

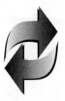

ISSUE 9

Should a Pregnant Woman Be Punished for Exposing Her Fetus to Risk?

YES: **Liles Burke**, from *Hope Elisabeth Ankrom v. State of Alabama* (May 26, 2011)

NO: **Lynn M. Paltrow**, from "Punishment and Prejudice: Judging Drug-Using Pregnant Women," in Julia A. Hanigsberg and Sara Ruddick, eds., *Mother Troubles: Rethinking Contemporary Maternal Dilemmas* (Beacon Press, 1999)

Learning Outcomes

After reading this issue, you should be able to:

- Discuss the implications of maternal responsibility during pregnancy.
- Discuss how environmental factors may affect a person's well-being and a person's responsibility for their behavior.
- Discuss how the debate about abortion is affecting public policy on other issues, including substance abuse and child welfare.

ISSUE SUMMARY

YES: Liles Burke sets out the majority opinion of the Alabama Court of Criminal Appeals in a case involving a pregnant woman who was found to have used cocaine while pregnant. Burke argues that Alabama law that forbids adults from exposing children to controlled substances applies in cases involving pregnant women and their fetuses.

NO: Attorney Lynn M. Paltrow argues that treating drug-using pregnant women as criminals targets poor, African American women while ignoring other drug usage and fails to provide the resources to assist them in recovery.

In 1989, fueled by the specter of an epidemic of drug use resulting in the birth of thousands of "crack babies," the Medical University of South Carolina established a program that required drug-using pregnant women to seek treatment and prenatal care or face criminal prosecution. This program applied only to patients attending the university's obstetric clinic, primarily poor black women, and not to private patients. Patients enrolled in the clinic saw a video and were given written information about the harmful effects of substance abuse during pregnancy. The information warned that the police, the court system, and child protective services in Charleston, South Carolina, might become involved if illegal drug use were detected.

Women who met certain criteria were required to undergo periodic urine screening for drugs. A patient who had a positive urine test or who failed to keep scheduled appointments for therapy or prenatal care could be arrested and placed in custody. If a woman delivered a baby who tested positive for drugs, she would be arrested immediately after her medical release and her newborn taken into protective custody. If the drug use was detected within the first 27 weeks of gestation, the patient was charged with possession of an illegal substance; after that date, the charge was possession and distribution of an illegal substance to a minor. If the drug use were detected during delivery, the woman would be charged with unlawful neglect of a child.

This stringent policy was developed as a result of clinicians' concern about the harmful effects of drug use on fetal development and prosecutors' desires to take a strong public stand condemning drug use. The Supreme Court of South Carolina upheld the law in a 1997 decision involving a woman, Cornelia Whitner, who admitted to using cocaine during pregnancy and whose baby was born with cocaine metabolites in his system. The court wrote that, "The abuse or neglect of a child at any time during childhood can exact a profound toll on the child herself as well as on society as a whole. However, the consequences of abuse or neglect that takes place after birth often pale in comparison to those resulting from abuse suffered by the viable fetus before birth."

Critics argued, however, that the law punished women without helping them correct their behavior. Although the law's stated goal was to get women into treatment, there were few places that women could receive treatment and the necessary support, such as transportation and child care. At the time, there was no women-only residential treatment center for substance-abusing pregnant women anywhere in the state.

The program was discontinued in September 1994 as the result of a settlement with the Civil Rights Division of the federal Department of Health and Human Services. By then, 42 pregnant women had been arrested. In recent years, however, similar cases have been tried in other states. In Alabama, prosecutors began filing charges against women under the state's 2006 chemical endangerment law, whose explicit goal was to prevent adults from bringing children to methamphetamine laboratories and other places where illegal substances are produced or distributed. Prosecutors argued that the law also applied to fetuses exposed to drugs while in the uterus. A long list of medical, legal, and public organizations filed legal briefs arguing against their interpretation of the law, but their prosecutors' position has been upheld by the Alabama Court of Criminal Appeals. Over 60 women have now been charged under the law.

In *Hope Elisabeth Ankrom v. State of Alabama*, Justice Liles Burke explains why a majority of the court's justices found that the state's chemical endangerment law includes a fetus within its definition of "child." Lynn Paltrow argues, however, that criminalization of drug use is a punitive response that rejects the humanity of the women who are denied treatment and support for recovering from their addiction.

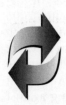

YES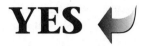

Liles Burke

⚸ Hope Elisabeth Ankrom v. State of Alabama

Hope Elisabeth Ankrom pleaded guilty to chemical endangerment of a child, a violation of [Section 26-15-3.2 of the Code of Alabama]. . . . The trial court sentenced Ankrom to three years in prison, but the court suspended that sentence and placed her on one year of supervised probation. Ankrom appealed her conviction. We affirm.

Facts and Procedural History

At the guilty-plea hearing, the parties stipulated to the following facts:

"On January 31, 2009, the defendant, Hope Ankrom, gave birth to a son, [B.W.], at Medical Center Enterprise. Medical records showed that the defendant tested positive for cocaine prior to giving birth and that the child tested positive for cocaine after birth.

"Department of Human Resources worker Ashley Arnold became involved and developed a plan for the care of the child. During the investigation the defendant admitted to Ashley that she had used marijuana while she was pregnant but denied using cocaine.

"Medical records from her doctor show that he documented a substance abuse problem several times during her pregnancy and she had tested positive for cocaine and marijuana on more than one occasion during her pregnancy."

On February 18, 2009, Ankrom was arrested and charged with chemical endangerment of a child. On August 25, 2009, the grand jury indicted Ankrom. The indictment stated that Ankrom "did knowingly, recklessly, or intentionally cause or permit a child . . . to be exposed to, to ingest or inhale, or to have contact with a controlled substance, chemical substance, or drug paraphernalia as defined in Section 13A–12–260 of the Code of Alabama. . . .

Discussion

Ankrom alleges that based on the facts of this case, she cannot be convicted of violating § 26–15–3.2(a)(1), Ala.Code 1975. . . . [T]he issue before this Court is whether a mother who ingested a controlled substance during her pregnancy, may be prosecuted under § 26–15–3.2(a)(1), Ala.Code 1975, if at birth

Circuit Court of Coffee County, 2011

175

the infant tests positive for the controlled substance. We answer that legal question in the affirmative, and we conclude that based on the facts of this case, Ankrom's conviction was proper. . .

Turning to the merits of the present case, § 26–15–3.2(a)(1), Ala.Code 1975, provides:

> "(a) A responsible person commits the crime of chemical endangerment of exposing a child to an environment in which he or she does any of the following:
>
> > "(1) Knowingly, recklessly, or intentionally causes or permits a child to be exposed to, to ingest or inhale, or to have contact with a controlled substance, chemical substance, or drug paraphernalia as defined in Section 13A–12–260. A violation under this subdivision is a Class C felony."

Ankrom alleges that the term "child" in § 26–15–3.2, Ala.Code 1975, does not include a viable fetus. The State responds that the plain meaning of the term "child," as used in the statute, includes an unborn child.

. . . The legislature has stated that "[t]he public policy of the State of Alabama is to protect life, born, and unborn. This is particularly true concerning unborn life that is capable of living outside the womb." . . . Chapter 15 of Title 26, Ala.Code 1975, does not define the term "child." However, Chapters 14 and 16 of Title 26, Ala.Code 1975, define a "child" as a "person" under the age of 18 years. . . .

Also, the Alabama Supreme Court has interpreted the term "minor child" in Alabama's wrongful-death-of-minor statute to include a viable fetus that received prenatal injuries causing death before a live birth. . . . Specifically, the Court held that "the parents of an eight and one-half month old stillborn fetus [are] entitled to maintain an action for the wrongful death of the child"; thus, the Court explicitly recognized the viable fetus as a "child." Eich, 293 Ala. at 100, 300 So. 2d at 358.

Furthermore, the dictionary definition of a word provides the meaning ordinary people would give the word. . . . According to Merriam–Webster's Collegiate Dictionary 214 (11th ed.2003), the word "child" is defined as "an unborn or recently born person." The word "child" is defined in Black's Law Dictionary 254 (8th ed.2004), as "[a] baby or fetus.". . .

. . . [W]e do not see any reason to hold that a viable fetus is not included in the term "child," as that term is used in § 26–15–3.2, Ala.Code 1975. Not only have the courts of this State interpreted the term "child" to include a viable fetus in other contexts, the dictionary definition of the term "child" explicitly includes an unborn person or a fetus. In everyday usage, there is nothing extraordinary about using the term "child" to include a viable fetus. For example, it is not uncommon for someone to state that a mother is pregnant with her first "child." Unless the legislature specifically states otherwise, the term "child" is simply a more general term that encompasses the more specific term "viable fetus." If the legislature desires to proscribe conduct against only a "viable fetus," it is necessary to use that specific term. However, if the legislature desires to proscribe conduct against a viable fetus and all other persons under a certain age, the term "child" is sufficient to convey that meaning. In fact, proscribing conduct against a "child" and a "viable fetus" would be redundant.

The term "child" in § 26–15–3.2, Ala.Code 1975, is unambiguous; thus, this Court must interpret the plain language of the statute to mean exactly what it says and not engage in judicial construction of the language in the statute. Also, because the statute is unambiguous, the rule of lenity does not apply. We do not see any rational basis for concluding that the plain and ordinary meaning of the term "child" does not include a viable fetus.

Ankrom advances three main arguments against interpreting the term "child" in § 26–15–3.2, Ala.Code 1975, to include a viable fetus: (1) The legislature has specifically included the term "fetus" or "unborn child" in other statutes when the legislature's intent was for the statute to apply to a fetus; (2) most courts from other jurisdictions have held that mothers could not be criminally prosecuted for prenatal substance abuse on the statutory theories of child abuse/endangerment or drug distribution; and (3) the legislature has declined to amend § 26–15–3.2, Ala.Code 1975, to explicitly include an unborn child in the definition of the term "child." We will address each argument in turn.

Contrary to Ankrom's argument, the fact that the legislature has included the term "fetus" or "unborn child" in other statutes does not mean that the term "child" in § 26–15–3.2, Ala.Code 1975, does not include a viable fetus. Ankrom specifically points to § 26–23–3, Ala.Code 1975, as an example to support her argument. Section 26–23–3, Ala.Code 1975, provides: "Any physician who knowingly performs a partial-birth abortion within this state and thereby kills a human fetus shall be guilty of a Class C felony and upon conviction thereof shall be punished as prescribed by law." Ankrom states that "[t]here is no doubt in the plain meaning of that statute of which class it is designed to protect: human fetuses." . . . Ankrom then reasons that "[i]f the legislature had intended for § 26–15–3.2(a) to apply to a fetus, then the legislature would have specifically included that language as it has in other statutes." . . . However, the flaw in Ankrom's reasoning is that she misses the distinction between the use of the more specific term "human fetus" and the more general term "child." As stated earlier, the general term "child" encompasses the more specific term "fetus." Statutes such as § 26–23–3 can only apply to a fetus or unborn child because it is impossible to perform an abortion after a live birth has been completed, so using the more general term "child" in such a statute would be nonsensical. On the other hand, statutes such as § 26–15–3.2 may proscribe conduct against born and unborn children; thus, the more general term "child" is necessary. Therefore, Ankrom's first argument is without merit.

Next, we acknowledge the many decisions from appellate courts in other states holding that a mother cannot be criminally prosecuted for prenatal substance abuse under those states' child abuse/endangerment or drug-distribution statutes. . . . However, we find that those cases are either distinguishable from the present case or unpersuasive.

Some of the cases from other jurisdictions involved prosecutions under statutes forbidding delivery of a controlled substance and, unlike the present case, depended on statutory construction of the term "deliver." . . . In other cases, the courts noted that their states' homicide statutes did not apply to a fetus, unlike Alabama's homicide statute, which does apply to unborn children. . . .

In Collins, the Texas Court of Appeals held that, divergent from Alabama, "the [Texas] Penal Code does not proscribe any conduct with respect to a fetus, and the Legislature, by its definitions of 'child,' 'person,' and 'individual,' has specifically limited the application of our penal laws to conduct committed against a human being who has been born and is alive." . . . Similarly, in Dunn, the Washington Court of Appeals held that "[n]o Washington criminal case has ever included 'unborn child' or fetus in its definition of person." . . .

In Gray, unlike the present case, the mother was prosecuted under a statute that stated, in relevant part: "No person, who is the parent of a child under eighteen years of age shall create a substantial risk to the health of safety of the child, by violating a duty of care, protection, or support." . . . Noting that criminal statutes must be strictly construed, the Ohio Supreme Court interpreted that statute by defining the terms "parent" and "child" to apply only to the relationship between mothers and fathers and their born infants. . . .

Other courts have worried about the implications of holding a mother criminally liable under a child-endangerment statute for conduct harmful to her fetus. Specifically, other courts have worried that holding a mother liable under such statutes would open the proverbial floodgates to prosecution of pregnant women who ingest legal toxins, such as alcohol or nicotine, or engage in any behavior that could conceivably injure the fetus. . . . In Wade, the Missouri Court of Appeals stated that the logic of allowing prosecutions to protect the interest of the fetus "would be extended to cases involving smoking, alcohol ingestion, the failure to wear seatbelts, and any other conduct that might cause harm to a mother's unborn child. It is a difficult line to draw and, as such, our legislature has chosen to handle the problems of pregnant mothers through social service programs instead of the court system." . . . However, in the present case, we need not worry about such unlimited extensions because we are not dealing with a general endangerment statute. Section 26–15–3.2(a)(1), Ala.Code 1975, the only statute we are asked to construe, concerns only conduct involving controlled substances or drug paraphernalia. It does not concern conduct involving smoking, alcohol ingestion, failure to wear seatbelts, or any other potentially harmful conduct that does not involve controlled substances.

Other courts have examined policy issues, legislative history, or other extrinsic materials to reach their conclusions that a mother cannot be criminally prosecuted for prenatal substance abuse under those states' child-abuse/endangerment statutes. . . . However, we are not at liberty to engage in such a review because we hold that § 26–15–3.2(a)(1), Ala.Code 1975, is unambiguous on its face. See Pinigis v. Regions Bank, 977 So.2d 446, 451 (Ala.2007) (holding that "courts may examine extrinsic materials, including legislative history, to determine [legislative] intent" only "[i]f the statutory language is ambiguous").

Again, we find the cases from other states holding that a mother cannot be criminally prosecuted for prenatal substance abuse under those states' child-abuse/endangerment or drug-distribution statutes to be distinguishable from the present case. To the extent that they are not distinguishable, we find that their reasoning is unpersuasive.

Ankrom's final argument against interpreting the term "child" in § 26–15–3.2, Ala.Code 1975, to include a viable fetus alleges that we should not interpret the term "child" to include a viable fetus because the legislature recently attempted to amend § 26–15–3.2, Ala.Code 1975, to explicitly state that the term "child" includes a child in utero at any stage of development, but the amendment failed. However, " 'failed legislative proposals' are "a particularly dangerous ground on which to rest an interpretation of a prior statute." ' " ' Baney v. State, 42 So.3d 170, 174 (Ala.Crim.App.2009) . . . In the present case, we do not need to speculate as to why the proposed amendment failed. Again, we hold that § 26–15–3.2, Ala.Code 1975, is unambiguous on its face; thus, we must construe the statute to mean exactly what it says. . . .

Finally, Ankrom argues that § 26–15–3.2, Ala.Code 1975, as applied in the present case, is void for vagueness because, she says, the statute did not give her adequate notice that her conduct was proscribed. See Vaughn v. State, 880 So.2d 1178, 1195 (Ala.Crim.App.2003) (holding that "the void-for-vagueness doctrine requires that a penal statute define the criminal offense with sufficient definiteness that ordinary people can understand what conduct is prohibited and in a manner that does not encourage arbitrary and discriminatory enforcement," but "[t]his prohibition against excessive vagueness does not invalidate every statute which a reviewing court believes could have been drafted with greater precision" because "[m]any statutes will have some inherent vagueness, for [i]n most English words and phrases there lurk uncertainties"). Specifically, Ankrom alleges that "[t]he plain language of the statute does not give notice that its criminal sanctions apply to fetuses exposed to controlled substances, and for that reason, Ms. Ankrom is being deprived of her due process right to fair notice of what conduct is impermissible." . . . However, as we held above, the plain meaning of the term "child," as found in § 26–15–3.2, Ala.Code 1975, includes a viable fetus. Therefore, Ankrom had adequate notice that her conduct was proscribed; thus, her constitutional argument is without merit.

Lynn M. Paltrow

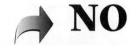

NO

Punishment and Prejudice: Judging Drug-Using Pregnant Women

The Villain Cocaine

In the late 1980s and into the 1990s newspapers, magazines, and television were full of stories documenting the devastating effects of cocaine and predicting a lost generation irredeemably damaged by the effects of their mothers' cocaine use. For example, in 1991 *Time* magazine ran a cover story on the subject.[1] Bold yellow letters read "Crack Kids" followed by the headline: "Their mothers used drugs, and now it's the children who suffer." The face of a tearful child filled the page beneath the words. . . .

The same year the *New York Times* ran a front page story entitled "Born on Crack and Coping with Kindergarten."[2] The story is accompanied by a photograph of a school teacher surrounded by young children. Underneath the caption reads: "I can't say for sure it's crack, said Ina R. Weisberg, a kindergarten teacher at P.S. 48 in the Bronx, but I can say that in all my years of teaching I've never seen so many functioning at low levels."

Throughout these years medical and popular journals, public school teachers and judges alike were willing to assume that if a child had a health or emotional problem and he or she had been exposed prenatally to cocaine, then cocaine and cocaine alone was the cause of the perceived medical or emotional problem. Rather than wait for careful research and evaluation of the drug's effect there was, as several researchers later criticized, a "rush to judgment" that blamed cocaine for a host of problems that the research simply has not borne out.[3]

Indeed, an article in the medical journal *Lancet* in 1989 found that scientific studies that concluded that exposure to cocaine prenatally had adverse effects on the fetus had a significantly higher chance of being published than more careful research finding no adverse effects.[4] The published articles, delineating the harmful effects on infants prenatally exposed to cocaine, reported brain damage, genito-urinary malformations, and fetal demise as just a few of the dire results of a pregnant woman's cocaine use. Infants that survived the exposure were described as inconsolable, unable to make eye contact, emitting a strange high-pitched piercing wail, rigid and jittery. These early studies, however, had numerous methodologic flaws that made generalization from them completely inappropriate. For example, these studies were based on individual case reports or on very small samples of women who used more than one drug. Researchers

From *Mother Troubles: Rethinking Contemporary Maternal Dilemmas,* Julia E. Hanigsberg and Sara Ruddick, eds. (Beacon Press, 1999). Copyright © 1999 by Lynn M. Paltrow. Reprinted by permission of the author.

often failed to control for the other drugs and problems the mother might have, and/or failed to follow up on the child's health.[5] The articles describing these studies were nevertheless relied upon to show that cocaine alone was the cause of an array of severe and costly health problems.

Like alcohol and cigarettes, using cocaine during pregnancy can pose risks to the woman and the fetus. More carefully controlled studies, however, are finding that cocaine is not uniquely or even inevitably harmful. For example, unlike the devastating and permanent effects of fetal alcohol syndrome, which causes permanent mental retardation, cocaine seems to act more like cigarettes and marijuana, increasing certain risks like low birth weight but only as one contributing factor and only in some pregnancies.[6] Epidemiological studies find that statistically speaking many more children are at risk of harm from prenatal exposure to cigarettes and alcohol. In fact, one recent publication on women and substance abuse has created the label "Fetal Tobacco Syndrome" to draw attention to the extraordinarily high miscarriage and morbidity rates associated with prenatal exposure to cigarette smoke.[7]

By the late 1980s it was already becoming clear to researchers in the field that the labels "crack babies" and "crack kids" were dangerous and counter-productive.[8] If one read far enough in the *Time* article—past the pictures of premature infants and deranged children—the story reported that

> [a]n increasing number of medical experts, however, vehemently chal-
> lenge the notion that most crack kids are doomed. In fact, they detest
> the term crack kids, charging that it unfairly brands the children and
> puts them all into a single dismal category. From this point of view,
> crack has become a convenient explanation for problems that are
> mainly caused by a bad environment. When a kindergartner from a
> broken home in the impoverished neighborhood misbehaves or seems
> slow, teachers may wrongly assume that crack is the chief reason, when
> other factors, like poor nutrition, are far more important.

Even the *New York Times* article about crack-exposed children in kinder-garten eventually revealed that researchers "after extensive interviews [found] the problems in many cases were traced not to drug exposure but to some other traumatic event, death in the family, homelessness, or abuse, for example."[9] And despite the fact that school administrators "rarely know who the children are who have been exposed to crack . . . and the effects of crack are difficult to diag-nose because they may mirror and be mixed up with symptoms of malnutri-tion, low birth-weight, lead poisoning, child abuse and many other ills that frequently afflict poor children," the article resorts to crack as the only reasonable explanation for an otherwise seemingly inexplicable phenomenon. . . .

The Public Responds

The public response to the media and medical journal reports was largely one of outrage. The harshest reaction was the call for the arrest of the preg-nant women and new mothers who used drugs. Numerous states considered legislation to make it a crime for a woman to be pregnant and addicted.[10] Although not a single state legislature passed a new law creating the crime of fetal abuse, individual prosecutors in more than thirty states arrested women whose infants tested positive for cocaine, heroin, or alcohol. Many of these women were arrested for child abuse, newly interpreted as "fetal" abuse. Others, like Jennifer Johnson in Florida, were charged with delivery of drugs to a minor.[11] In that case, the prosecutor argued that the drug delivery occurred through the umbilical cord after the baby was born but before the umbilical cord was cut. Still other women were charged with assault with a deadly weapon (the weapon being cocaine), or feticide (if the woman suffered a miscarriage), or homicide (if the infant, once born, died). Some women were charged with contributing to the delinquency of a minor.

While arrests were almost always the result of the action of an individual prosecutor, in the state of South Carolina there was unprecedented coordination between health care providers, the prosecutor's office, and the police.

In 1989, the city of Charleston, South Carolina, established a collaborative effort among the police department, the prosecutor's office, and a state hospital, the Medical University of South Carolina (MUSC), to punish pregnant women and new mothers who tested positive for cocaine. Under the policy, the hospital tested certain pregnant women for the presence of cocaine. Women were tested for the presence of cocaine to further criminal investigations, but the women never consented to these searches and search warrants were never obtained.

While the hospital refused to create a drug treatment program designed to meet the needs of pregnant addicts, or to put even a single trained drug counselor on its obstetrics staff, it did create a program for drug-testing certain patients, their in-hospital arrest, and removal to jail (where there was neither drug treatment nor prenatal care); the ongoing provision of medical information to the police and prosecutor's office; and tracking for purposes of ensuring their arrest. Some women were taken to jail while still bleeding from having given birth. They were handcuffed and shackled while hospital staff watched with approval. All but one of the women arrested were African American. The program itself had been designed by and entrusted to a white nurse who admitted that she believed that the "mixing of races was against God's will."[12] She noted in the medical records of the one white woman arrested that she lived "with her boyfriend who is a Negro."[13] . . .

Who Are These Mothers?

As a report from the Southern Regional Project on Infant Mortality observed:

> Newspaper reports in the 1980s sensationalized the use of crack cocaine and created a new picture of the "typical" female addict; young, poor, black, urban, on welfare, the mother of many children and addicted to crack. In interviewing nearly 200 women for this study, a very different picture of the "typical" chemically dependent woman emerges. She is most likely white, divorced or never married, age 31, a high school graduate, on public assistance, the mother of two or three children, and

addicted to alcohol and one other drug. It is clear from the women we interviewed that substance abuse among women is not a problem confined to those who are poor, black, or urban, but crosses racial, class, economic and geographic boundaries.[14]

African American women have been disproportionately targeted for arrest and punishment, not because they use more drugs or are worse mothers, but because, as Dorothy Roberts explains, "[t]hey are the least likely to obtain adequate prenatal care, the most vulnerable to government monitoring, and the least able to conform to the white middle-class standard of motherhood. They are therefore the primary targets of government control."[15]

Beyond the stock images and prejudicial stereotypes, the media has given the public little opportunity to meet or get to know the pregnant women on drugs. If we never learn who they are it is inevitable that their drug use will seem inexplicably selfish and irresponsible. Yet, if we could meet them and learn their history, we might be able to begin to understand them and the problems that need to be addressed.

Let me give an example. In the popular television show *NYPD Blue* we get to know the irascible Detective Sipowicz. While he is neither handsome nor charming, we come to care for him. We learn that he is an alcoholic who is able to stop drinking and improve his life. When he has a massive relapse and behaves outrageously, effectively abandoning his new wife and their newborn son, committing crimes of violence and countless violations of his responsibilities as a police officer, we nevertheless want to forgive him and give him another chance.

We are able to sympathize, at least in part because we have been given the information about why he has relapsed. His first son, whom he has finally reconnected with, is murdered, and Sipowicz, who can't handle it emotionally, turns back to the numbing, relief-giving effects of alcohol.

Sipowicz, in the end, is supported by his police colleagues who cover up for him and give him yet another chance. By contrast, when the same program did an episode involving a heroin-addicted pregnant woman, whose drug habit leads her two older sons to a life of crime, we never get to know why she has turned to drugs. We do not know as we did with Sipowicz what could have driven her to this behavior. The viewer can only assume that her drug use is purely selfish, stemming from a thoughtless hedonism. Thus, she is not entitled to understanding, sympathy, or the many second chances Sipowicz's character routinely gets.

But like Sipowicz, pregnant women who use drugs also have histories and complex lives that affect their behavior and their chances of recovery. We know that substance abuse in pregnancy is highly correlated with a history of violent sexual abuse.[16] In one study 70 percent of the pregnant addicted women were found to be in violent battering relationships. A hugely disproportionate number, compared to a control group, were raped as children. Drugs appear to be used as a means to numb the pain of a violent childhood and adulthood. Like Vietnam veterans who self-medicated with drugs for their post-traumatic stress disorders, at least some pregnant women also use drugs to numb the pain of violent and traumatic life experiences.[17]

Are their difficult childhoods or their experiences with violence an excuse for drug use? No. But the information begins to provide some idea of root causes that might need to be taken into consideration when trying to imagine the appropriate societal reaction. Will the threat of jail remove the trauma and pain that in many instances prompted the drug use and stands in the way of recovery? It is not that a woman who uses drugs is not responsible, but rather that we have to hold her responsible in a context that takes into account the obstacles, internal and external, that stand in the way of recovery. . . .

All pregnant women, not just poor ones, are routinely denied access to the limited drug treatment that exists in this country. In a landmark study in 1990, Dr. Wendy Chavkin surveyed drug treatment programs in New York City. She found that 54 percent flat out refused to take pregnant women.[18] Sixty-seven percent refused to take women who relied on Medicaid for payment, and 84 percent refused to take crack-addicted pregnant women.

One hospital in New York was sued for excluding women from drug treatment. The program argued that its exclusion of all women was justified and no different from its medical judgment to exclude all psychotics.[19] While New York State courts found that such exclusion violated state law, this did not automatically increase needed services. . . .

Other barriers also exist. [In the case of Jennifer Johnson, a pregnant Florida woman,] Judge Eaton ruled that "the defendant also made a choice to become pregnant and to allow those pregnancies to come to term." The prosecutor argued that "[w]hen she delivered that baby she broke the law." By saying this, the judge makes clear that it was having a child that was against the law. If Ms. Johnson had had an abortion she would not have been arrested—even for possessing drugs.[20] But this statement not only reveals a willingness to punish certain women for becoming mothers, it also reflects a host of widely held beliefs and assumptions about access to reproductive health services for women.

For example, implicit in this statement is the assumption that Ms. Johnson had sex and became pregnant voluntarily. Given the pervasiveness of rape in our society, assuming voluntary sexual relations may not be justified. Perhaps, though, the judge, like many others, simply thought that addicts have no business becoming pregnant in the first place. A South Carolina judge put it bluntly: "I'm sick and tired of these girls having these bastard babies on crack cocaine." Apparently concerned about his candor, he later explained: "They say you're not supposed to call them that but that's what they are . . . when I was a little boy, that's what they called them."[21]

On call-in radio talk shows someone inevitably asks why these mothers can't just be sterilized or injected with Depo Provera until they can overcome their drug problems and, while they are at it, their low socioeconomic status. The consistency of this view should not be surprising given our country's history of eugenics and sterilization abuse. Indeed, the U.S. Supreme Court has declared sterilization of men unconstitutional, but has never overturned its decision upholding the sterilization of women perceived to be a threat to society.[22]

The suggestion of sterilization, however, is particularly attractive if there is no explanation about why a pregnant woman with a drug problem would want to become pregnant or to have a child in the first place. But drug-using pregnant women become pregnant and carry to term for the same range of reasons all women do. Because contraception failed. Because they fell in love again and hoped this time they could make their family work. Because they are "prolife" and would never have an abortion. Because when they found out the beloved father of the baby was really already married, they thought it was too late to get a legal abortion. Because they do not know what their options might be. Because they have been abused and battered for so long they no longer believe they can really control any aspect of their lives including their reproductive lives. Because they wanted a child. Because their neighbors and friends, despite their drug use, had healthy babies and they believed theirs would be healthy too.

The threat of sterilization is just another punitive response that denies the humanity of the women themselves. Although Judge Eaton did not propose sterilization as part of the sentence he imposed on Ms. Johnson, as some judges in related cases have,[23] he undoubtedly assumed that Ms. Johnson could decide, once pregnant, whether or not to continue that pregnancy to term. Since 1976, however, the United States government has refused to pay for poor women's abortions and few states have picked up the costs.[24] In Florida, like most other states, the "choice" Judge Eaton spoke of does not exist for low-income women. . . .

Lack of access to abortion services is only one of the many barriers that exist for a drug-addicted pregnant woman who attempts to make responsible "choices." There are many other barriers that make it extremely difficult for pregnant women on drugs to get the kind of help and support they need. Access to services for drug-addicted women who are physically abused is also limited. For example, many battered women's shelters are set up to deal with women who have experienced violence, but are not equipped to support a woman who has become addicted to drugs as a way to numb the pain of the abuse.[25] Other barriers include lack of housing, employment, and access to prenatal care. As one of the few news stories to discuss these women's dilemmas explains:

> Soon after she learned she was pregnant, [Kimberly] Hardy [who was eventually prosecuted for delivery of drugs to a minor], convinced she had to get away from her crowd of crack users as well as her crumbling relationship with her [boyfriend] Ronald, took the kids home to Mississippi for the duration of her pregnancy. But by moving, she lost her welfare benefits, including Medicaid. Unable to pay for clinic visits, she had to go without prenatal care.[26]

And what about the men in their lives? Their contributions to the problem, physiologically and socially, are ignored or deliberately erased. Rarely in the media do we know what has happened to the potential fathers. Their drug use, abandonment, and battering somehow miraculously disappear from view.

Nevertheless, men often do play a significant role. For example, in California Pamela Rae Stewart was arrested after her newborn died. One of her alleged crimes contributing to the child's ultimate demise was having sex with her husband on the morning of the day of the delivery. Her husband, with whom she had had intercourse, was never arrested for fetal abuse. Indeed, the prosecutor's court papers argued that Ms. Stewart had "subjected herself to the rigors of intercourse," thereby totally nullifying the man's involvement or culpability.[27]

Prosecutors in South Carolina have also managed to ignore male culpability, even when it is the father who is supplying the pregnant woman with cocaine or other potentially harmful substances. Many women arrested in this state were not identified as substance addicted until after they had given birth, a point at which their drug use could not even arguably have a biological impact on the baby. Prosecutors argued that arrest was still justified because evidence of a woman's drug use during pregnancy is predictive of an inability to parent effectively. But fathers identified as drug users are not automatically presumed to be incapable of parenting. Indeed, when a man who happens to be a father is arrested for drunk driving, a crime that entails a serious lack of judgment and the use of a drug, he is not automatically presumed to be incapable of parenting and reported to the child welfare authorities. Prosecutors nevertheless rely on biological differences between mothers and fathers, arguing that a man's drug use could not have hurt the developing baby in the first place. However, studies indicate that male drug use can affect birth outcome: Studies on male alcohol use have demonstrated a relationship between male drinking and low birth weight in their children and a study of cocaine and men suggests that male drug use can also affect birth outcome.[28]

We continue to live in a society with double standards and extremely different expectations for men and women. Drug use by men is still glorified, while drug use by women is shameful, and by pregnant women a crime. This could not have been better demonstrated than by an advertising campaign by Absolut vodka. On Father's Day, as a promotional gimmick, Absolut sent 250,000 free ties to recipients of the *New York Times* Sunday edition. Scores of little sperm in the shape of Absolut vodka bottles swim happily on the tie's blue background. So while many call for arrest when a pregnant woman uses drugs or alcohol, fathers who drink are celebrated and, in effect, urged to "tie one on."

Of course, none of these arguments is made to suggest that women are not responsible for their actions or that they are unable to make choices that reflect free will. Rather, it is to say that popular expectations of what acting responsibly looks like and notions of "choice" have to be modified by an understanding of addiction as a chronic relapsing disease, of the degree to which our country has abandoned programs for poor women and children, and of the time, strength, and courage it takes for a drug-addicted woman to confront her history of drug use, violence, and abandonment. Compassion and significantly more access to coordinated and appropriate services will not guarantee that all of our mothers and children are healthy. But medical experts and both children's and women's rights advocates agree that such an approach is far more likely to improve health than are punishment and blame. . . .

The problem with treating the fetus as a person is that women will not simply continue to be less than equal, they will become nonpersons under the law. [To oppose the recognition of fetal personhood as a matter of law is not to deny the value and importance of potential life as a matter of religious belief, emotional conviction, or personal experience. Rather, by opposing such a new legal construct, we can avoid devastating consequences to women's health, prenatal health care, and women's hope for legal equality.—L.P.] No matter how much value we place on a fetus's potential life, it is still inside the woman's body. To pretend that the pregnant woman is separate is to reduce her to nothing more than, as one radio talk show host asserted, a "delivery system" for drugs to the fetus.

Notes

1. *Time Magazine* (13 May 1991).
2. Suzanne Dale, "Born on Crack and Coping with Kindergarten," *New York Times* (7 February 1991), A1.
3. Linda C. Mayes, R. H. Granger, M. H. Bornstein, and B. Zuckerman, "The Problem of Cocaine Exposure, A Rush to Judgment," *Journal of the American Medical Association* 267 (1992): 406.
4. Gideon Koren, Karen Graham, Heather Shear, and Tom Einarson, "Bias Against the Null Hypothesis: The Reproductive Hazards of Cocaine," *Lancet* (1989): 1, 1440–1442.
5. Mayes, "The Problem of Cocaine Exposure"; B. Lutiger, K. Graham, T. R. Einarson, and G. Koren, "Relationship Between Gestational Cocaine Use and Pregnancy Outcome: A Meta-Analysis," *Teratology* (1991): 44, 405–414.
6. Barry Zuckerman et al., "Effect of Maternal Marijuana and Cocaine Use on Fetal Growth," *New England Journal of Medicine* 320, no. 12 (23 March 1990): 762–768; Deborah A. Frank and Barry S. Zuckerman, "Children Exposed to Cocaine Prenatally: Pieces of the Puzzle," *Neurotoxicology and Teratology* 15 (1993): 298–300; Deborah A. Frank, Karen Breshahn, and Barry Zuckerman, "Maternal Cocaine Use: Impact on Child Health and Development," *Advances in Pediatrics* 40 (1993): 65–99.
7. Center on Addiction and Substance Abuse at Columbia University, *Substance Abuse and the American Woman* (1997); Joseph R. DiFranza and Robert A. Lew, "Effect of Maternal Cigarette Smoking on Pregnancy Complications and Sudden Death Syndrome," *Journal of Family Practice* 40 (1995): 385. Cigarette smoking has been linked to as many as 141,000 miscarriages and 4,800 deaths resulting from perinatal disorders, as well as 2,200 deaths from sudden infant death syndrome, nationwide.
8. American Academy of Pediatrics, Committee on Substance Abuse. Drug Exposed Infants, *Pediatrics* 86 (1990): 639.
9. Dale, "Born on Crack."
10. Allison Marshall, 1992, 1993, 1994 Legislative Update, in *National Association for Families and Addiction Research and Education Update* (Chicago, 1993, 1994, 1995).

11. *Johnson v. State,* 602 So.2d 1288 (Fla. 1992).

12. Brown Trial Transcript, *Ferguson et al. v. City of Charleston et al.,* U.S. District Court for the District of South Carolina, Charleston Division, C/A No. 2:93-2624-1 at 5:18–21 (Dec. 10, 1996).

13. Plaintiffs' Exhibit 119, *Ferguson et al. v. City of Charleston et al.,* U.S. District Court for the District of South Carolina, Charleston Division, C/A No. 2:93-2624-1.

14. Shelley Geshan, "A Step Toward Recovery, Improving Access to Substance Abuse Treatment for Pregnant and Parenting Women," *Southern Regional Project on Infant Mortality* (1993): 1.

15. Dorothy Roberts, "Punishing Drug Addicts Who Have Babies: Women of Color, Equality, and the Right of Privacy," *Harvard Law Review* 104, no. 7 (1991): 1419, 1422.

16. Dianne O. Regan, Saundra M. Ehrlich, and Loretta P. Finnegan, "Infants of Drug Addicts: At Risk for Child Abuse, Neglect, and Placement in Foster Care," *Neurotoxicology and Teratology* 9 (1987): 315–319.

17. Sheigla Murphy and Marsha Rosenbaum, *Pregnant Women on Drugs: Combating Stereotypes and Stigma* (New Brunswick, N.J.: Rutgers University Press, 1999).

18. Wendy Chavkin, "Drug Addiction and Pregnancy: Policy Crossroads," *American Journal of Public Health* 80, no. 4 (April 1990): 483–487.

19. *Elaine W. v. Joint Diseases North General Hospital Inc.,* 613 N.E.2d 523 (N.Y. 1993).

20. Lynn M. Paltrow, "When Becoming Pregnant Is a Crime," *Criminal Justice Ethics* 9, no. 1 (Winter–Spring 1990): 41–47.

21. *State v. Crawley,* Transcript of Record (Ct. Gen. Sess. Anderson Cnty., S.C., Oct. 17, 1994).

22. *Skinner v. Oklahoma,* 316 U.S. 535 (1942); *Buck v. Bell,* 274 U.S. 200 (1927); Stephen J. Gould, "Carrie Buck's Daughter," *Natural History* (July 1984).

23. *People v. Johnson,* No. 29390 (Cal.Super.Ct. Jan. 2, 1991).

24. *Harris v. McRae,* 448 U.S. 297 (1980).

25. Amy Hill, "Applying Harm Reduction to Services for Substance Using Women in Violent Relationships," *Harm Reduction Coalition* 6 (Spring 1998): 7–8.

26. Jan Hoffman, "Pregnant, Addicted and Guilty?" *New York Times Magazine* (19 August 1990): 53.

27. Shelly Geshan, "A Step Toward Recovery, Improving Access to Substance Abuse Treatment for Pregnant and Parenting Women" Southern Regional Project on Infant Mortality (1993): 1.

28. Dorothy Roberts, "Punishing Drug Addicts who have Babies: Women of Color, Equality, and the Right of Privacy," Harvard Law Review 104, no. 7, (1991): 1419, 1422.

EXPLORING THE ISSUE

Should a Pregnant Woman Be Punished for Exposing Her Fetus to Risk?

Critical Thinking and Reflection

1. The well-being of children is surely vitally important; how does the value attached to their well-being compare, as a matter of public policy, against the value of a woman's freedom and privacy?
2. Avoiding exposure to dangerous substances is about creating a good environment for the child; what is the responsibility of a person to make good decisions when environmental factors in their own life may not have helped them acquire good decision-making skills?
3. Does recognition that a child's well-being can be impaired by things that happen before the child is born lead one to conclude that a fetus is a person?
4. In your view, is protection of persons-to-be best achieved by criminalizing bad behavior or by fostering good behavior in mothers (and fathers)?

Is There Common Ground?

State policies similar to that developed by Alabama prosecutors remain highly contested. In New Mexico in May 2007, the Supreme Court struck down a law expanding the state's criminal child abuse law to drug-using pregnant women and fetuses. Courts in many other states have ruled similarly on this issue. However, according to the Guttmacher Institute, 15 states consider substance abuse during pregnancy to be child abuse under civil child-welfare statutes, and three consider it grounds for civil commitment. Some states also require health care professionals to report suspected prenatal drug abuse or to test for prenatal drug exposure if they suspect abuse. In 2012, *Ankrom v. State* and a similar case concerning a woman named Amanda Kimbrough were appealed from the Alabama Court of Criminal Appeals to the Supreme Court of Alabama. As of this writing, a ruling had not been issued.

Personhood laws have been introduced in a number of states. The measures have been struck down in Colorado, South Dakota, California, and Mississippi, but a bill signed into law in Oklahoma in February 2012 states that the laws of the state "shall be interpreted and construed to acknowledge on behalf of the unborn child at every stage of development all the rights, privileges, and immunities available to other persons, citizens, and residents of this state." Virginia lawmakers have suspended consideration of a similar law until at least 2013.

The approach tried in South Carolina to criminalize substance abuse in pregnancy has been limited by privacy concerns. In March 2001, the U.S. Supreme Court ruled in the case of *Ferguson v. City of Charleston* (121 S.C. 1281) that the Medical University of South Carolina's program to require drug-using pregnant women to seek treatment and prenatal care or face criminal prosecution was unconstitutional. The Court reversed the decision of the lower Fourth Circuit Court of Appeals and sent the case back to the circuit court for a factual determination of whether the women had actually consented to the search that led to their arrest and imprisonment. The circuit court had ruled that the searches were not "unreasonable searches" (prohibited under the Fourth Amendment to the Constitution) because of the "special need" to protect women and children from the consequences of cocaine use in pregnant women. The Supreme Court rejected this claim. But the Court's decision did not settle the public policy and ethical challenges that remain concerning drug use and pregnant women.

Additional Resources

An amicus brief filed in support of Hope Ankrom and Amanda Kimbrough on behalf of a list of organizations and individuals by the Drug Policy Alliance, National Advocates for Pregnant Women, and the Southern Poverty Law Center is available at http://advocatesforpregnantwomen.org/featured/in_the_alabama_supreme_court_1.php.

For information about the criminalization of substance abuse during pregnancy, see the Guttmacher Institute fact sheet, "Substance Abuse During Pregnancy," at www.guttmacher.org/statecenter/spibs/spib_SADP.pdf.

For more on the decision in Ferguson, see George Annas, "Testing Poor Pregnant Women for Cocaine: Physicians as Police Investigators," *The New England Journal of Medicine* (May 31, 2001) and Lawrence O. Gostin, "The Rights of Pregnant Women: The Supreme Court and Drug Use," *Hastings Center Report* (September–October, 2001).

For a book-length treatment of these issues, see Drew Humphries, *Crack Mothers: Pregnancy, Drugs, and the Media* (Ohio State University Press, 1999).

Internet References . . .

ProCon.org

This organization provides extensive resources on the debate over the death penalty and on physician involvement in it.

http://deathpenalty.procon.org/

The National Conference of State Legislatures

This organization monitors state legislative activity on conscience clause laws.

www.ncsl.org/

Professional Integrity

*P*robably one of the reasons bioethics is recognized as a distinct area of inquiry within the broader field of ethics is that many of the core issues in it are about the distinct role in society held by physicians and other medical professionals, and the special social relationships they have with people in need of their expertise and assistance. The questions are not just about how individuals should treat each other, but also about how individuals who have taken on the role of physician, nurse, or pharmacist should use their special knowledge to serve society. Physicians are often said to be healers—to have committed themselves to promoting health and saving life; is it acceptable, then, for a physician to hurt or even kill someone? Physicians and other medical professionals take on their social roles not merely because society asks them to, but because they are moral beings themselves and they wanted those roles; may society ask them to do something that conflicts with their own moral judgments? Several issues in this volume involve such questions. This unit explores a couple of them in detail.

- Should Physicians Be Allowed to Participate in Executions?
- Should Pharmacists Be Allowed to Deny Prescriptions on Grounds of Conscience?

ISSUE 10

Should Physicians Be Allowed to Participate in Executions?

YES: David Waisel, from "Physician Participation in Capital Punishment," *Mayo Clinic Proceedings* (September 2007)

NO: Atul Gawande, from "When Law and Ethics Collide—Why Physicians Participate in Executions," *The New England Journal of Medicine* (March 23, 2006)

Learning Outcomes

After reading this issue, you should be able to:

- Discuss the lethal injection method of execution in the United States, and explain the role of physicians in conducting them.
- Discuss whether the physician's medical role is consistent with participation in lethal injection executions.

ISSUE SUMMARY

YES: David Waisel, a professor of medicine, argues that if the state is to administer capital punishment, then physicians may honorably seek to help the condemned die as painlessly as possible.

NO: Physician and journalist Atul Gawande supports capital punishment but believes physicians, as healers, should play no role in it.

In France, during the reign of the Bourbon monarchs, the methods of execution included beheading with a sword or axe, hanging, burning at the stake, and being bludgeoned to death on the "breaking wheel." None of the methods were quick and painless; beheading often required multiple blows, and hanging takes several minutes when it works well. In 1791, during the French Revolution, Joseph-Ignace Guillotin, a physician who in 1789 had called for the reformation of capital punishment, devised a new beheading machine that allowed for quick and comparatively painless deaths. The machine proved, at least in one way, a great success: During the next few years, in the period

194

known as the Reign of Terror, tens of thousands of people were publicly executed using guillotines.

Guillotin's involvement is often cited in a contemporary debate that has arisen over whether physicians should participate in executions. It shows there is a long history of physician involvement in them, and it illustrates one of the primary reasons for involving physicians: a humanitarian belief that if people are to be executed, then they should be executed with as little suffering as possible. (Before Guillotin, execution was often specifically designed to cause suffering.)

The most common method of execution employed in the United States today is lethal injection, and physicians' expertise is especially useful in carrying it out. Execution by lethal injection was proposed in 1977 by the Oklahoma medical examiner, who (like Guillotin) sought a more humane method of killing the condemned. The method he developed consists of three drugs administered in sequence: a fast-acting barbiturate to put the condemned person to sleep, a paralytic to completely immobilize him, and potassium chloride to kill him. As the YES and NO selections document, much can still go wrong in administering the drugs, and when things do go wrong, the results can be very painful for the person being executed and horrific to witness. Physicians' understanding of the drugs and how they interact, and their expertise in starting the intravenous saline drip through which the drugs are administered, can help ensure that lethal injection is administered well.

The question of whether physicians should be allowed to participate in executions is usually handled separately from the question of whether capital punishment itself is permissible. The American Medical Association's position, for example, is that the permissibility of capital punishment is a personal moral decision but that whether physicians may participate in it follows from a proper understanding of the physician's special role in society. "A physician, as a member of a profession dedicated to preserving life when there is hope of doing so," declares Current Opinion 2.06 of the AMA's Code of Medical Ethics, "should not be a participant in a legally authorized execution." Physician participation in execution, continues the opinion, would include not merely causing the condemned to die, but also assisting or supervising someone who does. The physician is permitted by AMA policy to give a condemned person medical treatment before execution and to certify the person's death afterward.

The YES and NO selections, both by esteemed physicians affiliated with Harvard Medical School, offer contrasting positions on the permissibility of physician participation in execution. In the YES selection, David Waisel, professor of anesthesia at Boston Children's Hospital, argues that concern for the welfare of the condemned makes physician participation permissible. If executions are to occur, they should be done humanely and physicians not only may participate in them, but in fact it is honorable for them to participate. In the NO selection, Atul Gawande, a surgeon at Brigham and Women's Hospital in Boston and professor of surgery at Harvard Medical School, argues that physicians' special healing role in society is incompatible with assisting in executions.

195

YES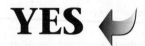

David Waisel

Physician Participation in Capital Punishment

If state administration of capital punishment is legal and ongoing, humane methods of execution should be sought and applied. In medieval times, the condemned and their families would bribe the executioner to make death quick and painless. In the 18th century, Dr Joseph-Ignace Guillotin proposed amending the French penal code to require executioners to use what is now known as the guillotine, believing that to be a more humane method of execution. In the United States, hanging was the predominant method of execution until electrocution was introduced as a more humane method in 1890.[1] One of the subtexts of electrocution was Thomas Edison's attempts to promote his direct current electricity by tainting the competing alternating current electricity through its association with the electric chair.[1] Cyanide gas was introduced in 1924.[2] Hanging, electrocution, and chemical asphyxiation were the primary methods of execution until the introduction of lethal injection in 1977.[2] Lethal injection has been the predominant form of execution in the 699 executions in the United States during the past 10 years.[3] Recent concerns about the technical issues surrounding legal execution, most specifically regarding drug delivery, have prompted some persons to suggest that physician participation in capital punishment would minimize these problems.

Opposing the involvement of physicians is the American Medical Association (AMA), which prohibits physician participation in legally authorized executions. According to the AMA's published position statements,[4] "An individual's opinion on capital punishment is the personal moral decision of the individual. A physician, as a member of a profession dedicated to preserving life when there is hope of doing so, should not be a participant in a legally authorized execution." The AMA further stated that physician participation in capital punishment "distorts the purpose and role of medicine and its professionals in the preservation of life. The use of physicians and medical technology in execution presents a conceptual contradiction for society and the public. The image of physician as executioner under circumstances mimicking medical care risks the general trust of the public."

The Code of Medical Ethics of the AMA prohibits physicians from "an action which would directly cause the death of the condemned [and] an action which would assist, supervise or contribute to the ability of another individual to directly cause the death of the condemned."[5] Prohibitions include nearly

From *Mayo Clinic Proceedings*, September 2007, pp. 1073–1080. Copyright © 2007 by Elsevier. Reprinted by permission via Rightslink.

all aspects of lethal injection such as "selecting injection sites; starting intra-venous lines as a port for a lethal injection device; prescribing, preparing, administering, or supervising injection drags or their doses or types; inspect-ing, testing, or maintaining lethal injection devices; and consulting with or supervising lethal injection personnel."[5]

In this commentary, I argue that poorly done executions needlessly hurt the condemned and that, in the case of lethal injections, the problems center not on the specific drugs chosen but on establishing and maintaining intra-venous access and assessing for anesthetic depth. I argue that it is honorable for physicians to minimize the harm to these condemned individuals and that organized medicine has an obligation to *permit* physician participation in legal execution. By participation, I mean to the extent necessary to ensure a good death. This includes designing protocols both in general and for specific con-demned persons and participating in the performance of these protocols, up to and including gaining intravenous access and giving drugs.

I will not address the policy of capital punishment. Although numerous issues surround capital punishment (appropriateness, fairness, and effective-ness as a crime deterrent, etc), they are beyond the scope of this article. The purpose of this commentary is to address physician participation in the ongo-ing practice of lethal injection.

The Need for Physician Participation

Lethal injection is the predominant form of execution in the United States, in part because it is considered more humane than hanging, electrocution, and chemical asphyxiation. In 1977, an anesthesiologist suggested a process that appeared to mimic a typical induction of anesthesia: sodium thiopental to cause unconsciousness, pancuronium bromide to paralyze the muscles, and (in the case of lethal injection) potassium chloride to stop the heart.[6]

In anesthetic practice, after a drug to induce anesthesia (like sodium thiopental) is given, anesthesiologists test for adequate depth of anesthesia, sometimes using a hands-on assessment like an eyelash reflex (touching the eyelashes to see if the eyelids flutter). A normal induction dose of 3 to 5 mg/kg of thiopental would be expected to produce unconsciousness in approxi-mately 30 seconds and peak respiratory depression in 1 to 1.5 minutes.[7] It is not uncommon for respiratory attempts to return shortly thereafter. Pancuro-nium bromide, a paralytic with no anesthetic properties, is given in a dose of 1 mg/kg and within 4 minutes [and] produces muscle relaxation to facilitate tracheal intubation.[8]

San Quentin Operational Procedure No. 770 describes how a typical lethal execution is to be done;[9] 2 intravenous lines are inserted, and saline flows through 1 of the lines. Individuals other than the condemned person leave the room. The door is sealed. Through injection ports located outside the room, 5 g of sodium thiopental (ie, 10 times the 500-mg induction of anesthesia dose for a man weighing 100 kg) is given in "[A] steady even flow . . . maintained with only a minimum amount of force applied to the syringe plunger." The intravenous line is then flushed with 20 cm^3 of normal saline. Two syringes of 50 mg of pancuronium bromide in 50 cm^3 of diluent (ie, a total of 100 mg, 10 times the 10-mg dose given for a man weighing 100 kg) are then "injected with slow, even pressure on the syringe plunger," and the intravenous line is flushed with 20 cm^3 of normal saline. Two syringes of 50 mEq of potassium chloride in 50 cm^3 of diluent (a total of 100 mEq of potassium chloride) are then injected.[9]

If this process is performed correctly, the inmate will be unconscious before receiving pancuronium bromide and potassium chloride.[7,10] These massive doses of sodium thiopental should both stop breathing and cause unconsciousness in 1 minute.[11] In the absence of a hands-on assessment of anesthetic depth, sustained apnea becomes a reasonable surrogate for adequate delivery of the massive doses of sodium thiopental. Sustained apnea guarantees a sufficient depth of anesthesia.

In contrast, spontaneous ventilation after sodium thiopental indicates that the desired dose of sodium thiopental was *not* delivered. Spontaneous ventilation does not indicate awareness, but it also does not confirm anesthesia.

The presence of apnea after administration of pancuronium bromide is not a guarantee that the sodium thiopental was delivered. A dose that is 3 times a normal intubating dose of pancuronium (ie, 30 mg instead of 10 mg in a man weighing 100 kg) will cause muscle relaxation within 1 minute.[8] Thus, only a fraction of the pancuronium bromide needs to be successfully administered to cause apnea. Apnea after pancuronium bromide, instead of after sodium thiopental, does not indicate that the inmate was anesthetized before the pancuronium bromide. If the inmate was not anesthetized before the administration of pancuronium bromide and potassium chloride, the inmate may have the sensation of paralysis without anesthesia (known as awareness) and may feel the burning of the highly concentrated potassium chloride.

One problem with lethal injection is obtaining venous access, leading to extensive and painful attempts, including placement of central venous access.[12] A more concerning problem is inadequate medication delivery during the execution. This can occur from technical errors and procedural errors (Table 1). For example, in 6 executions since 1999 in California, the condemned had reactions such as respirations and tachycardia, which may have been consistent with awareness or pain.[11] The possible patterns of successful and botched lethal injection are listed in Table 2 and Table 3.

Other problems exist with drug delivery. In 1994 in Illinois, with use of a machine to inject the sodium thiopental and pancuronium bromide, the intravenous catheter clogged, leaving the inmate snorting and his belly "heaving up and down with the breathing."[14] After the botched execution, the spokesman for the corrections department stated, "It looks like the two drugs just don't mix . . . they get tacky and don't flow when they come together."[18] The same problem had happened the only previous time the machine was used 4 years earlier.

In 1995 in Missouri, the arm restraint functioned as a tourniquet, prolonging the process and bringing into question the sensations of the condemned person.[21] The county coroner said that the heartbeat stopped several

Table 1

Sources of Error in Lethal Execution

Steps of execution	Sources of potential error
1. Prepare medications, including mixing sodium thiopental from powder	Improper and improvisational mixing of sodium thiopental[10,13]
2. Obtain intravenous access	Difficulty[14,15]
	Not placed intravascularly[16]
	Protocols do not address what should happen if obtaining peripheral venous access is not possible[9,15]
3. Inject sodium thiopental	Burning and blistering if injected into subcutaneous tissues[16,17]
	Human error[10,13]
4. Assess anesthetic depth	Not assessed, improperly assessed, false proxies of anesthesia[15]
	Individual not physically present to assess depth of anesthesia[10,13,15]
	Inadequate human skill[10,15]
5. Inject pancuronium bromide	Muscle relaxation may hide signs of inmate distress[10,13,15]
	Precipitation with sodium thiopental[15,18,19]
6. Repeat doses of pancuronium bromide and potassium chloride if necessary	Poorly designed protocols, no repeated doses of sodium thiopental[10,15]
7. Other problems	Deviation from protocols[15]
	Absence of written protocol[13]
	Inadequate records; no assessment of the quality of executions[10,15]
	No meaningful training, supervision, and oversight of the execution team[10,13,15,20]
	Inadequate lighting, overcrowded conditions and poorly designed facilities in which the execution team must work[10,13,15]
	Lack of respect for "solemn" task of executions[9]

minutes after the strap was loosened, suggesting that the sodium thiopental, pancuronium bromide, and potassium chloride entered the bloodstream at the same time, not giving the sodium thiopental time to work, and increasing the likelihood that the condemned person was aware while paralyzed or felt the burning from the potassium chloride. The inmate was "gasping, slightly convulsing" 7 minutes after initiation of the lethal injection.[21] The coroner declared that it was "a little error. It's not like the guy suffered."[21]

In 2006 in Ohio, after a difficult insertion of an intravenous line, the execution team chose not to insert a second intravenous line (as apparently called for by prison procedures)[22] and injected the drugs. The inmate appeared to have fallen asleep, with shallow breathing. But shortly thereafter, he "raised his head

Table 2

Proper and Improper Drug Administration Procedures for Lethal Injection*

Procedure	Consequence
Proper: STP→Apnea→P→KCL	Time is given for inmate to be anesthetized by sodium thiopental, as confirmed by apnea, then paralyzed, then given potassium chloride
Improper: STP→P→Apnea→KCL	Inmate is administered paralytic medication before becoming apneic, raising the possibility that insufficient sodium thiopental was delivered to the venous circulation. Inmate may be aware of being paralyzed and may feel the burning of potassium chloride. With 100 mg of pancuronium bromide being administered, even one-third of the intended dose would cause paralysis within 1 min
Improper: STP, P, KCL (at the same time)	No time is given for the sodium thiopental to work and no time is taken to assess whether the sodium thiopental has caused apnea
Improper: STP→P→KCL→→→P, KCL	In some protocols, the pancuronium bromide and potassium chloride are repeated at 10 min if the inmate is not dead. This indicates that the drugs were not delivered adequately (ie, insufficient doses) to the venous system (because if they had been, the inmate would be dead). Repeating pancuronium bromide and potassium chloride without the sodium thiopental increases the likelihood of awareness

*KCL = potassium chloride; P = pancuronium bromide; STP = sodium thiopental.

Table 3

Five Specific Cases of Lethal Injection in California*[11]

Inmate, year	Minutes										
	0	1	2	3	4	5	6	7	8	9	10
Siripongs, 1999	STP				P	Apnea					
Babbitt, 1999	STP			P		Apnea					
Rich, 2000	STP		P/apnea								
Anderson, 2002	STP		P			Apnea					
Allen, 2006	STP									P	Apnea

*All cases follow the example of STP→P→Apnea→KCL. One case, Williams, 2005, is not included because inadequate recordkeeping makes it unclear whether apnea occurred concurrent with the pancuronium bromide (6 min after sodium thiopental) or concurrent with the potassium chloride (12 min after sodium thiopental and 6 min after pancuronium bromide). KCL = potassium chloride; P = pancuronium bromide; STP = sodium thiopental.

and, frustrated, shook it back and forth, repeatedly declaring, 'it don't work.'"[22] The execution team obtained additional intravenous access, mistakenly connected the intravenous line to the failed intravenous catheter, administered the drugs, noticed a reaction by the inmate, subsequently reconnected the intravenous line to the correct catheter, and administered the drugs. The inmate "raised his head about a dozen times and appeared to try to speak"[22] before dying.

In 2006 in Florida, 2 intravenous catheters were placed in the condemned person, and it appears that both catheters infiltrated into the surrounding tissues, so that the drugs were injected into the tissues and not into the veins.[16] "More than 20 minutes after the first injection, [the inmate] appeared to be mouthing words, clenching his jaw, and grimacing."[23] The inmate received a second dose of drugs.[23] Likely as a result of the drugs entering the tissues instead of the vein, the inmate had footlong "chemical blisters on both of his arms."[16] An anesthesiologist familiar with the case testified that the accounts of the inmate breathing "like a fish out of water" were consistent with a "person who is partially paralyzed and struggling for breath."[16] This event led the Governor of Florida to declare a moratorium on state executions pending a report from a concurrently designated commission.

Attempts to tweak operating procedures for lethal injection are insufficient. The Morales Memorandum of Intended Decision reported that in February 2006, officials in California decided that "a continuous infusion of sodium thiopental during the administration of pancuronium bromide and potassium chloride would be added."[10] As in the 1994 case in Illinois, such an approach would lead to a precipitate being formed and subsequent clogging of the intravenous catheter.

If the problem is the delivery of the drugs and the assessment of anesthetic depth before injection of a paralytic and potassium chloride, then a person who is wholly competent at managing intravenous infusions and assessing for anesthetic depth is needed for humane lethal injection. Although nonphysicians *could* perform this procedure (as the AMA has argued), they would need to be trained by physicians to develop these skills. In the absence of extensive teaming and refresher courses for nonphysicians (which would seemingly fly in the face of the AMA statement), the most skilled individuals would be those who intravenously inject medications routinely to obtain an end result.

Arguments Regarding Roles of Physicians and the Government

Physicians have an obligation to be altruistic. Some interpret this obligation to prohibit physician participation in the execution of an unwilling individual (reports of condemned persons choosing to die rather than prolong their stay on death row notwithstanding[24]), even if the condemned person desires the aid of a physician to make death more humane. The AMA addresses this point directly: "While physician participation may potentially add some degree of humaneness to the execution of an individual, it does not outweigh the greater harm of causing death to the individual."[4]

Death, however, is not the sole issue. Physicians are permitted to let people die, such as in the withdrawal or withholding of care. Physicians are even permitted to be a proximate cause of death, in the sense that sometimes the medications needed to treat pain and discomfort unintentionally hasten death. Public policy has shifted in some countries and states to allow physicians to assist in the death of a patient. For example, from 1998 to 2002 in Oregon, 129 people self-administered legally prescribed lethal medications.[25] It is even becoming accepted that physicians may directly cause death. In the Netherlands, termination of life on request and assistance with suicide are not treated as criminal offenses if certain requirements are met.[26] The primary distinction is that in the aforementioned examples, death is considered in the best interest of the patient by the patient or concerned surrogate decisionmakers. In capital punishment, death is involuntary and is not in the best interest of the individual.

If one accepts the premise that physician participation will lead to more humane executions, does the fact that death is not in the inmate's best interest obviate a request for relief from suffering? Does physician participation mean that physicians are acting as tools of the government, helping the state carry out judicial punishment? More to the point, does acting in a manner concordant with the goals of the government make a physician a tool of the government?

Some argue that physician participation constitutes inappropriate use of physicians as a tool of the government.[27] Historically, when the government has used physicians to implement policies that did not benefit the individuals affected, the health of the society benefited. For example, physician participation in quarantine of individuals with infectious diseases, while limiting the freedom of movement of some individuals, resulted in an overall health benefit of minimizing the spread of disease. This societal health benefit legitimizes physician participation in quarantine, but physician participation in capital punishment provides no societal health benefit. According to Truog (Robert D. Truog, MD, Professor of Medical Ethics, Anesthesia, & Pediatrics, Harvard Medical School),[27] "A physician's participation in capital punishment does nothing to promote the moral community of medicine. Indeed, such participation offends the sense of community by prostituting medical knowledge and skills to serve the purposes of the state and its criminal justice system."[27] If the physician's primary role is to ensure a successful execution, such that a physician would be willing to do it in an inhumane way, then the physician is being used as a tool of the government to further state goals. But a legitimate question is whether the physician is acting as a tool of the individual to minimize suffering and further the individual's goals or whether the physician is acting as a tool of the government to ensure a successful execution. Although the outcome may be death, the act of the physician may be solely to provide comfort. In this case, a physician is not acting as a tool of the government; he is acting as a physician whose goals temporarily align with the goals of the government. Clearly, there are potential harms in permitting physicians to act in this way. But these harms need to be weighed against the benefits to the condemned. Physicians are responding to the immediate goals of the condemned. To prohibit this aid because the use of the physician as a tool for the individual (good reason) happens to occur in conjunction with the use of the physician as a tool for the government (bad reason) requires a compelling reason to forego our responsibilities to the individual. Indeed, a principled stance of prohibition regressively harms society's most vulnerable individuals. Consider this: a prison warden "testified that he believes a 'successful execution' is simply one where 'the inmate ends up dead at the end of the process.' When asked whether he considered a successful execution to mean anything else, he responded, 'I'm thinking not.'"[10] If you were to be executed, would you prefer to have a competent and caring individual obtain venous access quickly and minimize any chance of pain or awareness?

This argument, of course, is susceptible to comparison with the Nazi concentration camp physicians' argument that they were "morally neutral bystanders" who followed the law and who compassionately spared concentration camp "subhumans" from a slower and more painful death.[28] But I argue that this is too free an analogy. The process by which the laws are developed and the underlying intent of the laws (as well as can be surmised) [is] relevant in determining whether government authorization makes physician participation in capital punishment legitimate and permissible. We live in a society open to free speech and public protest, one in which citizens have a remarkable ability to participate in the development of laws and policies. Furthermore, capital punishment is public and avidly discussed, not hidden. Of importance, Nazi physicians thought "they were acting for the good of the whole nation and society."[28] Such notions of prioritizing the state (or even certain communities) over individuals often lead to harm. In Nazi Germany, the purpose of the government intervention (concentration camps, genocide, etc) was the actualization of political goals. In contrast, capital punishment does not advance a comprehensive political goal.

Slippery Slope Arguments Regarding Other Harms of Participation

Some worry that permitting physician participation in capital punishment will erode a physician's ability to be compassionate and independent, will make it easier to permit physicians to participate in government-sanctioned killing, and will harm public trust.[5,12,27,29] These arguments are rooted in the psychological slippery slope by claiming that one event will lead to another. The usefulness of the slippery slope argument is suspect.

We should always be concerned about permitting actions that would lead us down the psychological slippery slope to causing harm. However, the problem with many slippery slope arguments is that they do not precisely clarify how permitting the debated action will lead to another, often unspecified, action. In a different context, Burgess (John Burgess, BA, MA, DPhil, Faculty of Arts, University of Wollongong, New South Wales, Australia)[30] labeled this the One Great Slippery Slope Argument: "[I]f we adopt . . . a particular change in our practices it just might start a slide into a moral deterioration that ends with our committing Nazi-style atrocities." The argument that a slope exists is often used as a poor substitute for an argument about how the debated action will cause the slide down the slope. Furthermore, while uncritically accepting as legitimate the sketchy possibility that society could slide down the slope, slippery slope supporters often demand a detailed argument about how it could not occur.[30]

A good psychological slippery slope argument is detailed and modest.[30] The arguments connecting disaster with physician participation in capital punishment do not provide a clear and detailed account of how participation leads to calamity. Consider the most extreme and visceral argument, that permitting physician participation would be the first step down the slope to Nazi-like atrocities.[29,31] Such a descent would require a series of extraordinary events that culminate in a self-serving totalitarian regime and a dominant social group, whose primary concern is the health of the social organism and the exploitation of an identified other.[30] Perhaps most importantly, the Nazi premise of society as a biological organism led to the concept of medicalized killing as "killing as therapeutic imperative."[32] This medicalized view of society legitimized removing the disease (ie, killing) of those "unfit to live," just like antibiotics kill bacteria or a surgeon removes an appendix. This thinking provided a rationale for society (and thus physicians) to kill. There is no reason to believe that physician participation in capital punishment would lead to such a radical restructuring of society and society's views.

With that preamble, we will examine the claims. We do not know the effects of self-chosen participation in executions on a physician's ability to act with compassion and independence. We do have information on the effects on members of execution teams who carry out executions (eg, secure inmate, obtain intravenous access, inject medications) in 3 Southern states.[33] Individuals on execution teams use selective moral disengagement, moral justification, economic and security justification, dehumanization, and nonresponsibility to be able to perform executions. Executioners compartmentalize work and home life, construe participation in executions as a positive activity with "high moral and societal purposes," and become more desensitized as they participate in more executions. Lifton (Robert Jay Lifton, MD, is a psychiatrist who has studied and written extensively on mental adaptations to war, atrocities, and war crimes)[32] described compartmentalization in the context of Nazi physicians as the experience of the "doubling" of the self, in which the 2 selves are partitioned from each other. This mechanism of "doubling" enabled Nazi physicians to be evil at one moment and caring in the next moment and is what Lifton thought permitted specific individuals with what appeared to be relatively appropriate moral values to slide, incrementally, into performing atrocities. The concern is that compartmentalization by physicians participating in capital punishment could similarly harm physicians.

However, the application of this study of prison workers to physicians is unclear. Physicians participating in capital punishment have the ability to view their actions as helping the condemned. Indeed, to me, participation in a horrible detail to benefit another person is true altruism. Additionally, that article did not consider what sort of interventions may help those who participate in capital punishment (eg, caps on number of cases in which an individual participates, mandatory counseling). Even if a few willing physicians were harmed, it is hard to construct a detailed slippery slope argument that connects a few physicians undergoing compartmentalization with widespread societal harms. Furthermore, of importance, physicians will not be required to participate because most states have conscience clauses that permit caregivers to opt out of care they deem morally objectionable.[34]

Beyond the effect on specific physicians, there is concern that permitting physicians to appear to be tools of the government by participating in capital punishment will make it psychologically easier for physicians to be used in inappropriate ways.[27,29] Although this may be true, the possibility of an event is not the step-by-step connection between an event and a specified harm that constitutes evidence in a slippery slope argument. In addition, I argue that our society is more than capable of withstanding the psychological slippery slope.

One argument that supports the slippery slope claim is that physicians were prime leaders in Nazi Germany and if the physicians of that time had held the line and had not acquiesced in devaluing human life (as physicians in the United States would by aiding the process of capital punishment), it is unlikely that Nazi Germany would have happened.

The idea that protesting physicians could have been a bulwark against harm in Nazi Germany is speculative counterfactual history. Proponents of this argument highlight that physician participation in the Nazi party eclipsed other professions; 45% of doctors joined the party, a full 20% more than lawyers and teachers and greater than 35% more than the general population.[35] However, the many physicians who joined the party around 1937 tended to be unemployed. Their desire for participation most likely had to do with navigating the central bureaucracy of medicine and a craving for "enduring professional and socioeconomic security and desired recognition."[35] Thus, rather than lead change, most party physicians were "petty opportunists" who joined in response to the societal changes.[31]

Finally, it has been argued that physician involvement, even if or especially because of government imprimatur, will lead to a loss of public trust, perhaps leading patients to wonder about what these physicians and what medicine will do to them. Patients may wonder, for example, that if physicians are "used to killing" people, then what would hold physicians back from making recommendations not in the patient's best interests.

The concerns about how physician participation in capital punishment would lead to a loss of public trust would have to be explicated. To me, this can be no more harmful to the public trust than the 40-year Tuskegee Syphilis Study, in which the US Public Health Service withheld treatment from African American men to determine the effects of syphilis; the government radiation experiments, in which many were experimented on without their knowledge or consent; the Sunbeam fiasco, in which the AMA agreed to and then renounced a deal to endorse Sunbeam medical products that the AMA had no plans to test; and the inability of journal editors to police themselves for conflicts of interests and the withholding or fabrication of information such as with cloning.[36-40] These examples are not presented to say that one wrong should permit another. They are presented to say that, to me, these are likely more harmful to the public trust. The effects of these were more widespread. Yet organized medicine has weathered these events. If permitting physician participation in capital punishment is a matter of weighing the risks and benefits of participation, then using the argument of loss of public trust to prohibit participation would require that harm from the loss of public trust be substantial. No evidence suggests that physician participation in capital punishment would be more damaging to the public trust than these events. Indeed, organized medicine has already weathered physician participation in capital punishment "at every stage, whether preparing for, participating in, or monitoring executions."[41]

The Misapplied Argument of Palatability

A misplaced argument is that physician involvement will make executions smoother and thus more palatable, decreasing the likelihood of abolishing the death penalty.[41] Therefore, physicians, dedicated to improving the quality of life as the patient defines it, should not participate in any action that increases acceptance of capital punishment.[42] The implicit assumption is that physicians, by definition, should oppose capital punishment.[42] This connection, however, has no place in this discussion. It is organized medicine's obligation to lead, and organized medicine is free to make statements regarding the appropriateness of capital punishment. But to use participation as a stalking horse for abolition of capital punishment is disingenuous. This discussion is not about the appropriateness of capital punishment; this discussion is about physician participation in capital punishment.

The Value and Strength of Society

I have used the idea that our free and open society is a powerful bulwark against the potential harms of physician participation in capital punishment. I am fully aware that many enlightened and open societies have sunk into totalitarianism. It would be arrogant to suggest that our society is incapable of such a fall. But that does not mean it is likely that physician participation in capital punishment would be the tipping point or would even be contributory. I contend that, like the Nazi society, such a fall would be a function of widespread socioeconomic factors and that egregious medical abuse would follow, not precede, societal changes. I may be naive, but I believe our society has successfully weathered challenges, and I have faith in the strengths of our society and the sturdiness of its processes. In support of this argument, consider the experiences with physician aid-in-dying in Oregon and with euthanasia in the Netherlands, both of which some considered potential pathways to disaster.[43] In Oregon, the 5-year experience indicated no improprieties in physician aid-in-dying. In the Netherlands, the rate of uncommon improprieties, such as nonvoluntary euthanasia, has remained stable, with no indication of impending disaster.[44] In contrast, in an interview study, leaders in the Netherlands appeared disturbingly complacent about reports of euthanasia without explicit patient request.[45] Whether such unsettling attitudes will lead to future harms is unknown. Nonetheless, these 2 examples indicate that the presence of a slippery slope does not necessarily lead to descent down the slope. I argue that this stability is in large part due to society. In regard to analogies with Nazi Germany, we must be capable of and willing to make distinctions. To argue that the wanton torturing and killing of at least 11 million individuals is equivalent to the extensive processes of capital punishment is fallacious both by numbers and by process. Indeed, to me, comparisons to Nazi Germany are absurd, and if I had my way, this discussion would proceed without those analyses.

Is This Discussion Necessary?

Capital punishment could easily be performed without the use of venous access. The use of medications associated with treatment of humans for capital punishment is an accident, the result of a decision to ask a physician rather than a veterinarian for help. One can imagine, for example, that a veterinarian could provide an acceptable alternative, such as subcutaneous administration of etorphine hydrochloride (a synthetic opioid) and acepromazine maleate (a phenothiazine) to effectively cause cardiopulmonary arrest. Indeed, with subcutaneous injection, concerns about intravenous lethal injection would be nonexistent, and most of the problems discussed in this article would be moot. Although the literature is sparse, I imagine a number of combinations could be delivered subcutaneously or intramuscularly that would anesthetize an inmate before causing death.

Recommendations

The current AMA policy increases the chances of a botched execution. It seems cruel to permit capital punishment but not to permit participation of those who are capable of performing it humanely. If capital punishment is a reality in the United States, then for the sake of the condemned organized medicine should address how it should be performed. The AMA statement should be revised to address complex issues, some of which I briefly discuss.

Astute readers will note that I have avoided the use of the term *patients* when referring to inmates. I now advocate for the use of the word *patient* in this context. I conceptualize physician participation in capital punishment as an altruistic practice of medicine. The future *patient* should request physician participation, and the physician should be licensed to practice medicine in that state. To emphasize the altruistic nature of the service, physicians should refuse payment for this service. Although the fact that physicians are performing capital punishment should be public knowledge, specific physicians who perform capital punishment should be permitted to remain anonymous. I do realize that this connotes shame, but anonymity is necessary to protect a physician and his or her family from retaliation. Physicians who serve this *patient* community should receive counseling, and studies should be implemented to determine whether there should be limitations, such as the number of executions that a physician may perform. Physicians should be permitted to be involved in other ways to improve the humaneness of capital punishment, such as publicly suggesting and debating protocols or initiating and managing databases. Indeed, permitting physician participation in developing protocols is likely the best way to achieve humane executions while enabling physicians not to directly participate in the act of lethal injection.[10]

One issue that has come to the forefront is whether the government should be able to mandate physician participation.[13] It would be hard to argue that the government's interest is altruistic, that is, focused on removing harm from the patient. The government's interest is better understood as being able to achieve capital punishment as easily as possible. Permitting the government to mandate physician participation is wrongheaded because it verges on making the physician a tool of the government, not of the patient.

Some have suggested that the appropriate physician to perform capital punishment is the anesthesiologist.[10,13] To be sure, there are superficial similarities in appearance between capital punishment and induction of anesthesia. But such similarities are an accident of history. Many physicians, including intensivists and emergency department physicians, have the ability to manage intravenous infusions and assess for anesthetic depth or suggest alternative drugs. Indeed, although this article is focused on physician participation, many of these arguments are equally valid for others who develop caregiver-patient relationships and have the requisite skills. Space does not allow a detailed analysis for different professions.

Physician participation in capital punishment does have associated harms. But the question is whether the harms outweigh the benefits. Because the potential benefits are sufficiently clear and the potential harms are poorly explicated, we should permit physician participation in capital punishment.

References

1. Jones GR. Judicial electrocution and the prison doctor. *Lancet.* 1990;335(8691):713–714.

2. Bohm RM. *Deathquests: An Introduction to the Theory and Practice of Capital Punishment in the United States.* Cincinnati, OH: Anderson Publishing; 1999.

3. Death Penalty Information Center. Execution database: years selected 1997–2006. Available at: www.deathpenaltyinfo.org/executions.php. Accessed July 3, 2007.

4. Council on Ethical and Judicial Affairs, American Medical Association. Physician participation in capital punishment. *JAMA.* 1993;270(3):365–368.

5. Council on Ethical and Judicial Affairs, American Medical Association. Capital punishment. In: *Code of Medical Ethics: Current Opinions with Annotations 2006–2007.* Chicago, IL: American Medical Association; 2006:E-2.06.

6. Denno DW. When legislatures delegate death: the troubling paradox behind state use of electrocution and lethal injection and what it says about us. *Ohio State Law J.* 2002;63:63–260.

7. Reves JG, Glass PSA, Lubarsky DA, McEvoy MD. Intravenous nonopioid anesthetics. In: Miller RD, ed. *Miller's Anesthesia*. 6th ed. Philadelphia, PA: Elsevier Churchill Livingstone; 2005:317–378.

8. Naguib M, Lien CA. Pharmacology of muscle relaxants and their antagonists. In: Miller RD, ed. *Miller's Anesthesia*. Vol 1.6th ed. Philadelphia, PA: Elsevier Churchill Livingstone; 2005:481–572.

9. California State Prison, San Quentin. San Quentin Operational Procedure No. 770. Revised date: 6/13/03. Available at: www.law.berkeley.edu/clinics/dpclinic/Lethal%20Injection%20Documents/California/Morales /Morales%20Dist%20Ct.Cp/Ex%20A%20to%20TRO%20 motion%20(Procedure%20 No.%20770).pdf. Accessed July 3, 2007.

10. *Morales v Tilton* 465 F Supp 2d 972 (ND Cal), December 15, 2006.

11. *Morales v Hickman* 415 F Supp 2d 1037 (ND Cal), February 14, 2006.

12. Gawande A. When law and ethics collide—why physicians participate in executions. *N Engl J Med.* 2006;354(12):1221–1229.

13. *Taylor v Crawford* 445 F3d 1095 (8th Cir 2006).

14. Chapman R. Witnesses describe killer's 'macabre' final few minutes. *Chicago Sun-Times*. May 11 , 1994:5.

15. Brief for Amicus Curiae, Darick Demorris Walker, Supporting Petitioner re *Hill v McDonough*, US 2006 WL 558286. Available at: www.law.berkeley.edu/clinics/dpclinic/Lethal%20Injection%20Documents/Florida/Hill2006.03.06%20amicus%20walker.pdf. Accessed July 5, 2007.

16. Tisch C. Doctor: execution flawed at start. *St. Petersburg Times*. February 13, 2007:1B.

17. Reich DL, Kaplan JA. Complications of cardiovascular access. In: Benumof JL, Saidman LJ, eds. *Anesthesia and Perioperative Complications*. St. Louis, MO: Mosby-Year Book Inc; 1992:16–37.

18. Fornek S. Bad drug mix delayed execution. *Chicago Sun-Times*. May 12, 1994:12.

19. Morton WD, Lerman J. The effect of pancuronium on the solubility of aqueous thiopentone. *Can J Anaesth.* 1987;34(l):87–89.

20. Executioner needs precise training in carrying out lethal injections. *Tampa Tribune*. February 13, 2007:10.

21. O'neil T. Too-tight strap hampered execution; coroner: chemical flow was impeded. *St. Louis Post-Dispatch*. May 5, 1995:1B.

22. Provance J, Hall C. Problems bog down execution of Clark. *Toledo Blade*. May 3, 2006:Al.

23. Whoriskey P, Geis S. Lethal injection is on hold in 2 states. *The Washington Post*. December 16, 2006:A1.

24. Overall M, Smith M. 22-year-old killer gets early execution; sped-up law adds witnesses. *The Tulsa World*. May 8, 1997:A1.

25. Hedberg K, Hopkins D, Kohn M. Five years of legal physician-assisted suicide in Oregon [letter]. *N Engl J Med.* 2003;348(10):961–964.

26. van der Maas PJ, van der Wal G, Haverkate I, et al. Euthanasia, physician-assisted suicide, and other medical practices involving the end of life in the Netherlands, 1990–1995. *N Engl J Med.* 1996;335(22):1699–1705.

27. Truog RD, Brennan TA. Participation of physicians in capital punishment. *N Engl J Med.* 1993;329(18):1346–1350.

28. Pellegrino ED, Thomasma DC. Dubious premises—evil conclusions: moral reasoning at the Nuremberg trials. *Comb Q Healthc Ethics.* Spring 2000; 9(2):261–274.

29. Freedman AM, Halpern AL. The erosion of ethics and morality in medicine: physician participation in legal executions in the United States. NY *Law Sch Law Rev.* 1996;41(1):169–188.

30. Burgess JA. The great slippery-slope argument. *J Med Ethics.* 1993;19 (3): 169–174.

31. Lerner BH, Rothman DJ. Medicine and the Holocaust: learning more of the lessons [editorial]. *Ann Intern Med.* 1995;122(10):793–794.

32. Lifton RJ. *The Nazi Doctors: Medical Killing and the Psychology of Genocide.* New York, NY: Basic Books; 1986:15–16.

33. Osofsky MJ, Bandura A, Zimbardo PG. The role of moral disengagement in the execution process. *Law Hum Behav.* 2005;29(4):371–393.

34. Charo RA. The celestial fire of conscience—refusing to deliver medical care. *N Engl J Med.* 2005;352(24):2471–2473.

35. Kater MH. Criminal physicians in the third reich: towards a group portrait. In: Nicosia FR, Huener J, eds. *Medicine and Medical Ethics in Nazi Germany.* New York, NY: Bergbahn Books; 2002:77–92.

36. Jones JH. *Bad Blood: The Tuskegee Syphilis Experiments.* New York, NY: The Free Press; 1993.

37. United States Advisory Committee on Human Radiation Experiments. *The Human Radiation Experiments.* New York, NY: Oxford University Press; 1996.

38. Broken deal costs A.M.A. $9.9 million. *New York Times.* August 3, 1998:A12.

39. Our conflicted medical journals [editorial]. *New York Times.* July 23, 2006;4:11.

40. Bosman J. Reporters find science journals harder to trust, but not easy to verify. *New York Times.* February 13, 2006:C1.

41. Emanuel LL, Bienen LB. Physician participation in executions: time to eliminate anonymity provisions and protest the practice [editorial]. *Ann Intern Med.* 2001;135(10):922–924.

42. Stop killing people who kill people [editorial]. *Lancet.* 2007;369:343.

43. Snyder L, Sulmasy DP, Ethics and Human Rights Committee, American College of Physicians-American Society of Internal Medicine. Physician-assisted suicide. *Ann Intern Med.* 2001;135(3):209–216.

44. Onwuteaka-Philipsen BD, van der Heide A, Koper D, et al. Euthanasia and other end-of-life decisions in the Netherlands in 1990, 1995, and 2001. *Lancet.* 2003;362(9381):395–399.

45. Cohen-Almagor R. Non-voluntary and involuntary euthanasia in The Netherlands: Dutch perspectives. *Issues Law Med.* Spring 2003;18(3):239–257.

Atul Gawande

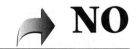

When Law and Ethics Collide— Why Physicians Participate in Executions

On February 14, 2006, a U.S. District Court issued an unprecedented ruling concerning the California execution by lethal injection of murderer Michael Morales. The ruling ordered that the state have a physician, specifically an anesthesiologist, personally supervise the execution, or else drastically change the standard protocol for lethal injections.[1] Under the protocol, the anesthetic sodium thiopental is given at massive doses that are expected to stop breathing and extinguish consciousness within one minute after administration; then the paralytic agent pancuronium is given, followed by a fatal dose of potassium chloride.

The judge found, however, that evidence from execution logs showed that six of the last eight prisoners executed in California had not stopped breathing before technicians gave the paralytic agent, raising a serious possibility that prisoners experienced suffocation from the paralytic, a feeling much like being buried alive, and felt intense pain from the potassium bolus. This experience would be unacceptable under the Constitution's Eighth Amendment protections against cruel and unusual punishment. So the judge ordered the state to have an anesthesiologist present in the death chamber to determine when the prisoner was unconscious enough for the second and third injections to be given—or to perform the execution with sodium thiopental alone.

The California Medical Association, the American Medical Association (AMA), and the American Society of Anesthesiologists (ASA) immediately and loudly opposed such physician participation as a clear violation of medical ethics codes. "Physicians are healers, not executioners," the ASA's president told reporters. Nonetheless, in just two days, prison officials announced that they had found two willing anesthesiologists. The court agreed to maintain their anonymity and to allow them to shield their identities from witnesses. Both withdrew the day before the execution, however, after the Court of Appeals for the Ninth Circuit added a further stipulation requiring them personally to administer additional medication if the prisoner remained conscious or was in pain.[2] This they would not accept. The execution was then postponed until at

From *The New England Journal of Medicine,* March 23, 2006, pp. 1221–1330. Copyright © 2006 by Massachusetts Medical Society. Reprinted by permission of Massachusetts Medical Society via Rightslink.

least May, but the court has continued to require that medical professionals assist with the administration of any lethal injection given to Morales.

This turn of events is the culmination of a steady evolution in methods of execution in the United States. On July 2, 1976, in deciding the case of *Gregg v. Georgia,* the Supreme Court legalized capital punishment after a decade-long moratorium on executions. Executions resumed six months later, on January 17, 1977, in Utah, with the death by firing squad of Gary Gilmore for the killing of Ben Bushnell, a Provo motel manager.

Death by firing squad, however, came to be regarded as too bloody and uncontrolled. (Gilmore's heart, for example, did not stop until two minutes afterward, and shooters have sometimes weakened at the trigger, as famously happened in 1951 in Utah when the five riflemen fired away from the target over Elisio Mares's heart, only to hit his right chest and cause him to bleed slowly to death.)[3]

Hanging came to be regarded as still more inhumane. Under the best of circumstances, the cervical spine is broken at C2, the diaphragm is paralyzed, and the prisoner suffocates to death, a minutes-long process.

Gas chambers proved no better: asphyxiation from cyanide gas, which prevents cells from using oxygen by inactivating cytochrome oxidase, took even longer than death by hanging, and the public revolted at the vision of suffocating prisoners fighting for air and then seizing as the hypoxia worsened. In Arizona, in 1992, for example, the asphyxiation of triple murderer Donald Harding took 11 minutes, and the sight was so horrifying that reporters began crying, the attorney general vomited, and the prison warden announced he would resign if forced to conduct another such execution.[4] Since 1976, only 2 prisoners have been executed by firing squad, 3 by hanging, and 12 by gas chamber.[5]

Electrocution, thought to cause a swifter, more acceptable death, was used in 74 of the first 100 executions after *Gregg.* But officials found that the electrical flow frequently arced, cooking flesh and sometimes igniting prisoners—postmortem examinations frequently had to be delayed for the bodies to cool—and yet some prisoners still required repeated jolts before they died. In Alabama, in 1979, for example, John Louis Evans III was still alive after two cycles of 2600 V; the warden called Governor George Wallace, who told him to keep going, and only after a third cycle, with witnesses screaming in the gallery, and almost 20 minutes of suffering did Evans finally die.[3] Only Florida, Virginia, and Alabama persisted with electrocutions with any frequency, and under threat of Supreme Court review, they too abandoned the method.

Lethal injection now appears to be the sole method of execution accepted by courts as humane enough to satisfy Eighth Amendment requirements—largely because it medicalizes the process. The prisoner is laid supine on a hospital gurney. A white bedsheet is drawn to his chest. An intravenous line flows into his or her arm. Under the protocol devised in 1977 by Dr. Stanley Deutsch, the chairman of anesthesiology at the University of Oklahoma, prisoners are first given 2500 to 5000 mg of sodium thiopental (5 to 10 times the recommended maximum), which can produce death all by itself by causing complete cessation of the brain's electrical activity followed by respiratory arrest and circulatory collapse. Death, however, can take up to 15 minutes or longer with thiopental alone, and the prisoner may appear to gasp, struggle, or convulse. So 60 to 100 mg of the paralytic agent pancuronium (10 times the usual dose) is injected one minute or so after the thiopental. Finally, 120 to 240 meq of potassium is given to produce rapid cardiac arrest.

Officials liked this method. Because it borrowed from established anesthesia techniques, it made execution like familiar medical procedures rather than the grisly, backlash-inducing spectacle it had become. (In Missouri, executions were even moved to a prison-hospital procedure room.) It was less disturbing to witness. The drugs were cheap and routinely available. And officials could turn to doctors and nurses to help with technical difficulties, attest to the painlessness and trustworthiness of the technique, and lend a more professional air to the proceedings.

But medicine balked. In 1980, when the first execution was planned using Dr. Deutsch's technique, the AMA passed a resolution against physician participation as a violation of core medical ethics. It affirmed that ban in detail in its 1992 Code of Medical Ethics. Article 2.06 states, "A physician, as a member of a profession dedicated to preserving life when there is hope of doing so, should not be a participant in a legally authorized execution," although an individual physician's opinion about capital punishment remains "the personal moral decision of the individual." It states that unacceptable participation includes prescribing or administering medications as part of the execution procedure, monitoring vital signs, rendering technical advice, selecting injection sites, starting or supervising placement of intravenous lines, or simply being present as a physician. Pronouncing death is also considered unacceptable, because the physician is not permitted to revive the prisoner if he or she is found to be alive. Only two actions were acceptable: provision at the prisoner's request of a sedative to calm anxiety beforehand and certification of death after another person had pronounced it.

The code of ethics of the Society of Correctional Physicians establishes an even stricter ban: "The correctional health professional shall . . . not be involved in any aspect of execution of the death penalty." The American Nurses Association (ANA) has adopted a similar prohibition. Only the national pharmacists' society, the American Pharmaceutical Association, permits involvement, accepting the voluntary provision of execution medications by pharmacists as ethical conduct.

States, however, wanted a medical presence. In 1982, in Texas, Dr. Ralph Gray, the state prison medical director, and Dr. Bascom Bentley agreed to attend the country's first execution by lethal injection, though only to pronounce death. But once on the scene, Gray was persuaded to examine the prisoner to show the team the best injection site.[6] Still, the doctors refused to give advice about the injection itself and simply watched as the warden prepared the chemicals. When he tried to push the syringe, however, it did not work. He had mixed all the drugs together, and they had precipitated into a clot of white sludge. "I could have told you that," one of the doctors reportedly said, shaking his head.[3] Afterward, Gray went to pronounce the prisoner dead but found him still alive. Though the doctors were part of the team now, they did nothing but suggest allowing time for more drugs to run in.

Today, all 38 death-penalty states rely on lethal injection. Of 1012 murderers executed since 1976, 844 were executed by injection.[5] Against vigorous opposition from the AMA and state medical societies, 35 of the 38 states explicitly allow physician participation in executions. Indeed, 17 require it: Colorado, Florida, Georgia, Idaho, Louisiana, Mississippi, Nevada, North Carolina, New Hampshire, New Jersey, New Mexico, Oklahoma, Oregon, South Dakota, Virginia, Washington, and Wyoming. To protect participating physicians from license challenges for violating ethics codes, states commonly provide legal immunity and promise anonymity. Nonetheless, several physicians have faced such challenges, though none have lost their licenses as yet.[7] And despite the promised anonymity, several states have produced the physicians in court to vouch publicly for the legitimacy and painlessness of the procedure.

States have affirmed that physicians and nurses—including those who are prison employees—have a right to refuse to participate in any way in executions. Yet they have found physicians and nurses who are willing to participate. Who are these people? And why do they do it?

It is not easy to find answers to these questions. The medical personnel are difficult to identify and reluctant to discuss their roles, even when offered anonymity. Among the 15 medical professionals I located who have helped with executions, however, I found 4 physicians and 1 nurse who agreed to speak with me; collectively, they have helped with at least 45 executions. None were zealots for the death penalty, and none had a simple explanation for why they did this work. The role, most said, had crept up on them.

Dr. A has helped with about eight executions in his state. He was extremely uncomfortable talking about the subject. Nonetheless, he sat down with me in a hotel lobby in a city not far from where he lives and told me his story.

Almost 60 years old, he is board certified in internal medicine and critical care, and he and his family have lived in their small town for 30 years. He is well respected. Almost everyone of local standing comes to see him as their primary care physician—the bankers, his fellow doctors, the mayor. Among his patients is the warden of the maximum-security prison that happens to be in his town. One day several years ago, they got talking during an appointment. The warden complained of difficulties staffing the prison clinic and asked Dr. A if he would be willing to see prisoners there occasionally. Dr. A said he would. He'd have made more money in his own clinic—the prison paid $65 an hour—but the prison was important to the community, he liked the warden, and it was just a few hours of work a month. He was happy to help.

Then, a year or two later, the warden asked him for help with a different problem. The state had a death penalty, and the legislature had voted to use lethal injection exclusively. The executions were to be carried out in the warden's prison. He needed doctors, he said. Would Dr. A help? He would not have to deliver the lethal injection. He would just help with cardiac monitoring. The warden gave the doctor time to consider it.

"My wife didn't like it," Dr. A told me. "She said, 'Why do you want to go there?'" But he felt torn. "I knew something about the past of these killers." One of them had killed a mother of three during a convenience-store robbery and then, while getting away, shot a man who was standing at his car pumping gas. Another convict had kidnapped, raped, and strangled to death an 11-year-old girl. "I do not have a very strong conviction about the death penalty, but I don't feel anything negative about it for such people either. The execution order was given legally by the court. And morally, if you think about the animal behavior of some of these people. . . . " Ultimately, he decided to participate, he said, because he was only helping with monitoring, because he was needed by the warden and his community, because the sentence was society's order, and because the punishment did not seem wrong.

At the first execution, he was instructed to stand behind a curtain watching the inmate's heart rhythm on a cardiac monitor. Neither the witnesses on the other side of the glass nor the prisoner could see him. A technician placed two IV lines. Someone he could not see pushed the three drugs, one right after another. Watching the monitor, he saw the sinus rhythm slow, then widen. He recognized the peaked T waves of hyperkalemia followed by the fine spikes of ventricular fibrillation and finally the flat, unwavering line of an asystolic arrest. He waited half a minute, then signaled to another physician who went out before the witnesses to place his stethoscope on the prisoner's unmoving chest. The doctor listened for 30 seconds and then told the warden the inmate was dead. Half an hour later, Dr. A was released. He made his way through a side door, past the crowd gathered outside, and headed home.

In three subsequent executions there were difficulties, though, all with finding a vein for an IV. The prisoners were either obese or past intravenous drug users, or both. The technicians would stick and stick and, after half an hour, give up. This was a possibility the warden had not prepared for. Dr. A had placed numerous lines. Could he give a try?

OK, Dr. A decided. Let me take a look.

This was a turning point, though he didn't recognize it at the time. He was there to help, they had a problem, and so he would help. It did not occur to him to do otherwise.

In two of the prisoners, he told me, he found a good vein and placed the IV. In one, however, he could not find a vein. All eyes were on him. He felt responsible for the situation. The prisoner was calm. Dr. A remembered the prisoner saying to him, almost to comfort him, "No, they can never get the vein." The doctor decided to place a central line. People scrambled to find a kit.

I asked him how he placed the line. It was like placing one "for any other patient," he said. He decided to place it in the subclavian vein, because that is what he most commonly did. He opened the kit for the triple-lumen catheter and explained to the prisoner everything he was going to do. I asked him if he was afraid of the prisoner. "No," he said. The man was perfectly cooperative. Dr. A put on sterile gloves, gown, and mask. He swabbed the man's skin with antiseptic.

"Why?" I asked.

"Habit," he said. He injected local anesthetic. He punctured the vein with one stick. He checked to make sure he had good, nonpulsatile flow. He threaded the guidewire, the dilator, and finally the catheter. All went smoothly. He flushed the lines, secured the catheter to the skin with a stitch, and put a clean dressing on, just as he always does. Then he went back behind the curtain to monitor the lethal injection.

Only one case seemed to really bother him. The convict, who had killed a policeman, weighed about 350 pounds. The team placed his intravenous lines without trouble. But after they had given him all three injections, the prisoner's heart rhythm continued. "It was an agonal rhythm," Dr. A said. "He was dead," he insisted. Nonetheless, the rhythm continued. The team looked to Dr. A. His explanation of what happened next diverges from what I learned from another source. I was told that he instructed that another bolus of potassium be given. When I asked him if he did, he said, "No, I didn't. As far as I remember, I didn't say anything. I think it may have been another physician." Certainly, however, all boundary lines had been crossed. He had agreed to take part in the executions simply to pronounce death, but just by being present, by having expertise, he had opened himself to being called on to do steadily more, to take responsibility for the execution itself. Perhaps he was not the executioner. But he was darn close to it.

I asked him whether he had known that his actions—everything from his monitoring the executions to helping officials with the process of delivering the drugs—violated the AMA's ethics code. "I never had any inkling," he said. And indeed, the only survey done on this issue, in 1999, found that just 3 percent of doctors knew of any guidelines governing their participation in executions.[8] The humaneness of the lethal injections was challenged in court, however. The state summoned Dr. A for a public deposition on the process, including the particulars of the execution in which the prisoner required a central line. His local newspaper printed the story. Word spread through his town. Not long after, he arrived at work to find a sign pasted to his clinic door reading, "THE KILLER DOCTOR." A challenge to his medical license was filed with the state. If he wasn't aware of the AMA's stance on the issue earlier, he was now.

Ninety percent of his patients supported him, he said, and the state medical board upheld his license under a law that defined participation in executions as acceptable activity for a physician. But he decided that he wanted no part of the controversy anymore and quit. He still defends what he did. Had he known of the AMA's position, though, "I never would have gotten involved," he said.

Dr. B spoke to me between clinic appointments. He is a family physician, and he has participated in some 30 executions. He became involved long ago, when electrocution was the primary method, and then continued through the transition to lethal injections. He remains a participant to this day. But it was apparent that he had been more cautious and reflective about his involvement than Dr. A had. He also seemed more troubled by it.

Dr. B, too, had first been approached by a patient. "One of my patients was a prison investigator," he said. "I never quite understood his role, but he was an intermediary between the state and the inmates. He was hired to monitor that the state was taking care of them. They had the first two executions after the death penalty was reinstated, and there was a problem with the second one, where the physicians were going in a minute or so after the event and still hearing heartbeats. The two physicians were doing this out of courtesy, because the facility was in their area. But the case unnerved them to the point that they quit. The officials had a lot of trouble finding another doctor after that. So that was when my patient talked to me."

Dr. B did not really want to get involved. He was in his 40s then. He'd gone to a top-tier medical school. He'd protested the Vietnam War in the 1960s. "I've gone from a radical hippie to a middle-class American over the years," he said. "I wasn't on any bandwagons anymore." But his patient said the team needed a physician only to pronounce death. Dr. B had no personal objection to capital punishment. So in the moment—"it was a quick judgment"—he said OK, "but only to do the pronouncement."

The execution was a few days later by electric chair. It was an awful sight, he said. "They say an electrocution is not an issue. But when someone comes up out of that chair six inches, it's not for nothing." He waited a long while before going out to the prisoner. When he did, he performed a systematic examination. He checked for a carotid pulse. He listened to the man's heart three times with a stethoscope. He looked for a pupil response with his pen light. Only then did he pronounce the man dead.

He thought harder about whether to stay involved after that first time. "I went to the library and researched it," and that was when he discovered the AMA guidelines. As he understood the code, if he did nothing except make a pronouncement of death, he would be acting properly and ethically. (This was not a misreading. The AMA only later distinguished between pronouncing death, which it now considers unethical, and certifying death after someone has made the initial pronouncement, which it considers ethical.)

Knowing the guidelines reassured him about his involvement and made him willing to continue. They also emboldened him to draw thicker boundaries around his participation. During the first lethal injections, he and another physician "were in the room when they were administering the drugs," he said. "We could see the telemetry. We could see a lot of things. But I had them remove us from that area. I said I do not want any access to the monitor or the EKGs. . . . A couple times they asked me about recommendations in cases in which there were venous access problems. I said, 'No. I'm not going to assist in any way.' They would ask about amounts of medicines. They had problems getting the medicines. But I said I had no interest in getting involved in any of that."

Dr. B kept himself at some remove from the execution process, but he would be the first to admit that his is not an ethically pristine position. When he refused to provide additional assistance, the execution team simply found others who would. He was glad to have those people there. "If the doctors and nurses are removed, I don't think [lethal injections] could be competently or predictably done. I can tell you I wouldn't be involved unless those people were involved."

"I agonize over the ethics of this every time they call me to go down there," he said. His wife knew about his involvement from early on, but he could not bring himself to tell his children until they were grown. He has let almost no one else know. Even his medical staff is unaware.

The trouble is not that the lethal injections seem cruel to him. "Mostly, they are very peaceful," he said. The agonizing comes instead from his doubts about whether anything is accomplished. "The whole system doesn't seem right," he told me toward the end of our conversation. "I guess I see more and more [executions], and I really wonder. . . . It just seems like the justice system is going down a dead-end street. I can't say that [lethal injection] lessens the incidence of anything. The real depressing thing is that if you don't get to these people before the age of three or four or five, it's not going to make any difference in what they do. They've struck out before they even started kindergarten. I don't see [executions] as saying anything about that."

The medical people most wary of speaking to me were those who worked as full-time employees in state prison systems. Nonetheless, two did agree to speak, one a physician in a Southern state prison and the other a nurse who had worked in a prison out West. Both were less uncertain about being involved in executions than Dr. A or Dr. B.

The physician, Dr. C, was younger than the others and relatively junior among his prison's doctors. He did not trust me to keep his identity confidential, and I think he worried for his job if anyone found out about our conversation. As a result, although I had independent information that he had participated in at least two executions, he would speak only in general terms about the involvement of doctors. But he was clear about what he believed.

"I think that if you're going to work in the correctional setting, [participating in executions] is potentially a component of what you need to do," he said. "It is only a tiny part of anything that you're doing as part of your public health service. A lot of society thinks these people should not get any care at all." But in his job he must follow the law, and it obligates him to provide proper care, he said. It also has set the prisoners' punishment. "Thirteen jurors, citizens of the state, have made a decision. And if I live in that state and that's the law, then I would see it as being an obligation to be available."

He explained further. "I think that if I had to face someone I loved being put to death, I would want that done by lethal injection, and I would want to know that it is done competently."

The nurse saw his participation in fairly similar terms. He had fought as a Marine in Vietnam and later became a nurse. As an Army reservist, he served with a surgical unit in Bosnia and in Iraq. He worked for many years on critical care units and, for almost a decade, as nurse manager for a busy emergency department. He then took a job as the nurse-in-charge for his state penitentiary, where he helped with one execution by lethal injection.

It was the state's first execution by this method, and "at the time, there was great naiveté about lethal injection," he said. "No one in that state had any idea what was involved." The warden had the Texas protocol and thought it looked pretty simple. What did he need medical personnel for? The warden told the nurse that he would start the IVs himself, though he had never started one before.

"Are you, as a doctor, going to let this person stab the inmate for half an hour because of his inexperience?" the nurse asked me. "I wasn't." He said, "I had no qualms. If this is to be done correctly, if it is to be done at all, then I am the person to do it."

This is not to say that he felt easy about it, however. "As a Marine and as a nurse . . . , I hope I will never become someone who has no problem taking another person's life." But society had decided the punishment and had done so carefully with multiple judicial reviews, he said. The convict had killed four people even while in prison. He had arranged for an accomplice to blow up the home of a county attorney he was angry with while the attorney, his wife, and their child were inside. When the accomplice turned state's evidence, the inmate arranged for him to be tortured and killed at a roadside rest stop. The nurse did not disagree with the final judgment that this man should be put to death.

The nurse took his involvement seriously. "As the leader of the health care team," he said, "it was my responsibility to make sure that everything be done in a way that was professional and respectful to the inmate as a human being." He spoke to an official with the state nursing board about the process, and although involvement is against the ANA's ethics code, the board said he could do everything except push the drugs.

So he issued the purchase request to the pharmacist supplying the drugs. He did a dry run with the public citizen chosen to push the injections and with the guards to make sure they knew how to bring the prisoner out and strap him down. On the day of the execution, the nurse dressed as if for an operation, in scrubs, mask, hat, and sterile gown and gloves. He explained to the prisoner exactly what was going to happen. He placed two IVs and taped them down. The warden read the final order to the prisoner and allowed him his last words. "He didn't say anything about his guilt or his innocence," the nurse said. "He just said that the execution made all of us involved killers just like him."

The warden gave the signal to start the injection. The nurse hooked the syringe to the IV port and told the citizen to push the sodium thiopental. "The inmate started to say, 'Yeah, I can feel . . . ' and then he passed out." They completed the injections and, three minutes later, he flatlined on the cardiac monitor. The two physicians on the scene had been left nothing to do except pronounce the inmate dead.

I have personally been in favor of the death penalty. I was a senior official in the 1992 Clinton presidential campaign and in the administration, and in that role I defended the President's stance in support of capital punishment. I have no illusions that the death penalty deters anyone from murder. I also have great concern about the ability of our justice system to avoid putting someone innocent to death. However, I believe there are some human beings who do such evil as to deserve to die. I am not troubled that Timothy McVeigh was executed for the 168 people he had killed in the Oklahoma City bombing, or that John Wayne Gacy was for committing 33 murders. The European Union refuses to participate in any way in the trial of Saddam Hussein because of the court's insistence on allowing the death penalty as a possible punishment, but given Hussein's role in the massacre of more than 100,000 people, the European position only puzzles me.

Still, I have always regarded involvement in executions by physicians and nurses as wrong. The public has granted us extraordinary and exclusive dispensation to administer drugs to people, even to the point of unconsciousness, to put needles and tubes into their bodies, to do what would otherwise be considered assault, because we do so on their behalf—to save their lives and provide them comfort. To have the state take control of these skills for its purposes against a human being—for punishment—seems a dangerous perversion. Society has trusted us with powerful abilities, and the more willing we are to use these abilities against individual people, the more we risk that trust. The public may like executions, but no one likes executioners.

My conversations with the physicians and the nurse I had tracked down, however, rattled both of these views—and no conversation more so than one I had with the final doctor I spoke to. Dr. D is a 45-year-old emergency physician. He is also a volunteer medical director for a shelter for abused children. He works to reduce homelessness. He opposes the death penalty because he regards it as inhumane, immoral, and pointless. And he has participated in six executions so far.

About eight years ago, a new jail was built down the street from the hospital where he worked, and it had an infirmary "the size of our whole emergency room." The jail needed a doctor. So, out of curiosity as much as anything, Dr. D began working there. "I found that I loved it," he said. "Jails are an underserved niche of health care." Jails, he pointed out, are different from prisons in that they house people who are arrested and awaiting trial. Most are housed only a few hours to days and then released. "The substance abuse and noncompliance is high. The people have a wide variety of medical needs. It is a fascinating population. The setting is very similar to the ER. You can make a tremendous impact on people and on public health." Over time, he shifted more and more of his work to the jail system. He built a medical group for the jails in his area and soon became an advocate for correctional medicine.

Three years ago, the doctors who had been involved in executions in his state pulled out. Officials asked Dr. D if his group would take the contract. Before answering, he went to witness an execution. "It was a very emotional experience for me," he said. "I was shocked to witness something like this." He had opposed the death penalty since college, and nothing he saw made him feel any differently. But, at the same time, he felt there were needs that he as a correctional physician could serve.

He read about the ethics of participating. He knew about the AMA's stance against it. Yet he also felt an obligation not to abandon inmates in their dying moments. "We, as doctors, are not the ones deciding the fate of this individual," he said. "The way I saw it, this is an end-of-life issue, just as with any other terminal disease. It just happens that it involves a legal process instead of a medical process. When we have a patient who can no longer survive his illness, we as physicians must ensure he has comfort. [A death-penalty] patient is no different from a patient dying of cancer—except his cancer is a court order." Dr. D said he has "the cure for this cancer"—abolition of the death penalty—but "if the people and the government won't let you provide it, and a patient then dies, are you not going to comfort him?"

His group took the contract, and he has been part of the medical team for each execution since. The doctors are available to help if there are difficulties with IV access, and Dr. D considers it their task to ensure that the prisoner is without pain or suffering through the process. He himself provides the cardiac monitoring and the final determination of death. Watching the changes on the two-line electrocardiogram tracing, "I keep having that reflex as an ER doctor, wanting to treat that rhythm," he said. Aside from that, his main reaction is to be sad for everyone involved—the prisoner whose life has led to this, the victims, the prison officials, the doctors. The team's payment is substantial—$18,000—but he donates his portion to the children's shelter where he volunteers.

Three weeks after speaking to me, he told me to go ahead and use his name. It is Dr. Carlo Musso. He helps with executions in Georgia. He didn't want to seem as if he was hiding anything, he said. He didn't want to invite trouble, either. But activists have already challenged his license and his membership in the AMA, and he is resigned to the fight. "It just seems wrong for us to walk away, to abdicate our responsibility to the patients," he said.

There is little doubt that lethal injection can be painless and peaceful, but as courts have recognized, this requires significant medical assistance and judgment—for placement of intravenous lines, monitoring of consciousness, and adjustments in medication timing and dosage. In recent years, medical societies have persuaded two states, Kentucky and Illinois, to pass laws forbidding physician participation in executions. Nonetheless, officials in each of these states intend to continue to rely on medical supervision, employing nurses and nurse-anesthetists instead. How, then, to reconcile the conflict between government efforts to ensure a medical presence and our ethical principles forbidding it? Are our ethics what should change?

The doctors' and nurse's arguments for competence and comfort in the execution process do have some force. But however much they may wish to be there for an inmate, it seems clear that the inmate is not really their patient. Unlike genuine patients, an inmate has no ability to refuse the physicians' "care"—indeed, the inmate and his family are not even permitted to know the physician's identity. And the medical assistance provided primarily serves the government's purposes—not the inmate's needs as a patient. Medicine is being made an instrument of punishment. The hand of comfort that more gently places the IV, more carefully times the bolus of potassium, is also the hand of death. We cannot escape this truth. The ethics codes seem right.

It is this truth that persuades me that we should seek a legal ban on the participation of physicians and nurses in executions. And if it turns out that executions cannot then be performed without, as the courts put it, "unconstitutional pain and cruelty," the death penalty should be abolished.

It is far from clear that a society that punishes its most evil murderers with life imprisonment is worse off than one that punishes them with death. But a society in which the government actively subverts core ethical principles of medical practice is patently worse off for it. The government has shown willingness to use medical skills against individuals for its own purposes—having medical personnel assist in the interrogation of prisoners, for example, place feeding tubes for force-feeding them, and help with executing them. As medical abilities advance, government interest in our skills will only increase. Preserving the integrity of our ethics could not be more important.

The four physicians and the nurse I spoke to all acted against long-standing principles of their professions. Their actions have made our ethics codes effectively irrelevant in society. Yet, it must be said, most took their moral duties seriously. It is worth reflecting on this truth as well.

The easy thing for any doctor or nurse is simply to follow the written rules. But each of us has a duty not to follow rules and laws blindly. In medicine, we face conflicts about what the right and best actions are in all kinds of areas: relief of suffering for the terminally ill, provision of narcotics for patients with chronic pain, withdrawal of care for the critically ill, abortion, and executions, to name just a few. All have been the subject of professional rules and government regulation, and at times those rules and regulations will be wrong. We will then be called on to make a choice. We must do our best to choose intelligently and wisely.

Sometimes, however, we will be wrong—as I think the doctors and nurses are who have used their privileged skills to make possible 844 deaths by lethal injection thus far. We each should then be prepared to accept the consequences. Unlike Dr. Musso, however, nearly all these doctors and nurses have sought to keep their actions hidden in order not to face the consequences. In the final analysis, I think this is what makes their actions seem particularly troubling. We cannot blame them for their impulse to hide. But we cannot admire them either.

References

1. Michael Angelo Morales v. Roderick Q. Hickman, No. C 06 219 JF, (Dist. Ct. Northern Dist. of Cal. February 14, 2006).
2. Michael Angelo Morales v. Roderick Q. Hickman, No. CV 06 00926 JF (9th Cir. February 20, 2006).
3. Trombley S. The execution protocol: inside America's capital punishment industry. New York: Crown, 1992.
4. Solotaroff I. The last face you'll ever see: the private life of the American death penalty. New York: HarperCollins, 2001:7.
5. Death Penalty Information Center execution database. Accessed March 1, 2006, at http://www.deathpenaltyinfo.org/executions.php.
6. Breach of trust: physician participation in executions in the United States. Philadelphia: American College of Physicians, 1994.
7. Norbut M. Complaint cites Georgia doctors who took part in executions. American Medical News. July 4, 2005:1.
8. Farber NJ, Aboff BM, Weiner J, Davis EB, Boyer EG, Ubel PA. Physicians' willingness to participate in the process of lethal injections for capital punishment. Ann Intern Med 2001;135:884–8.

EXPLORING THE ISSUE

Should Physicians Be Allowed to Participate in Executions?

Critical Thinking and Reflection

1. How do you understand the physician's social role, and do you think it would be undermined by allowing physicians to participate in executions? Why or why not?
2. How morally important is it to conduct executions in such a way that the condemned do not suffer, and if that goal is important, what is the best way to accomplish it? Is physician participation necessary or helpful? Are there ways physicians might participate that would be more appropriate to their social role?

Is There Common Ground?

It is natural to think that moral debates should be solved by moral arguments. But what if the moral arguments have all been marshaled and articulated in the best way possible, and still there is disagreement? The hope that good moral argument should always eventually lead to moral agreement is what the philosopher Norman Daniels once called the philosopher's dream. In place of that dream, Daniels proposes that we must fall back on a political solution: We must organize our public institutions in such a way that personal differences can be allowed to continue. We should compromise. For Daniels, permitting such individual differences of opinion is part of the task of a liberal state.

Of course, whether a political compromise is possible or desirable on the issue of physician participation in lethal injection executions is itself controversial. In February 2010, the American Board of Anesthesiology declared that it would no longer provide board certification to anesthesiologists who participate in capital punishment. Losing board certification undermines a physician's ability to practice medicine, since board certification is an important professional credential.

In a recent, controversial paper, Lawrence Nelson and Brandon Ashby argue against the ABA's stance and for political compromise on this issue. They argue that there are "principled and morally serious arguments" behind both the pro and the con positions on permitting physicians to participate in execution by lethal injection, and that individual physicians should therefore be allowed to make their own decisions about participation. Nelson and Ashby believe that professional medical organizations "should not impose organizational sanctions that significantly impede or destroy physicians' ability to practice medicine."

Additional Resources

The paper by Lawrence Nelson and Brandon Ashby is "Rethinking the Ethics of Physician Participation in Lethal Injection Execution," *Hastings Center Report* (May–June 2011). The position of the American Board of Anesthesiology is found in "Anesthesiologists and Capital Punishment," at www.theaba.orgpdfCapitalPunishmentCommentary.pdf.

The position of the American Medical Association is found in, "Code of Medical Ethics Opinion 2.211—Physician-Assisted Suicide," at www .ama-assn.orgamapubphysician-resourcesmedical-ethicscode-medical-ethicsopinion2211.shtml.

The New England Journal of Medicine featured a roundtable discussion on physician participation in execution. Atul Gawande, Deborah W. Denno, Robert D. Truog, and David Waisel, "Physicians and Execution—Highlights from a Discussion of Lethal Injection," *The New England Journal of Medicine* (vol. 358, January 31, 2008). Video of the roundtable discussion is available at www.nejm.org/doi/full/10.1056/NEJMp0800378.

For a forceful argument against permitting physician participation, see L.L. Emanuel and L.B. Bienen, "Physician Participation in Executions: Time to Eliminate Anonymity and Protest the Practice," *Annals of Internal Medicine* (vol. 135, no. 10, 2001).

Ty Alper offers insight into physicians' views about lethal injection executions and their willingness to participate them in "The Truth about Physician Participation in Lethal Injection Executions," *North Carolina Law Review* (vol. 88, 2010).

Deborah Deno provides a study of lethal injection protocols around the United States. Deno argues that states have produced "grossly inadequate protocols that severely restrict sufficient understanding of how executions are performed and heighten the likelihood of unconstitutionality." Deborah Deno, "The Lethal Injection Quandary: How Medicine Has Dismantled the Death Penalty," *Fordham Law Review* (vol. 76, 2007).

ISSUE 11

Should Pharmacists Be Allowed to Deny Prescriptions on Grounds of Conscience?

YES: **Donald W. Herbe**, from "The Right to Refuse: A Call for Adequate Protection of a Pharmacist's Right to Refuse Facilitation of Abortion and Emergency Contraception," *Journal of Law and Health* (2002/2003)

NO: **Julie Cantor and Ken Baum**, from "The Limits of Conscientious Objection—May Pharmacists Refuse to Fill Prescriptions for Emergency Contraception?" *The New England Journal of Medicine* (November 4, 2004)

Learning Outcomes

After reading this issue, you should be able to:

- Discuss the considerations in favor and against granting pharmacists a right to refuse to fill a prescription if they believe the drug will be used in a way they find deeply objectionable on moral or religious grounds.
- Explain the use of mifepristone (RU-486) to produce a very early abortion.
- Explain the concepts of "conscience clause" and a "right of conscience."

ISSUE SUMMARY

YES: Law student Donald W. Herbe asserts that pharmacists' moral beliefs concerning abortion and emergency contraception are genuinely fundamental and deserve respect. He proposes that professional pharmaceutical organizations lead the way to recognizing a true right of conscience, which would eventually result in universal legislation protecting against all potential ramifications of choosing conscience.

NO: Julie Cantor, a lawyer, and Ken Baum, a physician and lawyer, reject an absolute right to object, as well as no right to object, to these prescriptions but assert that pharmacists who cannot or will not dispense a drug have a professional obligation to meet the needs of their customers by referring them elsewhere.

U nder U.S. law and practice, a person who objects on grounds of conscience or religious belief to performing certain acts has considerable protections. To force someone to perform an act totally forbidden by his or her religion would be a profound violation of ethical and human rights. But there are limits to exercising this right. Right now there is no military draft in the United States; however, all young men must register with the Selective Service Agency on their 18th birthday. If there were to be a military draft, a conscientious objector would have to demonstrate that he has a strongly held religious or moral belief, not just a political one, against participation in the military. Conscientious objectors could request alternative community service, such as caring for the elderly, or serving in the military as a noncombatant, for example, as a medic. In the Vietnam War, some conscientious objectors were jailed for their refusal to serve.

Conscientious objection has ethical implications for medical personnel as well. Physicians, for example, may refrain from performing procedures that are legal but repugnant to them on moral grounds. Just as in the military example, there are limits. Physicians cannot ethically refuse to provide life-saving or emergency treatment to a person on the grounds that the individual is a murderer or has committed an act that violates the physician's religion. They can refuse to perform abortions on grounds of conscience, but ethical codes require them to refer patients to another provider. Nurses have less discretion than physicians because they are employees of hospitals and are subject to disciplinary action. Nevertheless, they too can establish grounds for refusing to assist in an abortion procedure, sterilization, or the withdrawal of life-sustaining treatment.

The issue is murkier, however, when it comes to pharmacists, who are generally self-employed, or pharmacy employees. They do not directly participate in the acts they find objectionable, but they make those acts possible by dispensing medications. What are their options and obligations?

Birth control pills and emergency contraception medications, which are basically high doses of regular birth control pills taken to prevent pregnancy after unprotected sexual intercourse, have been on the market for years. Some pharmacists object to dispensing these medications. The issue became much more controversial when in September 2000 the Food and Drug Administration (FDA) approved the drug mifepristone as safe and effective. This drug, formerly known as RU-486 after Russel Uclaf, its initial French manufacturer, had been marketed in Europe for several years. Mifepristone is a synthetic steroid that blocks progesterone, preventing an implanted fertilized egg from developing. It must be taken within 49 days of conception and followed within 48 hours by a second drug, misoprostol, related to the hormone prostaglandin. Taken together, the two drugs act as a chemical form of early abortion. Emergency contraception, on the other hand, is not a form of abortion, since no conception has taken place.

And it is here that some pharmacists have drawn the line. Believing strongly that abortion is immoral, they want the legal right to exercise their religious beliefs and ethical right by refusing to dispense the drugs for this purpose and to be protected from losing their jobs, or other repercussions. Should they be allowed to do so and without referring women to another, more willing pharmacist?

The YES and NO selections present different points of view. Donald Herbe sees the exercise of conscientious objection as fundamental to pharmacists' human rights and calls for legislation to protect them from any kind of repercussions or discrimination. While recognizing that pharmacists have a legitimate interest in avoiding conflicts of conscience, Julie Cantor and Ken Baum believe that because pharmacists are licensed and have a professional obligation to serve the public, they must make alternative options available to customers who seek legal prescription drugs they find objectionable.

YES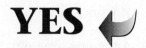

Donald W. Herbe

The Right to Refuse: A Call for Adequate Protection of a Pharmacist's Right to Refuse Facilitation of Abortion and Emergency Contraception

Introduction

The ability to convince an individual, through the art of honest persuasion, of the righteousness of a belief is celebrated; however, in failure of such persuasion, compelling that person to act contradictory to their retained ideal is detestable. The free will to reject a movement or disagree with a practice is the sort of liberty this Nation was founded upon, yet today the potential exists that many in the pharmaceutical profession will be forced into behaviors repugnant to their basic standards of goodness and morality. The proliferation of abortive and contraceptive drug therapies has thrust many pharmacists into roles as facilitators of practices they oppose on fundamental levels without a corresponding ability to opt out of such action.

When a patient desires drug therapies that, in the eyes of the pharmacist, are likely to destroy an unborn human life, the pro-life pharmacist is left in an unsettling position: accommodate the patient and breach basic moral principles *or* adhere to conscience and risk liability and disciplinary action.

Section I: Anti-Reproduction Pills and the Pharmacist's Role

The Pills

On September 28, 2000, the Food and Drug Administration (FDA) approved the drug mifepristone, formerly known as RU-486, for use in the United States as an abortifacient. Mifepristone had previously been approved and is currently used in some European countries, including France, England, and Sweden. Although mifepristone has other potential uses, such as postcoital contraception and daily-use birth control, its FDA approved use is as an early pregnancy abortifacient.

From *Journal of Law and Health*, vol. 17, issue 1, 2002/2003, excerpts from 77–103. Copyright © 2003 by Donald W. Herbe. Reprinted by permission of the author.

Mifepristone acts as an anti-hormone and precludes a woman's uterus from retaining an *implanted* fertilized egg. The drug blocks progesterone, an essential hormone in the acceptance and retention of an implanted egg within a woman's uterus; and, when taken in concurrence with misoprostol, induces a spontaneous abortion. The fact that the mifepristone abortion regimen acts to destroy an implanted egg as opposed to a fertilized yet not implanted egg, is what distinguishes it from emergency contraception.

Drugs used post-coitally with the intent to prevent the development of a pregnancy are referred to as emergency contraception. This labeling as emergency contraception is a bit conclusory, as the definition of whether use of such drugs is contraception or abortion lies at the heart of the controversy over them. However, for purposes of convenience and clarity, this Note will refer to drug regimens consumed post-intercourse for the purpose of preventing the onset or continuance of pregnancy as emergency contraception (EC), as that is the term that has been attached to them in modern medical, social, and political arenas.

Notwithstanding this controversy, the physical and biological effects of orally administered EC, often referred to as the morning-after pill, are not in dispute. EC may prevent the development of a pregnancy by inhibiting any of four successive biological events, either pre or post fertilization, necessary to establish and maintain a pregnancy. EC works before fertilization by either suppressing ovulation, like regular birth-control pills, or preventing fertilization of an egg by inhibiting the movement of the sperm or the egg. If an egg becomes fertilized, then EC may disrupt transport of the fertilized egg to the uterus or, if the transport through the fallopian tube is complete, prevent the implantation of the fertilized egg in the woman's uterus. EC is most effective when used up to seventy-two hours after unprotected intercourse and becomes completely ineffective after implantation occurs, usually six or seven days after intercourse.

The Pharmacist's Role

During the past twenty years emergency contraception pills (ECPs) have been available to and used by American women. During this time frame non-emergency oral contraceptives (those taken as a daily pre-intercourse regimen) were used off-label as emergency contraception and were distributed as such "primarily in hospital emergency rooms, reproductive health clinics, and university health centers." These medical facilities would repackage oral contraceptives for use as emergency contraception; pharmacies associated with certain clinics would repackage oral contraceptives into EC regimens and label them as such; and private physicians would instruct patients to take a larger dosage of their regular birth control pills as EC.

In 1998 the FDA approved the Preven Emergency Contraceptive Kit, an EC based on the Yuzpe regimen. In 1999, the FDA also approved Plan B, another EC regimen. While different regimens of oral contraceptives had been distributed and used before 1998 as emergency contraceptives, Preven and Plan B are the first regimens specifically approved by the FDA as safe and effective emergency contraceptives, to be packaged and marketed as such. Additionally, modified doses of oral contraceptives, not specifically packaged for use as an EC, can still be prescribed in doses that would effect emergency contraception if doctor and patient desire such a method.

Emergency contraception pills are classified as prescription drugs, and "states are delegated the power and responsibility of determining which health care professionals . . . have prescriptive authority." Currently, many states have authorized collaborative practices that have expanded the role of pharmacists. These collaborative practices generally authorize greater independence of the pharmacist to initiate drug therapies not specifically prescribed by a patient's physician or other authorized health care professional. In other words, some patients may not require a prescription from their doctor before being distributed certain medications or drugs from a pharmacist. However, with the exception of Washington, California, and Alaska, states do not authorize this expanded pharmacist role in the distribution of ECPs. Pharmacists are generally limited to dispensing ECPs specifically prescribed by some other authorized health care professional. Other general duties of a pharmacist in the distribution of ECPs may include counseling and educating women on EC use at the time the prescription is filled.

In Washington, California, and Alaska, pharmacists have the dual authority to prescribe *and* dispense ECPs under each state's respective collaborative practices. Generally speaking, the pharmacist may dispense ECPs in accordance with "standardized procedures or protocols developed by the pharmacist and an authorized prescriber[.]" Thus, a woman need not receive authorization from her doctor prior to buying ECPs; the pharmacist acts not as a third party or indirect provider of ECPs, but as a direct provider in accordance with a general collaborative protocol.

If pro-choice groups and the American Medical Association have their way, pharmacists will have no future role in ECPs. This is because these groups support an FDA reclassification of ECPs as over-the-counter (OTC) drugs, rather than prescription. Many pro-choice groups claim as a top goal the persuasion of the FDA to reclassify ECPs as OTC. If OTC status were granted, then "women would be able to get ECPs without encountering any type of health care provider."

OTC status for ECPs is not generally supported by pharmacists however, and is not likely in today's political climate. Advocates on both sides of the issue believe the Bush administration, with its influence on the FDA, will delay or negate a switch in classification from prescription to OTC. The behavioral and social policy concerns raised by ECPs "may make switching ECPs to OTC status a politically unpopular move." In any event, ECPs are currently available only by prescription.

Many restrictions have been imposed by the FDA in the use and distribution of mifepristone. First, the drug can only be used during the first forty-nine days after a woman's last menstrual cycle. Also, the drug is distributed to women directly from doctors and certain health clinics. Mifepristone "is not and will not be available in pharmacies[.]" Thus, under the current FDA restrictions, pharmacists have no role in mifepristone-induced abortions.

While current mifepristone use is much lower than expected since its FDA approval and subsequent availability to the public, some signals suggest that future use or access may become more widespread. A survey of doctors by the Kaiser Family Foundation discovered that twenty-three percent of doctors said they were "likely" to offer mifepristone in 2002; up from the seven percent that actually provided the drug since its approval. Also, health centers offering mifepristone have reported a ninety-nine percent rate of abortion in women who have taken the drug. An expected increase in availability, a near perfect rate of achieving the desired ends of abortion, together with continued efforts by pro-choice groups, such as Planned Parenthood, to increase accessibility to abortion, could be the impetus to pharmaceutical distribution of mifepristone in the future.

FDA approval of mifepristone and ECPs, such as Preven and Plan B, has made drug related reproductive therapy a real and potentially widespread option for women. Marketing campaigns by women's and abortion-rights groups and the drug manufacturers themselves will further introduce these drug options to women. This drug therapy revolution of sorts has expanded the pharmacist's role in the provision of emergency contraception, and perhaps, in the future, the provision of mifepristone.

The more women that are aware of and desire EC, the more involved and important pharmacists will become in the contraception process. One can imagine that if more and more states adopt the liberal EC distribution procedures of Washington and California, then pharmacists would become the primary providers of ECPs. And if mifepristone distribution restrictions are relaxed, pharmacists could feasibly become key players in the furnishing of abortion drugs as well. Whether they like it or not, pharmacists are being thrust into the role of common, everyday providers of controversial reproductive medications, and this position may put some pharmacists in the predicament of having to choose between their moral convictions regarding EC and abortion and the patient's wishes. . . .

The Pharmacist's Professional Ethical Obligations

Pharmacy is a profession, and much like the professions of medicine and law, entails a duty to assure and promote the patient's best interests. As professionals, pharmacists are expected to give priority to the patient's interests over their own immediate interests. As key players in the implementation of drug therapies, pharmacists are expected to withhold drugs "from those who have no authority to use them" and not to withhold "medications from those who do have authority to use them."

The patient's best interests are the pharmacist's primary commitment and concern. Among other things, pharmacists are expected to "help individuals achieve optimum benefit from their medications, to be committed to their welfare, and to maintain their trust"; to place "concern for the well-being of the patient at the center of professional practice" taking into consideration the "needs stated by the patient"; and to hold "the patient's welfare paramount." Further, patient autonomy and "personal and cultural differences among patients" must be respected by the pharmacist. These professional duties, and others, encompass the "collective conscience" of the pharmaceutical profession, and their implementation by each pharmacist is considered a moral obligation.

When presented with a validly authorized prescription for a legal medication, by a patient aware of the risks involved in taking the medication, and for whom the medication would be reasonably safe, the aforementioned principles and expectations leave the pharmacist with an ethical duty to fill and dispense the prescription. The duty to dispense in these circumstances may give rise to a serious conflict between the pharmacist's personal conviction concerning abortion and her professional duty to the patient.

In 1998, the American Pharmaceutical Association (APhA), and subsequently various other pharmaceutical organizations, eased the conflict between personal and professional morals by adopting policies recognizing a pharmacist's right to refuse dispensing medications based on the pharmacist's personal beliefs. However, if the pharmacist exercises her right of conscience and refuses to fill the prescription, the duty to the patient is not extinguished, and could be fulfilled by referring the patient to another pharmacist or distributor. In any event, "the patient should not be required to abide by the pharmacist's personal, moral decision." For many pharmacists, a referral would be no more than passive participation in the activity they initially refused to actively assist. Thus the dilemma, while transformed into whether to refer or not, is equally troublesome to the pharmacist.

Section II: The Potential Ramifications of Choosing Conscience

The pharmacist who ultimately decides that her moral convictions regarding abortion outweigh her professional obligation to the patient may refuse to fill the prescription and refer the patient to another pharmacist; or, the pharmacist with conscientious objection may refuse to dispense and refuse to refer. While the former decision will, in practical terms, shield the pharmacist from most negative consequences, the latter decision could have serious implications for the pharmacist, including employment termination or demotion, civil tort liability, or disciplinary action from the state pharmacy board. . . .

Legal protection must serve two purposes in order to appropriately ensure a pharmacist's right of conscientious refusal: 1) prevent and deter detrimental recriminatory action against the pharmacist; and 2) provide adequate remedies in the case that the pharmacist is sued or disciplined. The most efficient and effective means to these ends is the enactment of state and federal legislation.

The first step to successful enactment of pharmacist conscience legislation in each state and the United States is the cooperation of local, regional, and national pharmaceutical associations. The American Pharmaceutical Association took a large positive step when it adopted its pharmacist conscience clause. However, in the same pronouncement it rejected adoption of a policy encouraging enactment of state and national legal protection of the right of conscience. If pharmacists themselves, as represented by their professional associations and organizations, do not call for state and national legislative action, the road to adequate protection will be more difficult.

In any event, an effective conscience statute should take into consideration many complex issues including broad protection against recriminatory action, efficient administration of pharmacies, and accommodation of patients. First and foremost the conscience clause should serve its purpose stating clearly that no pharmacist shall be required to dispense abortion or EC drugs, nor shall any pharmacist be required to refer to another pharmacist who will dispense abortion or EC drugs. Although pharmacists currently have no role in the distribution of mifepristone, the abortion language should nonetheless be included as the potential for future pharmaceutical access exists. Next, the conscience statute should prohibit discrimination, civil liability, and professional disciplinary action that result from exercising the aforementioned rights of refusal. The statute should also encompass provisions prohibiting discrimination in the hiring process so as to preclude pharmacy-employers from screening applicants to avoid hiring pro-life pharmacists in the first place. Finally, the statute should provide adequate methods of deterrence. Employment discrimination could be deterred through its criminalization or by providing an express cause of action in tort as a remedy to the discriminatory hiring, firing, demotion, or promotion of pharmacists.

Employer and patient considerations should also exist in a pharmacist conscience clause. Prior notification of a pharmacist's beliefs regarding abortion and EC should be disclosed to the employer so as to enable efficient administration of the pharmacy. Further, patients should be put on notice in advance regarding when pharmacists with moral objections to abortion and EC will be on duty. For example, schedules could be posted conspicuously within a pharmacy as to when abortion and EC drugs will and will not be available to customer-patients. This will enable patients to avoid the hassle of going to a pharmacy and having their prescription refused. In any event, matters such as the aforementioned should be considered when drafting a pharmacist conscience clause.

Conclusion

Pharmacists, like other professionals such as physicians and attorneys, have a general duty to ensure their client's best interests, and thus must put the health of patients above all other considerations. Thus, it would seem to follow, when a pharmacist is presented with a valid prescription of what is safe for the patient to consume, the drugs should be distributed without dispute. However, to require that a pharmacist, or any professional, participate in what she would equate to the taking of a human life should never be a principle of professional ethics.

Certain issues, because of their inherent complexity and ambiguity, must be resolved, with guidance from religion, philosophy, and science, in the heart and mind of each individual. The commencement of human life and the relative sanctity of unborn life are issues that fall within this category of subjective individual determination. The thoughtful decision should be respected and free from vilifying recrimination. If a pharmacist, in her heart of hearts, concludes that accommodating prescriptions for abortive and EC medications is akin to directly facilitating the destruction of a precious human life, a refusal to accommodate such prescriptions should be protected under the law and within the profession. A safeguard of the right to refuse is imminently necessary as abortive drugs and EC become more widespread and risk of liability and loss of employment may compel many pharmacists to disregard their sacred beliefs or reap the consequences of their objections. Proactive acceptance of a pharmacist's conscientious objection to abortion and EC within the pharmaceutical community would pave the way to legislative protection already afforded doctors and nurses.

Julie Cantor and
Ken Baum

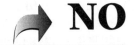 **NO**

The Limits of Conscientious Objection—May Pharmacists Refuse to Fill Prescriptions for Emergency Contraception?

Health policy decisions are often controversial, and the recent determination by the Food and Drug Administration (FDA) not to grant over-the-counter status to the emergency contraceptive Plan B was no exception. Some physicians decried the decision as a troubling clash of science, politics, and morality.[1] Other practitioners, citing safety, heralded the agency's prudence.[2] Public sentiment mirrored both views. Regardless, the decision preserved a major barrier to the acquisition of emergency contraception—the need to obtain and fill a prescription within a narrow window of efficacy. Six states have lowered that hurdle by allowing pharmacists to dispense emergency contraception without a prescription.[3–8] In those states, patients can simply bypass physicians. But the FDA's decision means that patients cannot avoid pharmacists. Because emergency contraception remains behind the counter, pharmacists can block access to it. And some have done just that.

Across the country, some pharmacists have refused to honor valid prescriptions for emergency contraception. In Texas, a pharmacist, citing personal moral grounds, rejected a rape survivor's prescription for emergency contraception.[9] A pharmacist in rural Missouri also refused to sell such a drug,[10] and in Ohio, Kmart fired a pharmacist for obstructing access to emergency and other birth control.[11] This fall, a New Hampshire pharmacist refused to fill a prescription for emergency contraception or to direct the patron elsewhere for help. Instead, he berated the 21-year-old single mother, who then, in her words, "pulled the car over in the parking lot and just cried."[12] Although the total number of incidents is unknown, reports of pharmacists who refused to dispense emergency contraception date back to 1991[13] and show no sign of abating.

Though nearly all states offer some level of legal protection for health care professionals who refuse to provide certain reproductive services, only Arkansas, Mississippi, and South Dakota explicitly protect pharmacists who refuse to dispense emergency and other contraception.[14] But that

From *The New England Journal of Medicine*, November 4, 2004, pp. 2008–2012. Copyright © 2004 by Massachusetts Medical Society. All rights reserved. Reprinted by permission.

list may grow. In past years, legislators from nearly two dozen states have taken "conscientious objection"—an idea that grew out of wartime tension between religious freedom and national obligation[15] and was co-opted into the reproductive-rights debate of the 1970s[16]—and applied it to pharmacists. One proposed law offers pharmacists immunity from civil lawsuits, criminal liability, professional sanctions, and employment repercussions.[17] Another bill, which was not passed, would have protected pharmacists who refused to transfer prescriptions.[18]

This issue raises important questions about individual rights and public health. Who prevails when the needs of patients and the morals of providers collide? Should pharmacists have a right to reject prescriptions for emergency contraception? The contours of conscientious objection remain unclear. This article elucidates those boundaries and offers a balanced solution to a complex problem. Because the future of over-the-counter emergency contraception is in flux, this issue remains salient for physicians and their patients.

Arguments in Favor of a Pharmacist's Right to Object

Pharmacists Can and Should Exercise Independent Judgment

Pharmacists, like physicians, are professionals. They complete a graduate program to gain expertise, obtain a state license to practice, and join a professional organization with its own code of ethics. Society relies on pharmacists to instruct patients on the appropriate use of medications and to ensure the safety of drugs prescribed in combination. Courts have held that pharmacists, like other professionals, owe their customers a duty of care.[19] In short, pharmacists are not automatons completing tasks; they are integral members of the health care team. Thus, it seems inappropriate and condescending to question a pharmacist's right to exercise personal judgment in refusing to fill certain prescriptions.

Professionals Should Not Forsake Their Morals as a Condition of Employment

Society does not require professionals to abandon their morals. Lawyers, for example, choose clients and issues to represent. Choice is also the norm in the health care setting. Except in emergency departments, physicians may select their patients and procedures. Ethics and law allow physicians, nurses, and physician assistants to refuse to participate in abortions and other reproductive services.[14, 20] Although some observers argue that active participation in an abortion is distinct from passively dispensing emergency contraception, others believe that making such a distinction between active and passive participation is meaningless, because both forms link the provider to the final outcome in the chain of causation.

Conscientious Objection Is Integral to Democracy

More generally, the right to refuse to participate in acts that conflict with personal ethical, moral, or religious convictions is accepted as an essential element of a democratic society. Indeed, Oregon acknowledged this freedom in its Death with Dignity Act,[21] which allows health care providers, including pharmacists, who are disquieted by physician-assisted suicide to refuse involvement without fear of retribution. Also, like the draftee who conscientiously objects to perpetrating acts of death and violence, a pharmacist should have the right not to be complicit in what they believe to be a morally ambiguous endeavor, whether others agree with that position or not. The reproductive-rights movement was built on the ideal of personal choice; denying choice for pharmacists in matters of reproductive rights and abortion seems ironic.

Arguments Against a Pharmacist's Right to Object

Pharmacists Choose to Enter a Profession Bound by Fiduciary Duties

Although pharmacists are professionals, professional autonomy has its limits. As experts on the profession of pharmacy explain, "Professionals are expected to exercise special skill and care to place the interests of their clients above their own immediate interests."[22] When a pharmacist's objection directly and detrimentally affects a patient's health, it follows that the patient should come first. Similarly, principles in the pharmacists' code of ethics weigh against conscientious objection. Given the effect on the patient if a pharmacist refuses to fill a prescription, the code undermines the right to object with such broadly stated objectives as "a pharmacist promotes the good of every patient in a caring, compassionate, and confidential manner," "a pharmacist respects the autonomy and dignity of each patient," and "a pharmacist serves individual, community, and societal needs."[23] Finally, pharmacists understand these fiduciary obligations when they choose their profession. Unlike conscientious objectors to a military draft, for whom choice is limited by definition, pharmacists willingly enter their field and adopt its corresponding obligations.

Emergency Contraception Is Not an Abortifacient

Although the subject of emergency contraception is controversial, medical associations,[24] government agencies,[25] and many religious groups agree that it is not akin to abortion. Plan B and similar hormones have no effect on an established pregnancy, and they may operate by more than one physiological mechanism, such as by inhibiting ovulation or creating an unfavorable environment for implantation of a blastocyst.[26] This duality allowed the Catholic Health Association to reconcile its religious beliefs with a mandate adopted by Washington State that emergency contraception must be provided to rape survivors.[27] According to the association, a patient and a provider who aim only to prevent conception follow Catholic teachings and state law. Also, whether one believes that pregnancy begins with fertilization or implantation, emergency contraception cannot fit squarely within the concept of abortion because one cannot be sure that conception has occurred.

Pharmacists' Objections Significantly Affect Patients' Health

Although religious and moral freedom is considered sacrosanct, that right should yield when it hinders a patient's ability to obtain timely medical treatment. Courts have held that religious freedom does not give health care providers an unfettered right to object to anything involving birth control, an embryo, or a fetus.[28, 29] Even though the Constitution protects people's beliefs, their actions may be regulated.[30] An objection must be balanced with the burden it imposes on others. In some cases, a pharmacist's objection imposes his or her religious beliefs on a patient. Pharmacists may decline to fill prescriptions for emergency contraception because they believe that the drug ends a life. Although the patient may disapprove of abortion, she may not share the pharmacist's beliefs about contraception. If she becomes pregnant, she may then face the question of abortion—a dilemma she might have avoided with the morning-after pill.

Furthermore, the refusal of a pharmacist to fill a prescription may place a disproportionately heavy burden on those with few options, such as a poor teenager living in a rural area that has a lone pharmacy. Whereas the savvy urbanite can drive to another pharmacy, a refusal to fill a prescription for a less advantaged patient may completely bar her access to medication. Finally, although Oregon does have an opt-out provision in its statute regulating assisted suicide, timing is much more important in emergency contraception than in assisted suicide. Plan B is most effective when used within 12 to 24 hours after unprotected intercourse.[31] An unconditional right to refuse is less compelling when the patient requests an intervention that is urgent.

Refusal Has Great Potential for Abuse and Discrimination

The limits to conscientious objection remain unclear. Pharmacists are privy to personal information through prescriptions. For instance, a customer who fills prescriptions for zidovudine, didanosine, and indinavir is logically assumed to be infected with the human immunodeficiency virus (HIV). If pharmacists can reject prescriptions that conflict with their morals, someone who believes that HIV-positive people must have engaged in immoral behavior could refuse to fill those prescriptions. Similarly, a pharmacist who does not condone extramarital sex might refuse to fill a sildenafil prescription for an unmarried man. Such objections go beyond "conscientious" to become invasive. Furthermore, because a pharmacist does not know a patient's history on the basis of a given prescription, judgments regarding the acceptability of a prescription may be medically inappropriate. To a woman with Eisenmenger's syndrome, for example, pregnancy may mean death. The potential for abuse by pharmacists underscores the need for policies ensuring that patients receive unbiased care.

Toward Balance

Compelling arguments can be made both for and against a pharmacist's right to refuse to fill prescriptions for emergency contraception. But even cogent ideas falter when confronted by a dissident moral code. Such is the nature of belief. Even so, most people can agree that we must find a workable and respectful balance between the needs of patients and the morals of pharmacists.

Three possible solutions exist: an absolute right to object, no right to object, or a limited right to object. On balance, the first two options are untenable. An absolute right to conscientious objection respects the autonomy of pharmacists but diminishes their professional obligation to serve patients. It may also greatly affect the health of patients, especially vulnerable ones, and inappropriately brings politics into the pharmacy. Even pharmacists who believe that emergency contraception represents murder and feel compelled to obstruct patients' access to it must recognize that contraception and abortion before fetal viability remain legal nationwide. In our view, state efforts to provide blanket immunity to objecting pharmacists are misguided. Pharmacies should follow the prevailing employment-law standard to make reasonable attempts to accommodate their employees' personal beliefs.[32] Although neutral policies to dispense medications to all customers may conflict with pharmacists' morals, such policies are not necessarily discriminatory, and pharmacies need not shoulder a heightened obligation of absolute accommodation.

Complete restriction of a right to conscientious objection is also problematic. Though pharmacists voluntarily enter their profession and have an obligation to serve patients without judgment, forcing them to abandon their morals imposes a heavy toll. Ethics and law demand that a professional's morality not interfere with the provision of care in life-or-death situations, such as a ruptured ectopic pregnancy.[29] Whereas the hours that elapse between intercourse and the intervention of emergency contraception are crucial, they do not meet that strict test. Also, patients who face an objecting pharmacist do have options, even if they are less preferable than having the prescription immediately filled. Because of these caveats, it is difficult to demand by law that pharmacists relinquish individual morality to stock and fill prescriptions for emergency contraception.

We are left, then, with the vast middle ground. Although we believe that the most ethical course is to treat patients compassionately—that is, to stock emergency contraception and fill prescriptions for it—the totality of the arguments makes us stop short of advocating a legal duty to do so as a first resort. We stop short for three reasons: because emergency contraception is not an absolute emergency, because other options exist, and because, when possible, the moral beliefs of those delivering care should be considered. However, in a profession that is bound by fiduciary obligations and strives to respect and care for patients, it is unacceptable to leave patients to fend for themselves. As a general rule, pharmacists who cannot or will not dispense a drug have an obligation to meet the needs of their customers by referring them elsewhere. This idea is uncontroversial when it is applied to common medications such as antibiotics and statins; it becomes contentious, but is equally valid, when it is applied to emergency contraception. Therefore, pharmacists who object should, as a matter of ethics and law, provide alternatives for patients.

Pharmacists who object to filling prescriptions for emergency contraception should arrange for another pharmacist to provide this service to customers promptly. Pharmacies that stock emergency contraception should ensure, to the extent possible, that at least one nonobjecting pharmacist is on duty at all times. Pharmacies that do not stock emergency contraception should give clear notice and refer patients elsewhere. At the very least, there should be a prominently displayed sign that says, "We do not provide emergency contraception. Please call Planned Parenthood at 800-230-PLAN (7526) . . . for assistance." However, a direct referral to a local pharmacy or pharmacist who is willing to fill the prescription is preferable. Objecting pharmacists should also redirect prescriptions for emergency contraception that are received by telephone to another pharmacy known to fill such prescriptions. In rural areas, objecting pharmacists should provide referrals within a reasonable radius.

Notably, the American Pharmacists Association has endorsed referrals, explaining that "providing alternative mechanisms for patients . . . ensures patient access to drug products, without requiring the pharmacist or the patient to abide by personal decisions other than their own."[33] A referral may also represent a break in causation between the pharmacist and distributing emergency contraception, a separation that the objecting pharmacist presumably seeks. And, in deference to the law's normative value, the rule of referral also conveys the importance of professional responsibility to patients. In areas of the country where referrals are logistically impractical, professional obligation may dictate providing emergency contraception, and a legal mandate may be appropriate if ethical obligations are unpersuasive.

Inevitably, some pharmacists will disregard our guidelines, and physicians—all physicians—should be prepared to fill gaps in care. They should identify pharmacies that will fill patients' prescriptions and encourage patients to keep emergency contraception at home. They should be prepared to dispense emergency contraception or instruct patients to mimic it with other birth-control pills. In Wisconsin, family-planning clinics recently began dispensing emergency contraception, and the state set up a toll-free hotline to help patients find physicians who will prescribe it.[34] Emergency departments should stock emergency contraception and make it available to rape survivors, if not all patients.

In the final analysis, education remains critical. Pharmacists may have misconceptions about emergency contraception. In one survey, a majority of pharmacists mistakenly agreed with the statement that repeated use of emergency contraception is medically risky.[35] Medical misunderstandings that lead pharmacists to refuse to fill prescriptions for emergency contraception are unacceptable. Patients, too, may misunderstand or be unaware of emergency contraception.[36] Physicians should teach patients about this option before the need arises, since patients may understand their choices better when they are not under stress. Physicians should discuss emergency contraception during office visits, offer prescriptions in advance of need, and provide education through pamphlets or the Internet. Web sites . . . allow users to search for physicians who prescribe emergency contraception by ZIP Code, area code, or address, and Planned Parenthood offers extensive educational information . . . , including details about off-label use of many birth-control pills for emergency contraception.

Our principle of a compassionate duty of care should apply to all health care professionals. In a secular society, they must be prepared to limit the reach of their personal objection. Objecting pharmacists may choose to find employment opportunities that comport with their morals—in a religious community, for example—but when they pledge to serve the public, it is unreasonable to expect those in need of health care to acquiesce to their personal convictions. Similarly, physicians who refuse to write prescriptions for emergency contraception should follow the rules of notice and referral for the reason previously articulated: the beliefs of health care providers should not trump patient care. It is difficult enough to be faced with the consequences of rape or of an unplanned pregnancy; health care providers should not make the situation measurably worse.

Former Supreme Court Chief Justice Charles Evans Hughes called the quintessentially American custom of respect for conscience a "happy tradition"[37]—happier, perhaps, when left in the setting of a draft objection than when pitting one person's beliefs against another's reproductive health. Ideally, conflicts about emergency contraception will be rare, but they will occur. In July, 11 nurses in Alabama resigned rather than provide emergency contraception in state clinics.[38] As patients understand their birth-control options, conflicts at the pharmacy counter and in the clinic may become more common. When professionals' definitions of liberty infringe on those they choose to serve, a respectful balance must be struck. We offer one solution. Even those who challenge this division of burdens and benefits should agree with our touchstone—although health professionals may have a right to object, they should not have a right to obstruct.

References

1. Drazen JM, Greene MF, Wood AJJ. The FDA, politics, and Plan B. N Engl J Med 2004;350:1561–2.
2. Stanford JB, Hager WD, Crockett SA. The FDA, politics, and Plan B. N Engl J Med 2004;350:2413–4.
3. Alaska Admin. Code tit. 12, § 52.240 (2004).
4. Cal. Bus. & Prof. Code § 4052 (8) (2004).
5. Hawaii Rev. Stat. § 461-1 (2003).
6. N.M. Admin. Code § 16.19.26.9 (2003).
7. Wash. Rev. Code § 246-863-100 (2004).
8. Me. Rev. Stat. Ann. tit.32, §§ 13821-13825 (2004).
9. Pharmacist refuses pill for victim. Chicago Tribune. February 11, 2004:C7.
10. Simon S. Pharmacists new players in abortion debate. Los Angeles Times. March 20, 2004:A18.

11. Sweeney JF. May a pharmacist refuse to fill a prescription? Plain Dealer. May 5, 2004:E1.

12. Associated Press. Pharmacist refuses to fill morning after prescription.

13. Sauer M. Pharmacist to be fired in abortion controversy. St. Petersburg Times. December 19, 1991:1B.

14. State policies in brief: refusing to provide health services. New York: Alan Guttmacher Institute, September 1, 2004.

15. Seeley RA. Advice for conscientious objectors in the armed forces. 5th ed. Philadelphia: Central Committee for Conscientious Objectors, 1998:1–2.

16. 42 U.S.C. § 300a-7 (2004).

17. Mich. House Bill No. 5006 (As amended April 21, 2004).

18. Oregon House Bill No. 2010 (As amended May 11, 1999).

19. Hooks Super X, Inc. v. McLaughlin, 642 N.E. 2d 514 (Ind. 1994).

20. Section 2.01. In: Council on Ethical and Judicial Affairs. Code of medical ethics: current opinions with annotations. 2002–2003 ed. Chicago: American Medical Association, 2002.

21. Oregon Revised Statute § 127.885 § 4.01 (4) (2003).

22. Fassett WE, Wicks AC. Is pharmacy a profession? In: Weinstein BD, ed. Ethical issues in pharmacy. Vancouver, Wash.: Applied Therapeutics, 1996:1–28.

23. American Pharmacists Association. Code of ethics for pharmacists: preamble.

24. Hughes EC, ed. Obstetric-gynecologic terminology, with section on neonatology and glossary of congenital anomalies. Philadelphia: F.A. Davis, 1972.

25. Commodity Supplemental Food Program, 7 C.F.R. § 247.2 (2004).

26. Glasier A. Emergency postcoital contraception. N Engl J Med 1997; 337:1058–64.

27. Daily reproductive health report: state politics & policy: Washington governor signs law requiring hospitals to offer emergency contraception to rape survivors. Menlo Park, Calif.: Kaisernetwork, April 2, 2002.

28. Brownfield v. Daniel Freeman Marina Hospital, 208 Cal. App. 3d 405 (Cal. Ct. App. 1989).

29. Shelton v. Univ. of Medicine & Dentistry, 223 F.3d 220 (3d Cir. 2000).

30. Tribe LH. American constitutional law. 2nd ed. Mineola, N.Y.: Foundation Press, 1988:1183.

31. Brody JE. The politics of emergency contraception. New York Times. August 24, 2004:F7.

32. Trans World Airlines v. Hardison, 432 U.S. 63 (1977).

33. 1997–98 APhA Policy Committee report: pharmacist conscience clause. Washington, D.C.: American Pharmacists Association, 1997.

34. Politics wins over science. Capital Times. May 13, 2004:16A.

35. Alford S, Davis L, Brown L. Pharmacists' attitudes and awareness of emergency contraception for adolescents. Transitions 2001;12(4):1–17.

36. Foster DG, Harper CC, Bley JJ, et al. Knowledge of emergency contraception among women aged 18 to 44 in California. Am J Obstet Gynecol 2004;191:150–6.

37. United States v. Macintosh, 283 U.S. 605, 634 (1931) (Hughes, C.J., dissenting).

38. Elliott D. Alabama nurses quit over morning-after pill. Presented on All Things Considered. Washington, D.C.: National Public Radio, July 28, 2004 (transcript). *Copyright © 2004 Massachusetts Medical Society.*

EXPLORING THE ISSUE

Should Pharmacists Be Allowed to Deny Prescriptions on Grounds of Conscience?

Critical Thinking and Reflection

1. How do you believe individual rights should be balanced against the social good? Individual freedom of speech and freedom to refuse vaccinations are typically thought to be limited in certain cases in which exercising those freedoms may lead to social harms; how does this balancing principle translate to the case of pharmacists filling prescriptions?
2. Does filling a prescription make a pharmacist complicit in the woman's use of the drug? Explain your reasoning.
3. If a pharmacist refuses to fill a prescription but helps a woman find someone else who will fill it, is the pharmacist as complicit in the woman's act as if he had filled the prescription himself? Explain your reasoning.

Is There Common Ground?

In November 2004, the FDA announced a labeling change for mifepristone. Because the FDA and the manufacturer Danco Laboratories had received reports of serious side effects, the warning label was changed to reflect this new information.

Both the U.S. federal government and the great majority of states have laws protecting conscientious objectors in health care. The Illinois Health Care Right of Conscience Act is particularly detailed and protects physicians, health care personnel, health care facilities, and health care payers who refuse to participate in services that are contrary to their conscience. In April 2005, however, Gov. Rod Blagojevich issued an emergency rule requiring pharmacies to fill prescriptions for birth control and mifepristone "without delay." Bills have been introduced that specifically include pharmacists in the Health Care Right of Conscience Act.

As of 2012, six states (Arizona, Arkansas, Georgia, Idaho, Mississippi, and South Dakota) have laws specifically recognizing a pharmacist's right of conscientious objection. A California law requires pharmacists to dispense these drugs unless the employer approves the refusal and the woman has another way of filling the prescription. A New Jersey law prohibits pharmacists from refusing to fill prescriptions on moral, religious, or ethical grounds.

Additional Resources

The National Conference of State Legislatures monitors state legislative activity on conscience clause laws. See www.ncsl.org/programs/health/conscienceclauses.htm.

A national survey of physicians found that physicians who were male, religious, and had moral objections to controversial but legal procedures like administering terminal sedation in dying patients or prescribing birth control to teenagers without parental approval were less likely to report that doctors must disclose information or refer patients for these medical procedures (Farr A. Curlin et al., "Religion, Conscience, and Controversial Clinical Practices," *The New England Journal of Medicine* [February 8, 2007]).

In "Pharmacies, Pharmacists, and Conscientious Objection," Mark R. Wicclair argues that the health needs of patients and the professional obligations of pharmacists limit the extent to which they may refuse to assist patients who have lawful prescriptions for medically indicated drugs (*Kennedy Institute of Ethics Journal* [vol. 16, no. 3, 2006]). On the other hand, Brian P. Knestout asserts that "conscience clauses" protect medical professionals who do not wish to perform or assist in procedures related to abortion, sterilization, or euthanasia ("An Essential Prescription: Why Pharmacist-Inclusive Clauses Are Necessary," *Journal of Contemporary Health Lawand Policy*, [Spring 2006]).

Adrienne Asch compares conscientious objections to health care practices to similar behavior in times of war and offers limited support for these exceptions to professional responsibility ("Two Cheers for Conscience Exceptions," *Hastings Center Report* [November–December 2006]).

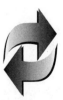

Internet References . . .

Presidential Commission for the Study of Bioethical Issues

The Web site of the commission provides access both to its own reports and to the work of many past presidential bioethics commissions.

www.bioethics.gov/

World Anti-Drug Doping Agency

This international organization has information for athletes, coaches, fans, and others about the use of drugs in sports.

www.wada-ama.org

The Woodrow Wilson International Center for Scholars

The Wilson Center offers a variety of resources about the ethical debate and government oversight of synthetic biology.

www.synbioproject.org/

The Development and Use of Biotechnology

*T*he growth of medical and biological science and technology has created enormous possibilities for understanding heredity and its influence on disease, for identifying and perhaps also treating people who are at risk for genetic diseases, and for changing human bodies in ways that have nothing to do with the treatment of disease. More, human understanding of the mysteries of life and mastery of techniques for controlling life put humans in the place, perhaps, of creating new forms of life—organisms specially designed to serve various human needs or wants. All scientific and technical breakthroughs bring unresolved questions, however. And the track record is not always great: The abuse of genetic information (much of it misinformation) in the past haunt efforts today to use this information wisely and compassionately. What impact will medical and biological knowledge and technology have on our lives and futures, and on the lives and futures of our children? These are some of the challenging issues raised in this unit.

- Is the Use of Medical Tools to Enhance Human Beings Morally Troubling?

- Should Performance-Enhancing Drugs Be Banned from Sports?

- May Doctors Offer Medical Drugs and Surgery to Stop a Disabled Child from Maturing?

- Should Scientists Create Artificial Organisms?

ISSUE 12

Is the Use of Medical Tools to Enhance Human Beings Morally Troubling?

YES: **President's Council on Bioethics,** from *Beyond Therapy: Biotechnology and the Pursuit of Happiness* (U.S. Government Printing Office, 2003)

NO: **Howard Trachtman,** from "A Man Is a Man Is a Man," *The American Journal of Bioethics* (May/June 2005)

Learning Outcomes

After reading this issue, you should be able to:

- Discuss a range of arguments for and against using medical technologies to enhance human bodies and behavior.
- Identify some claims commonly made about human nature in the debate about enhancement.

ISSUE SUMMARY

YES: The President's Council on Bioethics, a presidential body formed by President Bush, argues that biotechnological interventions for making people better than normal raise profound concerns about the relationship between humans and nature, human identity, and human happiness.

NO: Physician Howard Trachtman says that the medical community should embrace enhancement as a never-ending quest for health that recognizes that perfection can never be achieved.

$\mathbf{P}$erhaps more than any other people, Americans seem to be obsessed with self-improvement. Each year there is a flood of new books and television commercials promoting ways to be richer, thinner, smarter, happier, healthier, more successful, attractive, or all of the above. Whatever one's presumed character or bodily flaw, there is a remedy. And for parents, there is an additional opportunity (sometimes presented as an obligation) to make one's children richer, thinner, smarter, happier, or all of the above.

Traditionally, most of these strategies for improving ourselves or our children are activities or experiences—education, exercise, summer camps, yoga, and so on. But what if we could change that? What if the self-improvement could be achieved with much less work, or without real work at all—in effect dropping the kinds of activities that the term "self-improvement" brings to mind and more directly *enhancing* ourselves or our children? The most obvious targets for enhancement include physical form and functioning, cognitive functioning, and mood or temperament, but conceivably we could even go beyond the traditional targets of self-improvement and enhance such seeming givens of human life as lifespan, so that we lived hundreds of years or more.

Increasingly, if incrementally, biotechnologies seem to offer this promise. A biotechnological enhancement strategy that is by now relatively familiar is the use of pharmaceuticals, such as performance-enhancing drugs in sports (discussed in issue 13) or cognitive enhancers, such as Ritalin, in the classroom. Certain antidepressants are thought to have the ability to enhance mood. Surgery sometimes offers another familiar though limited route to enhancement, at least of bodily form.

Foreseeable sometime in the future is enhancement through genetic manipulation. This could happen by identifying genes that confer improved capabilities (which is much more difficult than news stories usually suggest, but may for at least some traits prove feasible) and transferring them into a person's somatic cells—into muscles to produce superior physical performance, for example—or into germline cells—that is, the cells that produce gametes—so that the changes would be passed from generation to generation. The first method would allow individuals to seek genetic enhancements for themselves or for their children, if the genes were transferred into their children's bodies, and the second would be a way of enhancing both one's children and subsequent generations.

The basic idea of genetic enhancement is arguably not new. Germline genetic enhancement has been practiced for centuries in animal husbandry and agriculture. By breeding for certain characteristics, animals and plants have been created to better meet human purposes. The largest Great Dane and the smallest Pekinese, and all the dog breeds in between, are descended from a handful of wolves tamed by humans in Asia nearly 15,000 years ago. Over the last 500 years, humans have practiced breeding techniques that account for vastly different appearances and characteristics of modern dogs.

Applying these techniques to humans—the theory of eugenics or "better genes"—also has a long but disastrous history. Its advocates, many of them in the United States in the twentieth century, advocated the elimination of "undesirable" people by preventing them from reproducing through involuntary sterilization. In the most malevolent form of eugenics, of course, the Nazi regime in Germany in the 1930s wanted to create a "master race" by encouraging reproduction among blonde, blue-eyed, tall Aryan types and eliminating from the gene pool by murdering those from other population groups, such as Jews and gypsies.

While these eugenics methods are not only barbarous and morally corrupt, the idea of enhancing one's capacities and those of future generations has been given new life by scientific advances in genetics. Being able to manipulate genes—the very core of human inheritance—opens up a new world of possibilities. Already animals like sheep and cows have been cloned, that is, their genomes were transferred into eggs to create animals that are genetically identical (although the animals are never entirely identical because of uterine and environmental differences). In principle, if the genetic contributions to traits can be identified, it might eventually be possible to use genetic enhancement to conduct a new eugenics—a "liberal eugenics"—in which the birth of people with desirable traits is promoted although people with undesirable traits are not targeted or suppressed.

Enhancement raises an assortment of ethical questions. Even if it is possible to enhance an individual's height, beauty, intelligence, or capacity for happiness, is it desirable? If these techniques proved to be safe and effective, would they be distributed fairly throughout society?

These questions are at the core of the selections that follow. The President's Council on Bioethics, a presidential commission formed during the administration of George W. Bush and chaired by the physician and philosopher Leon Kass, argues that there are a number of moral problems with enhancement, whether it is undertaken for one's own benefit or for one's children. Physician Howard Trachtman, on the other hand, accepts enhancement as a new way of expressing a natural desire to improve health and well-being. He believes that we should not fear progress or try to limit medical manipulations.

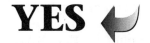
Beyond Therapy: Biotechnology and the Pursuit of Happiness

Before proceeding, we wish to reiterate our intention in this inquiry, so as to avoid misunderstanding. In offering our synopsis of concerns, we are not making predictions; we are merely pointing to possible hazards, hazards that become visible only when one looks at "the big picture." More important, we are not condemning either biotechnological power or the pursuit of happiness, excellence, or self-perfection. Far from it. We eagerly embrace biotechnologies as aids for preventing or correcting bodily or mental ills and for restoring health and fitness. We even more eagerly embrace the pursuits of happiness, excellence, and self-improvement, for ourselves, our children, and our society. Desires for these goals are the source of much that is good in human life. Yet, as has long been known, these desires can be excessive. Worse, they can be badly educated regarding the nature of their object, sometimes with tragic result: we get what we ask for only to discover that it is very far from what we really wanted. Finally, they can be pursued in harmful ways and with improper means, often at the price of deforming the very goals being sought. To guard against such outcomes, we need to be alert in advance to the more likely risks and the more serious concerns. We begin with those that are more obvious and familiar.

Familiar Sources of Concern

The first concerns commonly expressed regarding any uses of biotechnology beyond therapy reflect, not surprisingly, the dominant values of modern America: health and safety, fairness and equality, and freedom. The following thumbnail sketches of the issues should suffice to open the questions—though of course not to settle them.

A. Health: Issues of Safety and Bodily Harm

In our health-conscious culture, the first reason people worry about any biotechnical intervention, whatever its intended purpose, is safety. This will surely be true regarding "elective" uses of biotechnology that aim beyond therapy. Athletes who take steroids to boost their strength may later suffer premature heart disease. College students who snort Ritalin to increase their concentration may become addicted. Melancholics taking mood-brighteners to change

From the President's Council on Bioethics, October 2003.

their outlook may experience impotence or apathy. To generalize: no biological agent used for purposes of self-perfection or self-satisfaction is likely to be entirely safe. This is good medical common sense: anything powerful enough to enhance system A is likely to be powerful enough to harm system B (or even system A itself), the body being a highly complex yet integrated whole in which one intervenes partially only at one's peril. And it surely makes sense, ethically speaking, that one should not risk basic health pursuing a condition of "better than well."

Yet some of the interventions that might aim beyond therapy—for example, genetic enhancement of muscle strength, retardation of aging, or pharmacologic blunting of horrible memories or increasing self-esteem—may, indirectly, lead also to improvements in general health. More important, many good things in life are filled with risks, and free people—even if properly informed about the magnitude of those risks—may choose to run them if they care enough about what they might gain thereby. . . .

B. Unfairness

An obvious objection to the use of enhancement technologies, especially by participants in competitive activities, is that they give those who use them an unfair advantage: blood doping or steroids in athletes, stimulants in students taking the SATs, and so on. This issue . . . has been well aired by the International Olympic Committee and the many other athletic organizations who continue to try to formulate rules that can be enforced, even as the athletes and their pharmacists continue to devise ways to violate those rules and escape detection. Yet as we saw, the fairness question can be turned on its head, and some people see in biotechnical intervention a way to compensate for the "unfairness" of natural inequalities—say, in size, strength, drive, or native talent. Still, even if everyone had equal access to genetic improvement of muscle strength or mind-enhancing drugs, or even if these gifts of technology would be used only to rectify the inequalities produced by the unequal gifts of nature, an additional disquiet would still perhaps remain: The disquiet of using such new powers in the first place or at all, even were they fairly distributed. . . .

C. Equality of Access

A related question concerns inequality of access to the benefits of biotechnology, a matter of great interest to many Members of this Council. . . . The issue of distributive justice is more important than the issue of unfairness in competitive activities, especially if there are systemic disparities between those who will and those who won't have access to the powers of biotechnical "improvement." Should these capabilities arrive, we may face severe aggravations of existing "unfairnesses" in the "game of life," especially if people who need certain agents to treat serious illness cannot get them while other people can enjoy them for less urgent or even dubious purposes. If, as is now often the case with expensive medical care, only the wealthy and privileged will be able to gain easy access to costly enhancing technologies, we might expect to see an ever-widening gap between "the best and the brightest" and the rest. The emergence of a biotechnologically improved "aristocracy"—augmenting the already cognitively stratified structure of American society—is indeed a worrisome possibility, and there is nothing in our current way of doing business that works against it. Indeed, unless something new intervenes, it would seem to be a natural outcome of mixing these elements of American society: our existing inequalities in wealth and status, the continued use of free markets to develop and obtain the new technologies, and our libertarian attitudes favoring unrestricted personal freedom for all choices in private life.

Yet the situation regarding rich and poor is more complex, especially if one considers actual benefits rather than equality or relative well-being. The advent of new technologies often brings great benefits to the less well off, if not at first, then after they come to be mass-produced and massmarketed and the prices come down. (Consider, over the past half-century, the spread in the United States of refrigerators and radios, automobiles and washing machines, televisions and VCRs, cell phones and personal computers, and, in the domain of medicine, antibiotics, vaccines, and many expensive diagnostic and therapeutic procedures.) To be sure, the gap between the richest and the poorest may increase, but in absolute terms the poor may benefit more, when compared not to the rich but to where they were before. . . .

D. Liberty: Issues of Freedom and Coercion, Overt and Subtle

A concern for threats to freedom comes to the fore whenever biotechnical powers are exercised by some people upon other people. We encountered it in our discussion of "better children" (the choice of a child's sex or the drug-mediated alteration of his or her behavior . . .), as well as in the coerced use of anabolic steroids by the East German Olympic swimmers. . . . This problem will of course be worse in tyrannical regimes. But there are always dangers of despotism within families, as many parents already work their wills on their children with insufficient regard to a child's independence or long-term needs, jeopardizing even the "freedom to be a child." To the extent that even partial control over genotype—say, to take a relatively innocent example, musician parents selecting a child with genes for perfect pitch—would add to existing social instruments of parental control and its risks of despotic rule, this matter will need to be attended to. Leaving aside the special case of children, the risk of overt coercion does not loom large in a free society. On the contrary, many enthusiasts for using technology for personal enhancement are libertarian in outlook; they see here mainly the enlargement of human powers and possibilities and the multiplication of options for private choice, both of which they see as steps to greater human freedom. They look forward to growing opportunities for more people to earn more, learn more, see more, and do more, and to choose—perhaps several times in one lifetime—interesting new careers or avocations. And they look with suspicion at critics who they fear might want to limit their private freedom to develop and use new technologies for personal advancement or, indeed, for any purpose whatsoever. The coercion they fear comes not from advances in technology but from the state, acting to deny them their right to pursue happiness or self-improvement by the means they privately choose.

Yet no one can deny that people living in free societies, and even their most empowered citizens, already experience more subtle impingements on freedom and choice, operating, for example, through peer pressure. What is freely permitted and widely used may, under certain circumstances, become practically mandatory. If most children are receiving memory enhancement or stimulant drugs, failure to provide them for your child might be seen as a form of child neglect. If all the defensive linemen are on steroids, you risk mayhem if you go against them chemically pure. And, a point subtler still, some critics complain that, as with cosmetic surgery, Botox, and breast implants, many of the enhancement technologies of the future will very likely be used in slavish adherence to certain socially defined and merely fashionable notions of "excellence" or improvement, very likely shallow and conformist. If these fears are realized, such exercises of individual freedom, suitably multiplied, might compromise the freedom to be an individual.

This special kind of reduction of freedom—let's call it the problem of conformity or homogenization—is of more than individual concern. In an era of mass culture, itself the byproduct of previous advances in communication, manufacture, and marketing techniques, the exercise of uncoerced private choices may produce untoward consequences for society as a whole. Trends in popular culture lead some critics to worry that the self-selected nontherapeutic uses of the new biotechnical powers, should they become widespread, will be put in the service of the most common human desires, moving us toward still greater homogenization of human society—perhaps raising the floor but also lowering the ceiling of human possibility, and reducing the likelihood of genuine freedom, individuality, and greatness. . . .

Essential Sources of Concern

Our familiar worries about issues of safety, equality, and freedom, albeit very important, do not exhaust the sources of reasonable concern. When richly considered, they invite us to think about the deeper purposes for the sake of which we want to live safely, justly, and freely. And they enable us to recognize that even the safe, equally available, noncoerced and non-faddish uses of biomedical technologies to pursue happiness or self-improvement raise ethical and social questions, questions more directly connected with the essence of the activity itself: the use of technological means to intervene into the human body and mind, not to ameliorate their diseases but to change and improve their normal workings. Why, if at all, are we bothered by the voluntary self-administration of agents that would change our bodies or alter our minds? What is disquieting about our attempts to improve upon human nature, or even our own particular instance of it?

The subject being relatively novel, it is difficult to put this worry into words. We are in an area where initial revulsions are hard to translate into sound moral arguments. Many people are probably repelled by the idea of drugs that erase memories or that change personalities, or of interventions that enable seventy-year-olds to bear children or play professional sports, or, to engage in some wilder imaginings, of mechanical implants that would enable men to nurse infants or computer-brain hookups that would enable us to download the Oxford English Dictionary. But can our disquiet at such prospects withstand rational, anthropological, or ethical scrutiny? Taken one person at a time, with a properly prepared set of conditions and qualifications, it will be hard to say what is wrong with any biotechnical intervention that could improve our performances, give us (more) ageless bodies, or make it possible for us to have happier souls. Indeed, in many cases, we ought to be thankful for or pleased with the improvements our biotechnical ingenuity is making possible. . . .

A. Hubris or Humility: Respect for "the Given"

A common, man-on-the-street reaction to the prospects of biotechnological engineering beyond therapy is the complaint of "man playing God." If properly unpacked, this worry is in fact shared by people holding various theological beliefs and by people holding none at all. Sometimes the charge means the sheer prideful presumption of trying to alter what God has ordained or nature has produced, or what should, for whatever reason, not be fiddled with. Sometimes the charge means not so much usurping Godlike powers, but doing so in the absence of God-like knowledge: the mere playing at being God, the hubris of acting with insufficient wisdom. . . .

One revealing way to formulate the problem of hubris is what one of our Council Members has called the temptation to "hyper-agency," a Promethean aspiration to remake nature, including human nature, to serve our purposes and to satisfy our desires. This attitude is to be faulted not only because it can lead to bad, unintended consequences; more fundamentally, it also represents a false understanding of, and an improper disposition toward, the naturally given world. The root of the difficulty seems to be both cognitive and moral: the failure properly to appreciate and respect the "giftedness" of the world. Acknowledging the giftedness of life means recognizing that our talents and powers are not wholly our own doing, nor even fully ours, despite the efforts we expend to develop and to exercise them. It also means recognizing that not everything in the world is open to any use we may desire or devise. Such an appreciation of the giftedness of life would constrain the Promethean project and conduce to a much-needed humility. Although it is in part a religious sensibility, its resonance reaches beyond religion.

Human beings have long manifested both wondering appreciation for nature's beauty and grandeur and reverent awe before nature's sublime and mysterious power. . . . [A]ppreciating that the given world—including our natural powers to alter it—is not of our own making could induce a welcome attitude of modesty, restraint, and humility. Such a posture is surely recommended for anyone inclined to modify human beings or human nature for purposes beyond therapy.

Yet the respectful attitude toward the "given," while both necessary and desirable as a restraint, is not by itself sufficient as a guide. The "giftedness of nature" also includes smallpox and malaria, cancer and Alzheimer disease, decline and decay. Moreover, nature is not equally generous with her gifts, even to man, the most gifted of her creatures. Modesty born of gratitude for the world's "givenness" may enable us to recognize that not everything in the world is open to any use we may desire or devise, but it will not by itself teach us which things can be tinkered with and which should be left inviolate. Respect for the "giftedness" of things cannot tell us which gifts are to be accepted as is, which are to be improved through use or training, which are to be housebroken through self-command or medication, and which opposed like the plague. . . .

B. "Unnatural" Means: The Dignity of Human Activity

Until only yesterday, teaching and learning or practice and training exhausted the alternatives for acquiring human excellence, perfecting our natural gifts through our own efforts. But perhaps no longer: biotechnology may be able to do nature one better, even to the point of requiring less teaching, training, or practice to permit an improved nature to shine forth. As we noted earlier, the insertion of the growth-factor gene into the muscles of rats and mice bulks them up and keeps them strong and sound without the need for nearly as much exertion. Drugs to improve alertness (today) or memory and amiability (tomorrow) could greatly relieve the need for exertion to acquire these powers, leaving time and effort for better things. What, if anything, is disquieting about such means of gaining improvement?

The problem cannot be that they are "artificial," in the sense of having man-made origins. Beginning with the needle and the fig leaf, man has from the start been the animal that uses art to improve his lot by altering or adding to what nature alone provides. Ordinary medicine makes extensive use of similar artificial means, from drugs to surgery to mechanical implants, in order to treat disease. If the use of artificial means is absolutely welcome in the activity of healing, it cannot be their unnaturalness alone that disquiets us when they are used to make people "better than well."

Still, in those areas of human life in which excellence has until now been achieved only by discipline and effort, the attainment of similar results by means of drugs, genetic engineering, or implanted devices looks to many people (including some Members of this Council) to be "cheating" or "cheap." Many people believe that each person should work hard for his achievements. Even if we prefer the grace of the natural athlete or the quickness of the natural mathematician—people whose performances deceptively appear to be effortless—we admire also those who overcome obstacles and struggle to try to achieve the excellence of the former. This matter of character—the merit of disciplined and dedicated striving—is surely pertinent. For character is not only the source of our deeds, but also their product. As we have already noted, healthy people whose disruptive behavior is "remedied" by pacifying drugs rather than by their own efforts are not learning self-control; if anything, they may be learning to think it unnecessary. People who take pills to block out from memory the painful or hateful aspects of a new experience will not learn how to deal with suffering or sorrow. A drug that induces fearlessness does not produce courage.

Yet things are not so simple. Some biotechnical interventions may assist in the pursuit of excellence without in the least cheapening its attainment. And many of life's excellences have nothing to do with competition or overcoming adversity. Drugs to decrease drowsiness, increase alertness, sharpen memory, or reduce distraction may actually help people interested in their natural pursuits of learning or painting or performing their civic duty. Drugs to steady the hand of a neurosurgeon or to prevent sweaty palms in a concert pianist cannot be regarded as "cheating," for they are in no sense the source of the excellent activity or achievement. And, for people dealt a meager hand in the dispensing of nature's gifts, it should not be called cheating or cheap if biotechnology could assist them in becoming better equipped—whether in body or in mind.

Nevertheless, . . . there remains a sense that the "naturalness" of means matters. It lies not in the fact that the assisting drugs and devices are artifacts, but in the danger of violating or deforming the nature of human agency and the dignity of the naturally human way of activity. In most of our ordinary efforts at self-improvement, whether by practice, training, or study, we sense the relation between our doings and the resulting improvement, between the means used and the end sought. . . . In contrast, biotechnical interventions act directly on the human body and mind to bring about their effects on a passive subject, who plays little or no role at all.

C. Identity and Individuality

With biotechnical interventions that skip the realm of intelligible meaning, we cannot really own the transformations nor can we experience them as genuinely ours. And we will be at a loss to attest whether the resulting conditions and activities of our bodies and our minds are, in the fullest sense, our own as human. But our interest in identity is also more personal. For we do not live in a generic human way; we desire, act, flourish, and decline as ourselves, as individuals. To be human is to be someone, not anyone—with a given nature (male or female), given natural abilities (superior wit or musical talent), and— most important—a real history of attachments, memories, and experiences, acquired largely by living with others.

In myriad ways, new biotechnical powers promise (or threaten) to transform what it means to be an individual: giving increased control over our identity to others, as in the case of genetic screening or sex selection of offspring by parents; inducing psychic states divorced from real life and lived experience; blunting or numbing the memories we wish to escape; and achieving the results we could never achieve unaided, by acting as ourselves alone.

To be sure, in many cases, biomedical technology can restore or preserve a real identity that is slipping away: keeping our memory intact by holding off the scourge of Alzheimer disease; restoring our capacity to love and work by holding at bay the demons of self-destroying depression. In other cases, the effect of biotechnology on identity is much more ambiguous. By taking psychotropic drugs to reduce anxiety or overcome melancholy, we may become the person we always wished to be—more cheerful, ambitious, relaxed, content. But we also become a different person in the eyes of others, and in many cases we become dependent on the continued use of psychotropic drugs to remain the new person we now are. . . .

D. Partial Ends, Full Flourishing

Beyond the perils of achieving our desired goals in a "less-than-human way" or in ways "not fully our own," we must consider the meaning of the ends themselves: better children, superior performance, ageless bodies, and happy souls. Would their attainment in fact improve or perfect our lives as human beings? Are they—always or ever—reasonable and attainable goals?. . .

In many cases, biotechnologies can surely help us cultivate what is best in ourselves and in our children, providing new tools for realizing good ends, wisely pursued. But it is also possible that the new technological means may deform the ends themselves. In pursuit of better children, biotechnical powers risk making us "tyrants"; in pursuit of superior performance, they risk making us "artifacts." In both cases, the problem is not the ends themselves but our misguided idea of their attainment or our false way of seeking to attain them. And in both cases, there is the ubiquitous problem that "good" or "superior" will be reconceived to fit the sorts of goals that the technological interventions can help us attain. We may come to believe that genetic predisposition or brain chemistry holds the key to helping our children develop and improve, or that stimulant drugs or bulkier muscles hold the key to excellent human activity. If we are equipped with hammers, we will see only those things that can be improved by pounding.

The goals of ageless bodies and happy souls—and especially the ways biotechnology might shape our pursuit of these ends—are perhaps more complicated. The case for ageless bodies seems at first glance to look pretty good. The prevention of decay, decline, and disability, the avoidance of blindness, deafness, and debility, the elimination of feebleness, frailty, and fatigue, all seem to be conducive to living fully as a human being at the top of one's powers—of having, as they say, a "good quality of life" from beginning to end. . . . And, should aging research deliver on its promise of adding not only extra life to years but also extra years to life, who would refuse it?

But . . . there may in fact be many human goods that are inseparable from our aging bodies, from our living in time, and especially from the natural human life cycle by which each generation gives way to the one that follows it. Because this argument is so counterintuitive, we need to begin not with the individual choice for an ageless body, but with what the individual's life might look like in a world in which everyone made the same choice. We need to make the choice universal, and see the meaning of that choice in the mirror of its becoming the norm.

What if everybody lived life to the hilt, even as they approached an ever-receding age of death in a body that looked and functioned—let's not be too greedy—like that of a thirty-year-old? Would it be good if each and all of us lived like light bulbs, burning as brightly from beginning to end, then popping off without warning, leaving those around us suddenly in the dark? Or is it perhaps better that there be a shape to life, everything in its due season, the shape also written, as it were, into the wrinkles of our bodies that live it—provided, of course, that we do not suffer years of painful or degraded old age and that we do not lose our wits?. . .

Going against both common intuition and native human desire, some commentators have argued that living with full awareness and acceptance of our finitude may be the condition of many of the best things in human life: engagement, seriousness, a taste for beauty, the possibility of virtue, the ties born of procreation, the quest for meaning. . . .

What about the pursuit of [happiness], and especially of the sort that we might better attain with pharmacological assistance? Painful and shameful memories are disturbing; guilty consciences trouble sleep; low self-esteem, melancholy, and world-weariness besmirch the waking hours. Why not memory-blockers for the former, mood-brighteners for the latter, and a good euphoriant—without risks of hangovers or cirrhosis—when celebratory occasions fail to be jolly? For let us be clear: If it is imbalances of neurotransmitters that are largely responsible for our state of soul, would it not be sheer priggishness to refuse the help of pharmacology for our happiness, when we accept it guiltlessly to correct for an absence of insulin or thyroid hormone?

And yet, . . . there seems to be something misguided about the pursuit of utter and unbroken psychic tranquility or the attempt to eliminate all shame, guilt, and painful memories. Traumatic memories, shame, and guilt, are, it is true, psychic pains. In extreme doses, they can be crippling. Yet, short of the extreme, they can also be helpful and fitting. They are appropriate responses to horror, disgraceful conduct, injustice, and sin, and, as such, help teach us to avoid them or fight against them in the future. Witnessing a murder should be remembered as horrible; doing a beastly deed should trouble one's soul. Righteous indignation at injustice depends on being able to feel injustice's sting. And to deprive oneself of one's memory—including and especially its truthfulness of feeling—is to deprive oneself of one's own life and identity. . . .

Looking into the future at goals pursuable with the aid of new biotechnologies enables us to turn a reflective glance at our own version of the human condition and the prospects now available to us (in principle) for a flourishing human life. For us today, assuming that we are blessed with good health and a sound mind, a flourishing human life is not a life lived with an ageless body or an untroubled soul, but rather a life lived in rhythmed time, mindful of time's limits, appreciative of each season and filled first of all with those intimate human relations that are ours only because we are born, age, replace ourselves, decline, and die—and know it. It is a life of aspiration, made possible by and born of experienced lack, of the disproportion between the transcendent longings of the soul and the limited capacities of our bodies and minds. It is a life that stretches toward some fulfillment to which our natural human soul has been oriented, and, unless we extirpate the source, will always be oriented. It is a life not of better genes and enhancing chemicals but of love and friendship, song and dance, speech and deed, working and learning, revering and worshipping. If this is true, then the pursuit of an ageless body may prove finally to be a distraction and a deformation. And the pursuit of an untroubled and self-satisfied soul may prove to be deadly to desire, if finitude recognized spurs aspiration and fine aspiration acted upon is itself the core of happiness. Not the agelessness of the body, nor the contentment of the soul, nor even the list of external achievements and accomplishments of life, but the engaged and energetic being-at-work of what nature uniquely gave to us is what we need to treasure and defend.

Howard Trachtman 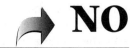 **NO**

A Man Is a Man Is a Man

Every field of human endeavor goes through a period of great anticipation in which the leading lights predict that the end of the discipline is near and that acquisition of new knowledge in the area is almost complete. Thus, at the end of the nineteenth century, physicists were confident that they had natural order of things under control and that mastery of the physical world was just a matter of time. A few decades later, David Hilbert and colleagues asserted that they were closing in on verification of the internal consistency and validity of mathematics and by inference all of philosophy (Goldstein 2005). In the early 1970s, as immunization practice and administration of antibiotics became standard and scourges of earlier eras like smallpox and polio were vanishing, specialists in infectious disease were sure that their field had things well in hand. Finally, after the fall of the Berlin Wall, Francis Fukuyama (1992) wrote confidently that history was at an end and that the global community was entering a phase of prosperity and harmony.

From the privileged vantage point of the early 21st century, we know how grandiose these predictions were. Einstein and his relativistic quanta, Godel and his incompleteness theorem, AIDS and Ebola, and the attack on the World Trade Center demonstrate that nothing ever goes quite exactly according to plan and that human beings still have plenty of work cut out for them.

In light of all of this sobering experience, it is surprising that physicians and bioethicists should have such unrealistic views and apprehensions about prospective therapeutic interventions that may arise from the remarkable advances in genetics or neurobiology. Michael Sandel's (2004) article is representative of this literature and Kamm's (2005) review is an insightful analysis of this position. However, I think it falls short on several practical points that should disarm anxious critics of enhancement.

Enhancement is a new term that is in vogue to describe what doctors have been doing since time immemorial, namely working to improve the lot of the patients they care for. Each medical advance from X-rays to imatinib has always been heralded as the advent of the new millennium only to be replaced by new problems or unexpected complications of old problems (Kantarjian et al. 2002). But, despite rapid approval and grand hopes, no enhancement or treatment has ever turned out to be all it was cracked up to be. Outcomes in real patients hardly ever live up to the exaggerated claims of the advanced sales

From *The American Journal of Bioethics*, vol. 5, no. 3, May–June 2005, pp. 31–33. Copyright © 2005 by Routledge/Taylor & Francis Group. Reprinted by permission via Rightslink. www.informaworld.com

pitch. With each answer that emerges from a clinical trial, there are even more questions that are raised about optimal efficacy, the best target population, and the appropriate balance of benefits and risks. Longer life spans means more cancer and dementia, more antibiotics mean more virulent organisms, improvements in neonatal care mean more damaged low birth weight survivors. Programs for medical enhancement will never deliver on all great expectations, either good or bad. As such there appears to be no inherent reason to fear enhancement or limit its application.

If enhancement represents the intrinsic nature of man to reach out and control his own fate by manipulating his environment and to reverse any adverse effects of his surroundings, then it is inappropriate to use the term mastery in describing this defining human capacity. Instead of considering enhancement an activity with automatic winners and losers, I suggest that it would clarify the discussion if it was viewed as a hard wired human trait that we all engage in. Some do it better than others but all of us try to enhance our lot in life as best as we can. It is undoubtedly true that knowledge can and will be misdirected and even abused by those interested in self-aggrandizement. However, again this is not a unique feature of the remarkable advances in genomics or imaging technology. The fact that there are Harry Limes in the world does not take away from the benefits of antibiotics. The abuse of erythropoietin by athletes does not detract from the qualitative improvement in the lives of patients with end stage renal disease who are treated with this drug (Schumacher et al. 2001).

Moreover, intent has always been a difficult barometer to gauge the behavior of any professional. Most patients are only interested in getting better or improving their health. They rarely concern themselves with the motivation of the care provider, be it money, fame, fortune, or an altruistic desire to help others. Similarly, physicians rarely question why people want to get better as long as they follow instructions and balance the risks and benefits reasonably in their health care judgments. Even in judging religious behavior, which must comply with extralegal concerns and varying standards of dogma, intent is usually implicitly assumed to be appropriate or ignored provided the outcome is not destructive to the individual or community. One would be hard pressed to see any advantage for the patients if individual doctors or the health profession as a whole got into the business of judging patients' intention when they seek a medical treatment to cure disease or enhance health. If there are any lessons to be drawn from the endless discussions about active and passive euthanasia, it may be that no one is served by making this fine distinction in clinical practice (Kamisar 1969).

Finally, the distinction that is being made between treatment which is justified and permissible *versus* enhancement which smacks of hubris and should be constrained may prove to be irrelevant in real life situations where the boundaries are blurred by rapid advances in medical therapeutics and the definition of disease itself. When is failure to concentrate a sign of disease worthy of treatment and when does it indicate a lazy student who is not willing to work hard enough in school? Is erectile dysfunction an ailment like salmonella enteritis or a failure to perform? If I can confidently help the patient with their problem safely and effectively, I for one would just as soon avoid categorizing their complaint into an acceptable *versus* unacceptable category.

Finally, what is intriguing is that those who frown upon physicians who would dispense treatments that enhance patients rather than treat a disease is the assumption that there will be near unanimous acceptance of the treatment and a groundswell of people requesting the therapy. However, a survey of the history of public health interventions indicates that people, at least in this country, are reluctant to take the words of doctors on faith. Although each advance reported in the press is greeted by the public with great fanfare and anticipation, in reality many treatments are rejected by large segments of the population. Think of the people who refuse immunizations for their child, who place greater credence in alternative medications instead of chemotherapy (Frederickson 2004). There will always be people in search for the quick fix to treat obesity, prevent dementia, or win an Olympic medal. But, I think it is contrary to experience to think that everyone will line up for each new genetic treatment or enhancement. Doctors would do well to remind themselves of how varied their patients really are and that application of any therapeutic advance will still begin with a sensitive dialogue between doctor and patient.

In conclusion, I would encourage the medical community to embrace enhancement as a never ending quest for health that will make us healthier but never perfect. We should not fear progress in diagnostics or try to limit medical manipulations. This is because experience teaches us that they will never meet their goals and always leave us striving for more. I endorse Kamm's proposal to promote education about appropriate utilization of advances in genetics and medical science, insure equitable use of these resources, and maintain surveillance for unanticipated and undesirable consequences. However, as it says in Ethics of the Fathers, "The day is short, the work is hard, the employees are tired, the reward is great, and the boss is pressing" (Babylonian Talmud, Ch. 2, Mishna, 20). But, at the end of the day, we will still be human and knowing that should give us the confidence to proceed.

Acknowledgement

The author wishes to thank Rachel Frank, R.N. for her thoughtful comments about this essay.

References

Frederickson, D. D., T. C. Davis, C. L. Arnould, et al. 2004. Childhood immunization refusal: Provider and parent perceptions. *Family Medicine* 36:431–439.

Fukuyama, F. 1992. *The end of history and the last man.* New York: Free Press.

Goldstein, R. 2005. *Incompleteness: The proof and paradox of Kort Godel.* New York: W.W. Norton & Co.

Kamisar, Y. 1969. Euthanasia legislation: Some non-religious objections. In *Euthanasia and the right to death,* ed. A. B. Downing, Los Angeles, CA: Nash Publishing Company.

Kamm, F. M. 2005. Is there a problem with enhancement? *Am. J. Bioethics* 5–14.

Kantarjian H., C. Sawyers, A. Hochhaus, et al. 2002. Hematologic and cytogenetic responses to imatinib mesylate in chronic myelogenous leukemia. *New England Journal of Medicine* 346:645–652.

Sandel, M. 2004. The case against perfection. *The Atlantic Monthly* 293(3): 51–62.

Schumacher, Y. O., A. Schmid, and T. Lenz. 2001. Blood testing in sports: Hematological profile of a convicted athlete. *Clinical Journal of Sport Medicine* 11:115–117.

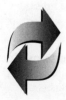

EXPLORING THE ISSUE

Is the Use of Medical Tools to Enhance Human Beings Morally Troubling?

Critical Thinking and Reflection

1. How does the President's Council connect the idea of human happiness to human finitude? Do you find the Council's reflections about this connection plausible?
2. The Council holds that imperfection is an important part of human nature, while Trachtman holds that enhancement is an important part of human nature. Do you agree with either one or both?
3. Sometimes people feel that human nature ought to be left alone because natural states of affairs are valuable in their own right. What do the Council and Trachtman say about this idea?

Is There Common Ground?

Discussions of new technologies easily lead into flights of fancy, to descriptions of futuristic scenarios entirely unlike anything we are familiar with today, and the debate about human enhancement is no different. Some proponents of human enhancement identify themselves as "transhumanists," and they call for developing and using enhancement technologies that allow us to transcend the human condition, to develop new abilities, to achieve near-immortality, perhaps even to shuck off this mortal coil altogether and become, as it were, software-based beings, who can be periodically upgraded and uploaded to new hardware. On the other side of the debate about enhancement are the many dystopias of literature and film, from Frankenstein and Brave New World to Gattaca and Eternal Sunshine of the Spotless Mind.

None of the genetic enhancements that arouse either fear or anticipation are possible with current technologies. Some say that they will never be possible, since the most desired and most unwelcome characteristics are not well understood and result from an uncontrollable interaction of genes and environment. Still, the future may bring still-undreamed-of possibilities, and even a limited power to enhance human bodies may raise some troubling questions. See issue 13.

Additional Resources

There are many Internet resources available to explore transhumanism. The philosopher Nick Bostrom sets out his view in the article "Human Genetic Enhancements: A Transhumanist Perspective," at www.nickbostrom

.com/ethics/genetic.html. The article was originally published in the *Journal of Value Inquiry,* vol. 37, no. 4 (2003). Bostrom's "A History of Transhumanist Thought," originally published in *Journal of Evolution and Technology* (vol. 14, no. 1, April 2005), is available at www.nickbostrom.com/papers/history.pdf. A variety of resources and documents can also be found at the Web site of humanity plus, an organization dedicated to promoting enhancement technologies; http://humanityplus.org/.

The issue of *The American Journal of Bioethics* (vol. 5, no. 3, 2005), from which Howard Trachtman's essay is drawn, also contains several other articles on enhancement. The lead article by Frances M. Kamm, "Is There a Problem with Enhancement?" analyzes Sandel's article from a philosophical perspective.

Michael Sandel develops a book-length but accessible argument against enhancement in *The Case Against Perfection: Ethics in the Age of Genetic Engineering* (Belknap Press, 2007).

Allen Buchanan is skeptical of arguments against enhancement in *Beyond Humanity?* (Oxford University Press, 2011).

See Jonathan Glover, *Choosing Children: Genes, Disability, and Design* (Oxford University Press, 2008) for a perspective incorporating the viewpoints of people with disabilities.

Julian Savulescu argues that we have a moral obligation to enhance human beings and that "to be human is to strive to be better" ("New Breeds of Humans: The Moral Obligation to Enhance," *Reproductive Medicine Online* [March 2005]).

See also Erik Parens, "Authenticity and Ambivalence: Toward Understanding the Enhancement Debate," *Hastings Center Report* (May–June 2005).

On the Web: "Genetic Enhancement" from the National Human Genome Research Institute, www.genome.gov/10004767.

ISSUE 13

Should Performance-Enhancing Drugs Be Banned from Sports?

YES: **Thomas H. Murray**, from "Making Sense of Fairness in Sports," *Hastings Center Report* (March/April 2010)

NO: **Julian Savulescu, Bennett Foddy, and Megan Clayton**, from "Why We Should Allow Performance Enhancing Drugs in Sport," *British Journal of Sports Medicine* (December 2004)

Learning Outcome

After reading this issue, you should be able to:

- Outline different kinds of arguments for and against permitting athletes to improve their performance through the use of drugs and other medical technologies.

ISSUE SUMMARY

YES: Social psychologist Thomas H. Murray contends that the ban on performance-enhancing drugs should continue because it furthers the true meaning of sports—which is to compare athletes on their natural talent and abilities.

NO: Philosopher Julian Savulescu and research colleagues Bennett Foddy and Megan Clayton argue that legalizing drugs in sport may be fairer and safer than banning them.

In sports, there are winners and losers. But for many athletes, winning is not enough. Elite athletes want to set records or exceed their prior performances. Athletes of less than elite status aspire to reach that higher level. And even ordinary competitors who know they will never jump as high as Michael Jordan or hit a hockey puck as precisely as Wayne Gretsky want to go farther than their natural talent and motivation might take them. The potential rewards are enormous, not just in personal gratification but also in prestige, career opportunities, and financial success.

For all these different types of sports figures, there is a strong tempta-tion to enhance their performance through the use of drugs. And increas-ingly they can find some drugs that may help them do it. Drug use in sports is not a new phenomenon. Athletes in the original Greek Olympics are believed to have used mushrooms and herbs to make them stronger and faster. In the nineteenth century, French cyclists drank Vin Mariani, a combination of wine and coca leaf extract called "the wine of athletes." Coca leaf, the source of cocaine, made it easier for them to endure the prolonged exertion of cycling.

These potions, however, were mild compared to the modern pharma-copeia available to athletes. In addition to natural substances, prescription drugs used in megadoses, and illegal substances like cocaine and marijuana, there are synthesized forms of human hormones and "designer drugs" for particular purposes.

Concern about drug use in sports in modern times is relatively recent. Steroid use first emerged in the 1964 Olympics. Anabolic androgenic steroids are compounds synthesized from the hormone testosterone, which is present in normal amounts in males. ("Anabolic" means "to build," and "androgenic" means "masculinizing.") Physicians prescribe such steroids to repair damaged tissue, but the doses that athletes use are many times greater than therapeutic ones. Because anabolic steroids build muscle mass, weight lifters, hammer throwers, and other athletes whose performance depends on muscle power are most likely to use them. In females, the results may be not just muscle mass but masculinizing features. In the Montreal Olympics in 1976, East German women swimmers were able to swim faster than other competitors, but they also had deep voices and body hair.

Stimulants such as amphetamines serve a different purpose; they give ath-letes unusually high levels of alertness, energy, and aggressiveness, characteristics particularly appealing to football players. Other kinds of medical intervention to enhance performance include "blood doping"—storing some of a cyclist's own blood and injecting it before a race to give the maximum number of oxygen-carrying red blood cells. A synthetic substance—erythropoetin (EPO), prescribed to treat anemia in cancer patients—can also be used in this way.

What has been the response of official sports organizations to this growing use of drugs? The World Anti-Doping Agency, an offshoot of the International Olympic Committee, has a nine-page list of banned substances (available at www.wada-ama.org). The major categories are anabolic agents, hormones and related substances (such as EPO and human growth hormone), beta-2 ago-nists (substances that relieve breathing stress, except for athletes who have asthma), agents with antiestrogenic activity (substances that enhance femi-nine characteristics), and diuretics and other agents that might mask the presence of drugs by depleting the body urine. In addition, blood doping, chemical and physical manipulation, and gene doping—a new addition to the armamentarium—are prohibited. Some substances are prohibited in competi-tions, including stimulants, narcotics, cannabinoids (marijuana and hashish), and other steroids. Certain sports prohibit alcohol or beta-blockers (drugs that lower blood pressure).

Is all this antidrug activity warranted, or is it an unacceptable invasion of privacy and a losing battle? Why should adults for whom sports is a primary value not be allowed to do whatever they choose to enhance their performance? Can drugs and sport coexist? The YES and NO selections take opposite views. Thomas H. Murray contends that drug use violates the integrity of sport and deprives it of its essential value and meaning. Julian Savulescu, Bennett Foddy, and Megan Clayton, on the other hand, argue that there is nothing inherently wrong in athletes' using drugs to perform at higher levels, and it would be better for all if drug use were legalized and controlled for athletes' safety.

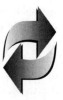

YES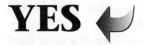

Thomas H. Murray

Making Sense of Fairness in Sports

From the steroid scandals of major league baseball to analysis of Oscar Pistorius's cheetahs to the sex-verification test of Caster Semenya, questions today about what constitutes fairness in sports are wide-ranging and varied.

It's easier to see what's unfair in sports. Suppose that the judges award the Olympic figure skating gold medal in Vancouver because of the skaters' wacky costumes—all feathers, sequins, and teasing glimpses of skin. Or that they choose based on their views on the skaters' countries of origin, or because they were bribed, or by tossing a coin.

All these are unfair (and some have been documented, or at least suspected, in past competitions). How do we know they're unfair? Because everyone who understands figure skating—or alpine skiing, or bobsledding, or, for that matter, baseball, cycling, or any other competitive sport—knows what's supposed to separate winners from also-rans. Among the countless differences between competitors, from eye color to favorite food, only certain differences are meant to be highlighted in each particular sport.

Successful short-track speed skaters possess explosive strength, finely honed technique, and the courage to face the possibility of serious injury from razor-sharp blades. Nordic skiers must have astonishing stamina. Each sport calls upon its particular mix of physical talents. Every sport requires the commitment to perfect those talents and to learn how to employ them skillfully and strategically. It may not be easy to say exactly what fairness means, but the ease with which we can call out unfairness suggests that the task is worthwhile and far from hopeless.

A match that should never happen is a one-on-one basketball game between LeBron James and me. When LeBron trounces me—as he assuredly will—it may be uninteresting, probably comical, perhaps even YouTubeable, but it will not be unfair. He is simply a superior player, not merely to me but probably to every other person living on this planet. (Kobe Bryant is likely to disagree.) The playing field, or court, is level. Talent and dedication determine the winner.

Then there are times when we choose to level the playing field by multiplying it. In the 2008 Paralympics there were thirteen distinct finals for the men's one-hundredmeter dash, twelve for the women's. The varieties and degrees of impairment among Paralympians in no way detract from the talents and dedication that competitors bring to the games. But the variety also

Murray, Thomas H. From *Hastings Center Report*, March–April 2010, pp. 13–15. Copyright © 2010 by The Hastings Center. Reprinted by permission of Wiley-Blackwell.

requires that the playing field be made level so that every athlete is competing against people with similar levels of impairment. In that way, talent and the many things we admire about dedicated athletes are on display and shape each athlete's performance.

The first thing to note is that a fair sports competition does not require that athletes be equal in every imaginable respect. Some basketball players are taller, stronger, quicker, or more agile than others. No one—well, almost no one—regards such differences in natural talents as unjust or unfair. Some have better coaches or more favorable training environments. At what point such differences cross the line from inevitable and acceptable to iniquitous and deplorable is something to be debated and settled by the people who participate in, understand, and love that sport—not by distant and disinterested philosophers. Debates such as this go on regularly in sports over new equipment, rules, strategies, and the like. Take the recent kerfuffle over the super-slippery, buoyant full-body swimsuits. After initial dithering, the Fédération Internationale de Natation (FINA)—the international governing body for swimming—[in 2009] banned many suits on the grounds that they changed the nature of the sport by allowing bulky athletes to float on top of the water rather than having to push through it. Whatever one thinks of FINA's ruling, it was right to focus on the meaning of the sport and on what characteristics lead to excellence and success.

Then again, the most gifted, hardest-working athlete or team does not always win. A random bounce, a slip, a hesitation can give victory to the side that might lose nine of ten matches. That's why we play the game.

When it comes to performance-enhancing drugs, gene doping, and the panoply of manipulations banned widely in sports, the challenge is less about fairness than about meaning. If the rules ban performance-enhancing drugs, then using those drugs to gain an advantage over athletes who refuse to cheat is unfair. Simple enough. Antidoping skeptics, however, often proclaim that the problem isn't with the drugs, but with the ban on drugs. It would be fairer, they argue, to give all competitors access to the same drugs. If everyone had ample supplies of anabolic steroids, erythropoietin, growth hormone, or whatever drugs boosted performance in their sport, then—they claim—unfairness would be eliminated along with the nuisances of drug testing, adjudication, and enforcement.

One response to the skeptics is to ask a different question: Is it not unfair to put the athletes who want to compete without drugs or gene doping at a competitive disadvantage by permitting everything—to tilt the playing field in favor of the drug users?

Any serious ethical commentary on the uses of performance-enhancing technology in sports must confront two compelling realities. First, sports science has provided a great deal of information about how to optimize training and performance. It has also led to a plethora of technologies and methods to enhance performance, from altitude chambers that allow athletes to gain the benefits of "training low, living high," to ice-filled vests runners can wear before a long race to cool their core temperatures, to esoteric measurements of muscle and organ function. Why, the skeptics ask, should we distinguish between these technologies of performance enhancement on the one hand and drugs like steroids on the other?

Part of the answer to this challenge is to recognize that sports are about what can be accomplished under specific limitations. Soccer players, other than goal tenders, may not use their hands or arms to direct the ball, even when that would be far more convenient and accurate than one's foot or head. Golf imposes strict limits on balls and clubs. Marathon runners may not use wheels, whether attached to their shoes or, as Rosie Ruiz did, to subway cars.

The other piece of the answer requires an understanding of what that particular sport values. What makes a great weight lifter does not make a great distance runner. Bodies that possess massive explosive strength are rarely the lithe, sinewy bodies best suited to run great distances. The limitations each sport chooses for itself reflect a shared understanding of what that sport is meant to display and reward. The rules of sports are arbitrary in the sense that they could be otherwise, and, in practice, sports modify their rules in response to changes in equipment, tactics, and athletes' abilities. But in another sense, the rules and the changes wrought in them are far from arbitrary: they must pass muster with the community of those who play and love that sport. The community must be satisfied that the new rules keep alive what it values, what natural talents enable athletes to excel, and what, in the end, is meaningful about participating and winning.

The second reality is the ineluctably comparative nature of sports. Athletes compete against other athletes. Winners and losers may be separated by fractions of a second. A drug that gives a 1 or 2 percent performance boost can be decisive. When some athletes use such technologies, all athletes feel the pressure to use them, merely to avoid losing ground. So the notion that we should just leave it up to each athlete to decide whether to use drugs is naive. When the lid is blown off, all athletes will feel the pressure to dope.

One proposed solution is to continue to ban some drugs—those deemed to be particularly harmful—but allow athletes free reign to use all others. Consider what is likely to happen. We'll continue to need drug testing and enforcement to deter athletes from using the substances on the banned list, so all the complaints about the inconvenience and intrusiveness of testing will remain. And now athletes will feel pressured to take ever more drugs, often at higher dosages, in untested and possibly dangerous combinations. It's hard to see that scenario as progress.

Whether performance-enhancing drugs or gene doping should be permitted in sports is, in the end, a matter to be decided by the communities of athletes and those who understand and love each sport. The dynamics of competition mean that, if doping were permitted, athletes would confront a terrible choice: refrain from drugs and give up an edge that will often be decisive, or join in an ever-rising spiral of drug use. I fear a public health catastrophe in the making if we choose the second path. I also would grieve for all those athletes who desire to compete without doping but who will mostly lose to their pharmacologically amped competitors.

Opening the doors of sports to drug use will also accelerate the dominance of doping gurus over the athletes who succumb to their sales pitches. An athlete's performance will become more and more a function of expert manipulations, and less of the athlete's talents or dedication. I cannot see that as a good thing for athletes, for sports, or for all of us who care about them.

Julian Savulescu, Bennett
Foddy, and Megan Clayton

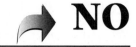 **NO**

Why We Should Allow Performance Enhancing Drugs in Sport

In 490 BC, the Persian Army landed on the plain of Marathon, 25 miles from Athens. The Athenians sent a messenger named Feidipides to Sparta to ask for help. He ran the 150 miles in two days. The Spartans were late. The Athenians attacked and, although out-numbered five to one, were victorious. Feidipides was sent to run back to Athens to report victory. On arrival, he screamed "We won" and dropped dead from exhaustion.

The marathon was run in the first modern Olympics in 1896, and in many ways the athletic ideal of modern athletes is inspired by the myth of the marathon. Their ideal is superhuman performance, at any cost.

Drugs in Sport

The use of performance enhancing drugs in the modern Olympics is on record as early as the games of the third Olympiad, when Thomas Hicks won the marathon after receiving an injection of strychnine in the middle of the race.[1] The first official ban on "stimulating substances" by a sporting organisation was introduced by the International Amateur Athletic Federation in 1928.[2]

Using drugs to cheat in sport is not new, but it is becoming more effective. In 1976, the East German swimming team won 11 out of 13 Olympic events, and later sued the government for giving them anabolic steroids.[3] Yet despite the health risks, and despite the regulating bodies' attempts to eliminate drugs from sport, the use of illegal substances is widely known to be rife. It hardly raises an eyebrow now when some famous athlete fails a dope test.

In 1992, Vicky Rabinowicz interviewed small groups of athletes. She found that Olympic athletes, in general, believed that most successful athletes were using banned substances.[4]

Much of the writing on the use of drugs in sport is focused on this kind of anecdotal evidence. There is very little rigorous, objective evidence because the athletes are doing something that is taboo, illegal, and sometimes highly dangerous. The anecdotal picture tells us that our attempts to eliminate drugs from sport have failed. In the absence of good evidence, we need an analytical argument to determine what we should do.

Condemned to Cheating?

We are far from the days of amateur sporting competition. Elite athletes can earn tens of millions of dollars every year in prize money alone, and millions more in sponsorships and endorsements. The lure of success is great. But the penalties for cheating are small. A six month or one year ban from competition is a small penalty to pay for further years of multimillion dollar success.

Drugs are much more effective today than they were in the days of strychnine and sheep's testicles. Studies involving the anabolic steroid androgen showed that, even in doses much lower than those used by athletes, muscular strength could be improved by 5–20%.[5] Most athletes are also relatively unlikely to ever undergo testing. The International Amateur Athletic Federation estimates that only 10–15% of participating athletes are tested in each major competition.[6]

The enormous rewards for the winner, the effectiveness of the drugs, and the low rate of testing all combine to create a cheating "game" that is irresistible to athletes. Kjetil Haugen[7] investigated the suggestion that athletes face a kind of prisoner's dilemma regarding drugs. His game theoretic model shows that, unless the likelihood of athletes being caught doping was raised to unrealistically high levels, or the payoffs for winning were reduced to unrealistically low levels, athletes could all be predicted to cheat. The current situation for athletes ensures that this is likely, even though they are worse off as a whole if everyone takes drugs, than if nobody takes drugs.

Drugs such as erythropoietin (EPO) and growth hormone are natural chemicals in the body. As technology advances, drugs have become harder to detect because they mimic natural processes. In a few years, there will be many undetectable drugs. Haugen's analysis predicts the obvious: that when the risk of being caught is zero, athletes will all choose to cheat.

The recent Olympic games in Athens were the first to follow the introduction of a global anti-doping code. From the lead up to the games to the end of competition, 3000 drug tests were carried out: 2600 urine tests and 400 blood tests for the endurance enhancing drug EPO.[8] From these, 23 athletes were found to have taken a banned substance—the most ever in an Olympic games.[9] Ten of the men's weightlifting competitors were excluded.

The goal of "cleaning" up the sport is unattainable. Further down the track the spectre of genetic enhancement looms dark and large.

The Spirit of Sport

So is cheating here to stay? Drugs are against the rules. But we define the rules of sport. If we made drugs legal and freely available, there would be no cheating.

The World Anti-Doping Agency code declares a drug illegal if it is performance enhancing, if it is a health risk, or if it violates the "spirit of sport."[10]

They define this spirit as follows.[11] The spirit of sport is the celebration of the human spirit, body, and mind, and is characterised by the following values:

- ethics, fair play and honesty
- health
- excellence in performance
- character and education
- fun and joy
- teamwork
- dedication and commitment
- respect for rules and laws
- respect for self and other participants
- courage
- community and solidarity[11]

Would legal and freely available drugs violate this "spirit"? Would such a permissive rule be good for sport?

Human sport is different from sports involving other animals, such as horse or dog racing. The goal of a horse race is to find the fastest horse. Horses are lined up and flogged. The winner is the one with the best combination of biology, training, and rider. Basically, this is a test of biological potential. This was the old naturalistic Athenian vision of sport: find the strongest, fastest, or most skilled man.

Training aims to bring out this potential. Drugs that improve our natural potential are against the spirit of this model of sport. But this is not the only view of sport. Humans are not horses or dogs. We make choices and exercise our own judgment. We choose what kind of training to use and how to run our race. We can display courage, determination, and wisdom. We are not flogged by a jockey on our back but drive ourselves. It is this judgment that competitors exercise when they choose diet, training, and whether to take drugs. We can choose what kind of competitor to be, not just through training, but through biological manipulation. Human sport is different from animal sport because it is creative. Far from being against the spirit of sport, biological manipulation embodies the human spirit—the capacity to improve ourselves on the basis of reason and judgment. When we exercise our reason, we do what only humans do.

The result will be that the winner is not the person who was born with the best genetic potential to be strongest. Sport would be less of a genetic lottery. The winner will be the person with a combination of the genetic potential, training, psychology, and judgment. Olympic performance would be the result of human creativity and choice, not a very expensive horse race.

Classical musicians commonly use blockers to control their stage fright. These drugs lower heart rate and blood pressure, reducing the physical effects of stress, and it has been shown that the quality of a musical performance is improved if the musician takes these drugs.[12] Although elite classical music is arguably as competitive as elite sport, and the rewards are similar, there is no stigma attached to the use of these drugs. We do not think less of the violinist or pianist who uses them. If the audience judges the performance to be improved with drugs, then the drugs are enabling the musician to express him or herself more effectively. The competition between elite musicians has rules—you cannot mime the violin to a backing CD. But there is no rule against the use of chemical enhancements.

Is classical music a good metaphor for elite sport? Sachin Tendulkar is known as the "Maestro from Mumbai." The Associated Press called Maria Sharapova's 2004 Wimbledon final a "virtuoso performance."[13] Jim Murrary[14] wrote the following about Michael Jordan in 1996:

> You go to see Michael Jordan play for the same reason you went to see Astaire dance, Olivier act or the sun set over Canada. It's art. It should be painted, not photographed.
>   It's not a game, it's a recital. He's not just a player, he's a virtuoso. Heifetz with a violin. Horowitz at the piano.

Indeed, it seems reasonable to suggest that the reasons we appreciate sport at its elite level have something to do with competition, but also a great deal to do with the appreciation of an extraordinary performance.

Clearly the application of this kind of creativity is limited by the rules of the sport. Riding a motorbike would not be a "creative" solution to winning the Tour de France, and there are good reasons for proscribing this in the rules. If motorbikes were allowed, it would still be a good sport, but it would no longer be a bicycle race.

We should not think that allowing cyclists to take EPO would turn the Tour de France into some kind of "drug race," any more than the various training methods available turn it into a "training race" or a "money race." Athletes train in different, creative ways, but ultimately they still ride similar bikes, on the same course. The skill of negotiating the steep winding descent will always be there. . . .

Test for Health, Not Drugs

The welfare of the athlete must be our primary concern. If a drug does not expose an athlete to excessive risk, we should allow it even if it enhances performance. We have two choices: to vainly try to turn the clock back, or to rethink who we are and what sport is, and to make a new 21st century Olympics. Not a super-Olympics but a more human Olympics. Our crusade against drugs in sport has failed. Rather than fearing drugs in sport, we should embrace them.

In 1998, the president of the International Olympic Committee, Juan-Antonio Samaranch, suggested that athletes be allowed to use non-harmful performance enhancing drugs. This view makes sense only if, by not using drugs, we are assured that athletes are not being harmed.

Performance enhancement is not against the spirit of sport; it is the spirit of sport. To choose to be better is to be human. Athletes should be given this choice. Their welfare should be paramount. But taking drugs is not necessarily cheating. The legalisation of drugs in sport may be fairer and safer.

References

1. House of Commons, Select Committee on Culture, Media and Sport. 2004. Seventh Report of Session 2003–2004, UK Parliament, HC 499–1.

2. House of Commons, Select Committee on Culture, Media and Sport. 2004. Seventh Report of Session 2003–2004, UK Parliament, HC 499–1.

3. Longman J. 2004. East German Steroids' toll: 'they killed Heidi', *New York Times* 2004 Jan 20, sect D:1.

4. Rabinawicz V. Athletes and drugs: a separate pace? *Psychol Today* 1992;25:52–3.

5. Hartgens F, Kuipers H. Effects of androgenic-anabolic steroids in athletes. *Sport Med* 2004;34:513–54.

6. IAAF, 2004. . . .

7. Haugen KK. The performance-enhancing drug game. *Journal of Sports Economics* 2004;5:67–87.

8. Wilson S. *Boxer Munyasia fails drug test in Athens*. Athens: Associated Press, 2004 Aug 10.

9. Zinser L. With drug-tainted past, few track records fall. *New York Times* 2004 Aug 29, Late Edition, p. 1.

10. WADA. World Anti-Doping Code, Montreal. World Anti-Doping Agency, 2003:16.

11. WADA. World Anti-Doping Code, Montreal. World Anti-Doping Agency, 2003:3.

12. Brantigan CO, Brantigan TA, Joseph N. Effect of beta blockade and beta stimulation on stage fright. *Am J Med* 1982;72:88–94.

13. Wilson S. *Sharapova beats Williams for title. Associated Press,* 2004 Jul 3, 09:10am.

14. Murray J. It's basketball played on a higher plane. *Los Angeles Times* 1996 Feb 4 1996, sect C:1.

EXPLORING THE ISSUE

Should Performance-Enhancing Drugs Be Banned from Sports?

Critical Thinking and Reflection

1. What does Murray mean when he says that the challenge posed by doping is "less about fairness than about meaning"? What does the meaning of sports have to do with "what can be accomplished under specific limitations" and "what that particular sport values"? How could unlimited use of technology change the meaning, for example, of the 100-meter sprint?
2. What, according to Savulescu, Foddy, and Clayton, is the true meaning of sports, and why does that account lead them to argue for permitting enhancement? Would you personally find sports more or less compelling to watch if doping were not limited? Why or why not?
3. Does an exploration of sports doping shed light on the larger debate about human enhancement? What kind of account would you expect the authors of these selections to give of doping or other enhancement technologies in, say, musical performance, the military, or medical surgical techniques?

Is There Common Ground?

In 2012, the United States Anti-Doping Agency charged that Lance Armstrong had doped his way to seven Tour de France titles, making him easily the highest profile American to be tarnished by a doping scandal. Armstrong initially fought the charge, and then decided not to contest it, meaning that all of his bicycling titles in that period would be stripped from him. In 2008, Marion Jones, who won five medals in track and field at the 2000 Sydney Olympics, admitted that she had used steroids and had lied to federal investigators. The Beijing and London Olympics in August 2008 passed without a major doping scandal, but testing was ever more strenuous and athletes were stripped of medals at both events.

Internationally, the Olympics and professional cycling have the toughest drug-testing rules and penalties. Until recently, major American sports have not acknowledged the problem. In 2005, Major League Baseball Commissioner Bud Selig announced a tougher policy for drug use, with suspensions of increasing times for violations. This action averted congressional action. In December 2007, a committee chaired by former Senate Majority Leader George Mitchell issued a report asserting that Major League Baseball has a "serious drug culture" in which steroid use is "widespread." The drugs of choice include steroid and increasingly human growth hormone, which cannot be detected by standard urine tests. Mitchell named many current and former well-known baseball players, including Roger Clemens, Miguel Tejada, Andy Pettitte, and Barry Bonds. The report blames all levels of baseball management and players' unions, as well as club owners, for ignoring the problem.

The first global treaty against doping in sports became effective February 2007, after 30 nations ratified an international agreement. (The United States ratified the agreement in 2008.) The treaty allows governments to take action against the illegal manufacture and supply of doping substances, among other provisions.

Additional Resources

Much information about doping in sports and the potential problems with it can be found at the Web sites of the World Anti-Doping Agency (www.wada-ama.org/) and the U.S. Anti-Doping Agency (www.usantidoping .org/). WADA also provides a list of drugs and techniques that are prohibited in international track and field, swimming, and other Olympic sports.

See D.H. Catlin, K.D. Fitch, and A. Ljungqvist, "Medicine and Science in the Fight Against Doping in Sport," *Journal of Internal Medicine* (August 2008), for a recent review of testing regimens.

Genetic enhancement to improve performance in sports is often rumored but not yet a reality, according to Thomas H. Murray in "Gene Doping and Olympic Sport," *Play True* (no. 1, 2005). He points to the dangers of untested technologies to alter genetic makeup. For a fuller exposition of Murray's views, see his chapter, "The Ethics of Drugs in Sport," in *Drugs & Performance in Sports*, edited by Richard H. Strauss (W. B. Saunders, 1987).

Joseph M. Saka argues that Congress can still address performance-enhancing drugs if voluntary action fails ("Back to the Game: How Congress Can Help Sports Leagues Shift the Focus from Steroids to Sports," *Journal of Contemporary Health Law and Policy* [2007]).

More information about the global treaty against doping is available at www.unesco.org/en/antidoping.

Norman Fost, a pediatrician, says appeals to ban drugs are paternalistic and caused more by a displeasure at the loss of innocence in sports than by actual harm ("Banning Drugs in Sports: A Skeptical View," *Hastings Center Report* [August 1986]).

An unsigned "Opinion" essay in *The Economist* (August 5, 2004) argues that an inflexible antidoping attitude is unsustainable in a society that uses performance-enhancing drugs so freely for other reasons.

See also Gary Wadler and Brian Hainline, *Drugs and the Athlete* (F.A. Davis, 1989) and David R. Mottram, ed., *Drugs in Sport*, 3rd ed. (Routledge, 2002).

ISSUE 14

May Doctors Offer Medical Drugs and Surgery to Stop a Disabled Child from Maturing?

YES: **Sarah E. Shannon**, from "In Support of the Ashley Treatment," *Pediatric Nursing* (March/April 2007)

NO: **Teresa A. Savage**, from "In Opposition of the Ashley Treatment," *Pediatric Nursing* (March/April 2007)

Learning Outcomes

After reading this issue, you should be able to:

- Evaluate the kinds of considerations that parents and physicians should weigh in thinking about how to use medical technology to care for children with disabilities.
- Outline some of the social issues that should be borne in mind when developing public policy concerning the treatment of people with disabilities.
- Discuss some of the concerns that disability advocates have about the treatment of cognitively disabled people.

ISSUE SUMMARY

YES: Nurse Sarah E. Shannon believes that ethically and legally parents have the right and duty to make decisions and to care for their family members who are unable to do so themselves and that we should not abandon parents of severely developmentally disabled children to the harsh social and economic realities that are barriers to good care.

NO: Nurse Teresa A. Savage believes that children like Ashley should have independent advocates, preferably persons with disabilities, to weigh the risks and benefits of proposed interventions.

Ashley (her real name) was born in 1997 with a severe brain impairment condition called static encephalopathy. She will never progress beyond the developmental level of an infant. At the age of 7, she was already showing signs of early puberty. Her parents wanted to keep her at home, but felt that as she grew older and bigger, and matured physically, it would be difficult to manage. They were concerned that the quality of life of the child they called their "pillow angel" would be diminished. In 2004, the parents and doctors at the Children's Hospital in Seattle devised a new treatment, which came to be called the "Ashley treatment."

This treatment included the administration of high-dose estrogen (sex steroid) therapy, which would stunt her growth; a hysterectomy (removal of her reproductive organs), which would prevent menstruation and make her infertile; and removal of her breast buds to prevent normal breast development. Before embarking on this treatment, the doctors consulted the hospitals' ethics committee, which met with the parents, Ashley herself, and her physicians. The committee agreed that the requests for estrogen therapy and hysterectomy were ethical in this case but should be considered in future patients only after review by an interdisciplinary panel.

This was not the first time that medical technology had been used to alter children's bodies. In "Tall Girls: The Social Shaping of a Medical Therapy," Joyce M. Lee and Joel D. Howell describe the practice in the second half of the twentieth century of prescribing estrogen therapy to otherwise healthy girls to keep them from growing too tall (*Archives of Pediatric and Adolescent Medicine*, October 2006). The definition of "too tall" was determined by societal beliefs about what it meant to be tall and female—not a good thing in those days.

As early as the 1940s, scientists observed that abnormal hormone levels influenced growth patterns both by prematurely closing long-bone growth plates (leading to short stature) and by keeping growth plates open over a prolonged time (leading to acromegaly, or extreme height). Through the 1950s and 1960s, articles appeared in medical journals attesting to the success of estrogen therapy in preventing girls from growing too tall, a condition that made them "self-conscious" and "embarrassed."

Lee and Howell assert that parents wanted to keep their girls shorter in order to improve their marriage prospects, since marriage was at that time thought to be a prerequisite for a successful life for a woman. As social norms changed toward the end of the twentieth century, scientific and medical interest in keeping girls from growing to their natural height diminished. And even among doctors who continued to treat girls, the expected height to which they might grow also increased. In 1956, a girl expected to reach 5'9" might be offered treatment, while by 1999 only girls who might grow to 6'2" would be in that category.

On the other hand, the use of growth hormone for very short but otherwise healthy boys has increased. The reasons are also socially determined. Tall men achieve more in society, it is believed, and have a greater choice of mates.

Ashley's treatment raises somewhat different questions. She has an underlying medical condition that means she will always be dependent on caregivers. In modifying her body, too, the goal was not to keep her normal, but to make her more abnormal—to prevent her from becoming fully adult. Ashley's parents hoped that, by preventing her from becoming sexually mature and from reaching a normal adult height, they could make it easier to care for her. They also thought that it would be easier for her not to have a mature woman's body.

In 2007, her parents created a blog (www.pillowangel.org) in order to tell her story. They believed parents of other children in similar circumstances should be able to consider using the "Ashley Treatment" for their children.

The YES and NO selections lay out the issues. Nurse Sarah E. Shannon believes that Ashley's parents' desire to care for her at home is their ethical and legal right, and that they should be able to make decisions in what they understand as Ashley's best interest. Nurse Teresa A. Savage argues that children like Ashley should have independent advocates to weigh the risks and benefits so that perceptions of "quality of life" from a disability perspective are included.

YES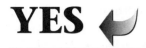

In Support of the Ashley Treatment

The news about Ashley, a severely cognitively and developmentally delayed child whose parents chose to medically limit her physical size, grabbed the attention of all of us. What if this was my child? Would I want to make my child smaller so that she would always be able to be cared for in a home, by family members? Growth attenuation treatment for children such as Ashley challenges us to think beyond our initial reactions. Ashley has the developmental and cognitive capacity of a young infant (Gunther & Diekema, 2006). She cannot hold up her head, roll or otherwise change her body position. She moves her arms and legs but cannot sit unsupported. Ashley responds positively to music and is able to vocalize but cannot talk (Parents' blog, 2006). She is alert to her environment but it is not clear that she recognizes people, including her own family. Ashley cries to express her frustration or discomfort. Currently, she lives at home with her parents and two siblings and is cared for by extended family.

Ashley's parents chose to attenuate Ashley's growth—to make her smaller—through the use of high dose estrogen therapy. In addition, Ashley's parents requested, and her physicians agreed, to remove her uterus and breast buds (Gunther & Diekema; Parents' blog; 2006). These three choices were made for separate therapeutic reasons. Growth attenuation through high dose estrogen therapy hastens the normal impact of puberty on girls' height. With puberty, estrogen levels rise and growth plate maturation occurs (Gunther & Diekema, 2006). High dose estrogen therapy takes advantage of this normal effect by stimulating growth plate maturation to occur prematurely. Therapy usually lasts for several years and, while data in developmentally delayed young children is sparse, the major risks appear similar to those for birth control pills, including uterine bleeding, breast development, and a small increased risk of deep vein thrombosis (DVT). Once puberty begins or growth attenuation is achieved, estrogen is stopped. The younger the child, the greater will be the effect on height. Ashley's physicians predict that "treatment beginning in a 5-year-old boy of average height and weight might result in a reduction in final length of as much as 24 inches (60 cm) and in weight of more than 100 pounds (45 kg)." (Gunther & Diekema, 2006, p. 1015).

Reprinted from *Pediatric Nursing Journal*, vol. 33, no. 2, April 2007, pp. 175–178. Reprinted with permission of the publisher, Jannetti Publications, Inc., East Holly Avenue, Box 56, Pitman, NJ 08071-0056; (856) 256-2300; fax: (856) 589-7463; Web site: www.pediatricnursing.net; for a sample copy of the journal, please contact the publisher.

Hysterectomy raises the issue of sterilization and whether this procedure was done primarily for birth control. Ashley has the mental capacity of an infant however making any possibility of consensual sex or parenthood impossible. Conversely, there are several health benefits resulting from removal of the uterus. First, it allows the high dose estrogen therapy to be administered without progesterone, reducing the risk of DVT (Gunther & Diekema, 2006). Second, hysterectomy avoids future hormone therapy to control menses. Menses can be a significant source of discomfort and a hygiene challenge that can aggravate skin breakdown when mobility is already impaired. For these reasons, a significant number of disabled women receive depot medroxyprogesterone acetate (DepoProvera) to suppress menstrual bleeding. However recent research has found that this increases their fracture risk 2.4 times above disabled women not on this medication (Watson, Lentz, & Cain, 2006). Hence, hysterectomy is being reconsidered as a more appropriate treatment for long-term control of menses. Third, a hysterectomy removes the cervix, alleviating the need to do routine PAP smears for health maintenance. For a woman as profoundly disabled as Ashley, the personal invasion and discomfort of a routine PAP smear can be intolerable (Brakman & Amari-Vaught, 1999).

The third procedure was breast bud removal, done while Ashley was under anesthesia for the hysterectomy. Was this cosmetic? An effort on the part of Ashley's parents to keep her child-like? How could removal of her breasts possibly benefit Ashley? Ashley's maternal lineage includes large and often, fibrocystic breasts, a painful condition (Parents' blog, 2006). Due to her profound developmental disability, Ashley is unable to sit up without chest support such as a chest strap, which puts pressure on breast tissue. This is a potential source of skin breakdown and discomfort aggravated by large breasts. Breast bud removal is a relatively simple procedure to remove the small subcutaneous breast tissue while retaining the nipple and areola. It is true that if Ashley's breast size becomes problematic later, she could have breast reduction surgery done. However, this is a much more complicated, painful and risky procedure.

Ashley's parents believe that the two biggest challenges Ashley faces in life are discomfort and boredom (Parents' blog, 2006). Avoiding discomfort in persons such as Ashley is a complex goal involving the entire multidisciplinary team. Ashley is fortunate to not suffer from any chronic health problems. However, persons with profound limitations in mobility have a lifetime risk of increased skin breakdown, a major cause of discomfort and morbidity. This risk is increased through factors that include increased body weight, body morphology (such as large breasts), and poor nutritional status and is decreased through actions such as frequent repositioning, optimal hygiene, and good nutritional status. Having a smaller body size minimizes the potential for skin breakdown. A smaller size also increases the opportunity that caregivers can reposition a person more frequently and effectively. Ashley's parents have argued that having Ashley remain small affords other benefits to her. Her grandparents can physically continue to provide care for her. She can continue to use a stroller that she seems to prefer and allows her to be moved around the home to hear and watch family activities, as is often done with an infant. She will continue to fit into a standard bathtub. She will be able to be picked up and held on a parent's lap. She will be kept at home to be cared for within a family environment.

Yet should we change Ashley to fit the home, or change the home to fit Ashley? We could insure that caregivers who are large and strong be available to families to provide care for profoundly disabled persons. We could redesign homes to accommodate persons with disabilities so that their wheelchairs could fit through doorways, their bodies into bathtubs. Yet this utopian view of care would require a level of public financing that is currently unavailable. Americans currently tolerate having 46 million of their neighbors, co-workers, and the strangers they walk past on the sidewalk living without heath care insurance (Hoffman, 2007). Custodial care, such as Ashley needs, is not covered by even the most generous of health care plans. After a few weeks, care at home must be provided by non-paid family caregivers, or helpers paid out-of-pocket, or those paid for through long-term care insurance that the adult person obtained prior to the event, or paid for by public assistance through the Medicaid program after the person (and their spouse) have exhausted their personal finances (U.S. Department of Health and Human Services, 2007). For the elderly who require assistance with activities of daily living, for example after suffering a stroke, finding homecare is difficult. For disabled infants and children it may be nearly impossible. Catlin (2007) described the plight of parents who are trying to secure home health nursing for fragile children. Pediatric-trained caregivers willing to work for the low wages paid in home care settings are in short supply. Reimbursement is nearly non-existent. Equipment for pediatric patients is in short supply. Ashley does not live in a utopian world. By allowing parents of severely developmentally disabled children to have access to growth attenuation treatment, we do not abandon them to these harsh social and economic realities.

The last criticism to address is that Ashley's parents have attenuated her growth for their own convenience. We are disquieted by the thought that Ashley's parents might have decided to keep her small, a 'pillow angel' as they call her, without regard for her dignity or safety. Perhaps it is this last point that disturbs us most deeply. Yet in most healthcare settings, across all age groups, we are witnesses to family decision-making for loved ones who lack decision-making capacity: the distraught family in the intensive care setting making choices for a seriously ill or injured loved one, the exhausted family in mental health making choices for the acutely mentally ill person, the young parents in the NICU making choices for the babies who came too soon and too small. Families approach these decisions without medical training, often in crisis, and with multiple demands on their care giving and financial means. Ethically and legally, we invest in the family the right and duty to make decisions and to care for family members who are unable to do so themselves. Why? Because families do the best they can and it is better than we, as professionals, could do for them. Sometimes we are called upon to protect our patients in situations of abuse or neglect. But most often, we are asked to simply bear witness to the daily sacrifices and acts of love that constitute family caregiving and to humbly guide these families in their decision-making. Ashley's parents, physicians and the multidisciplinary ethics committee have allowed us to share, and judge, their thoughtful deliberations (Gunther & Diekema; Parents' blog; 2006). Each of us can learn from their decisions and benefit from their generosity. So ask yourself again, what if this were my child—who I loved dearly and desperately wanted to ensure would always be able to be cared for in a home setting, by family members? What would I do?

References

Brakman S.V., & Amari-Vaught E. (1999). *Resistance and refusal. Hastings Center Report, 29*(1), 22.

Catlin A.J. (2007). Home care for the high-risk neonate: success or failure depends on home health nurse funding and availability. *Home Healthcare Nurse, 25*(2), 1–5.

Gunther D.F., & Diekema D.S. (2006). Attenuating growth in children with profound developmental disability: A new approach to an old dilemma. *Archives of Pediatrics & Adolescent Medicine, 160*(10), 1013–1017.

Hoffman C.B. (2007). Simple truths about America's uninsured. *American Journal of Nursing, 107*(1), 40–3, 46–47.

Parents' Blog: Ashley's Mom and Dad. (2006). The "Ashley Treatment", toward a better quality of life for "Pillow Angels." . . .

U.S. Department of Health and Human Services, *Medicare: The Official U.S. Government Site for People with Medicare. Long-term Care.* . . .

Watson K.C., Lentz M.J., & Cain K.C. (2006). Associations between fracture incidence and use of depot medroxyprogesterone acetate and anti-epileptic drugs in women with developmental disabilities. *Womens Health Issues 16*(6), 346–52.

Teresa A. Savage 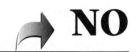 **NO**

In Opposition of the Ashley Treatment

Ashley, at age 6 years, had surgery to remove her uterus and breast buds and after recovering from surgery, was placed on high doses of estrogen for 3 years to permanently stunt her linear growth; her parents refer to the surgeries and hormonal medication as the "Ashley treatment." Her parents believed the surgery and medication would improve their daughter's quality of life by keeping her from reaching adult growth in height and weight. Ashley is permanently disabled from a static encephalopathy. She is reported to have the cognitive abilities arrested at a 3-month level. She is unable to move out of the position in which she is placed and prefers not to be in a sitting position but in a lying position. Her parents are devoted to their daughter and say that they made the decision for the "Ashley treatment" in order to keep her at home. They fear that if she grew an anticipated adult height of 5'6" and adult weight, they would be unable to move and carry her and include her in family gatherings.

Her parents described their reasoning in choosing the "Ashley treatment" in their blog (http://ashleytreatment.spaces.live.com/). Within their blog, there are certain assumptions that underlie their reasoning. I challenge these assumptions.

Assumption 1: Keeping Ashley small will improve her quality of life. Her parents listed "bedsores," "pneumonia," and "bladder infection" as reasons for keeping her small and therefore less likely to be "bedridden" and susceptible to those three complications of immobility.

In my experience in caring for premature infants, who are the smallest human beings ex utero, if you do not re-position them, they will get skin breakdown. If you do not use appropriate bedding, they will get skin breakdown. If you do not re-position them and perform pulmonary hygiene, they will get pneumonia. If you do not keep them adequately hydrated with appropriate nourishment, they are at risk for bladder infections. Size is less important as attention to positioning, bedding materials, pulmonary hygiene, nutrition, and elimination.

Ashley will still require total care and keeping her smaller will make it easier to provide her care. Keeping her small makes it physically easier to care for her, which will positively impact the quality of her life. If she was not kept

Reprinted from *Pediatric Nursing Journal*, vol. 33, no. 2, April 2007, pp. 175–178. Reprinted with permission of the publisher, Jannetti Publications, Inc., East Holly Avenue, Box 56, Pitman, NJ 08071-0056; (856) 256-2300; fax: (856) 589-7463; Web site: www.pediatricnursing.net; for a sample copy of the journal, please contact the publisher.

small, she could still have a "good" quality of life, but her care may require more effort. Caregiver effort is no minor factor in Ashley's quality of life; it is perhaps the most critical factor in her quality of life, so I don't think her parents should deny that it was a motivating factor in the decision to use high dose estrogen to stunt her growth.

Assumption 2: *Ashley will never bear children so she doesn't need her uterus. It is anticipated that menstrual hygiene will pose a caregiver problem and she may have menstrual cramps.*

Do the risks of a hysterectomy outweigh the potential for monthly cramps and bleeding? One might argue that she will be wearing diapers all her life, so what difference does it make if there is urine, stool, or blood in the diaper? She may have discomfort with her periods or she may not. Do the known and real risks of a hysterectomy outweigh the potential risks of her monthly periods?

If she does have skin problems associated with her menses, or she has discomfort that cannot be relieved with medication, she can be treated as any woman is treated—with hormonal therapy to relieve symptoms or to reduce or eliminate menstrual flow. If conservative therapy fails, she could have endometrial ablation or a hysterectomy. Why is it necessary to make this decision at age 6?

Some parents believe that a hysterectomy will protect their child from sexual abuse. A hysterectomy will protect against pregnancy but not molestation, rape, or sexually transmitted diseases.

Assumption 3: *Ashley will have large breasts because there is a family history of large breasts, fibrocystic disease, and breast cancer. [It is unclear if she tested positive for the BRCA1/2 gene. If she has the gene, she's at a greater than average risk for ovarian cancer, so why weren't her ovaries removed too?] Therefore, she is better off having her breast buds removed.*

Large breasts can be uncomfortable, although there are many women with large breasts who do not choose to have them removed or even reduced. Her parents worry that her breasts will create difficulties in strapping her into her adaptive seating. A penis and scrotum may present difficulties when positioning boys with the same type and degree of disability as Ashley's, but it has not been suggested that the penis and scrotum be removed because of ease in positioning. A boy with the same disability will not reproduce and can void through a shortened urethra, much like a girl's urethra, and surgery may require minimal cutting. So the same argument about justifying removal of the uterus and breasts could be made to remove a disabled boy's penis and scrotum, but that sounds more like mutilation.

Her parents' blog also maintained that large breasts could "invite" abuse. Parents of children with this level of disability worry about vulnerability to sexual molestation. No surgery or hormonal medicating can prevent molestation, and large breasts do not "invite" abuse. Opportunity and lack of supervision invite abuse. Only close supervision of anyone coming in contact with the vulnerable person can protect against abuse.

Assumption 4: *High dose estrogen will cause the growth plates to close, thereby stopping linear growth and concomitant weight gain.*

Are the long-term risks of high dose estrogen in a 6-year old girl known? Is it known whether or not the high dose estrogen will reduce growth to the degree that is desired? (Were the breast buds removed because of the possibility for breast cancer with high dose estrogens?) Again, it is disturbing to have healthy tissue removed in anticipation of a problem.

Assumption 5: *Adults with a mental age of an infant are undignified.*

Adults with profound intellectual disability often do not look like the rest of the population. Their features may be coarse; they may have open mouths, protruding tongues, and drooling. They are often the subject of ridicule by unkind, cruel people. Do the attitudes and behavior of uncouth people warrant surgery and hormonal medicating of the recipient of the bad behavior? The stigma toward people with disabilities has persisted despite community integration, mainstream education, independent living, and the Americans with Disabilities Act. The parents' view of dignity, keeping Ashley's appearance more consistent with her intellectual level, differs from the view of dignity from people in the disability communities. The parents quote a passage in their blog that says "The estrogen treatment is not what is grotesque. Rather, it is the prospect of having a full-grown and fertile woman endowed with a mind of a baby." It is regrettable if her parents capitulate to the stigma and believe growth attenuation is necessary to preserve their daughter's dignity.

Disability groups have responded to the "Ashley treatment" with a fervor. They view the choices these parents made as a failure of society to provide the support to people with disabilities and their families (American Association on Intellectual and Developmental Disabilities, 2007; Disability Rights Education & Defense Fund, 2007; Not Dead Yet, 2007; Dick Sobsey [parent of a child with a disability and Director of the John Dossetor Health Ethics Centre, University of Alberta], 2007; Feminists Response in Disability Activism, 2007; ADAPT Youth, 2007r; TASH, 2007). They criticize the medical establishment for offering drastic interventions with unknown long-term risks instead of advocating for social changes that would support Ashley and her family.

I have a colleague who talks about "holding families hostage to the revolution." It's unfair to malign this family who acted with medical endorsement in choosing interventions that many people in the disability community find repugnant. They were doing what they thought was best for Ashley and their family and were extremely brave in publicly sharing their experience. However, before the revolution is over, and to afford children like Ashley all the protections that a human being should have, due process should occur when interventions like the "Ashley treatment" is recommended. The child should have an independent advocate to weigh the risks and benefits of the proposed intervention. Preferably, the advocate should be a person with a disability who is better able to envision from a disability perspective what able-bodied parents can never know—what it is like to live with a disability. Albrecht and Devlieger (1999) describe the disability paradox where people with moderate to severe disabilities report a good or excellent quality of life. The parents' projection of Ashley's quality of life may be conflated with the projection of their own or their family's quality of life. They fear the effects of the "unending work" (to borrow from Corbin and Strauss, 1988) on their lives and, in turn, believe it will adversely affect Ashley's quality of life. It seems the vast majority of disability activists strongly oppose the "Ashley treatment." I wonder if her parents viewed it as the lesser of two evils.

References

ADAPT Youth. (2007). ADAPT Youth appalled at parents surgically keeping disabled daughter childlike. . . .

Albrecht, G. L., & Devlieger, P. J. (1999). The disability paradox: High quality of life against all odds. *Social Science & Medicine, 48,* 977–988.

American Association on Intellectual and Developmental Disabilities. (2007). Unjustifiable non-therapy: A response to Gunther & Diekema (2006), and to the issue of growth attenuation for young people on the basis of disability. . . .

Corbin, J., & Strauss, A. (1988). *Unending work and care: Managing chronic illness at home.* San Francisco: Jossey-Bass publishers.

Disability Rights Education and Defense Fund. (2007). Modify the system, not the person. . . .

Feminists Response in Disability Activism (FRIDA). (2007). FRIDA demands ethics and accountability from the AMA. . . .

Gunther, D. F., & Diekema, D. S. (2006). Attenuating growth in children with profound developmental disability: A new approach to an old dilemma. *Archives of Pediatric & Adolescent Medicine, 160,* 1013–1017.

Not Dead Yet. (2007). *Not Dead Yet statement on "Growth Attenuation" experimentation.* . . .

Sobsey, D. (2007). Growth attenuation and indirect-benefit rationale. *Ethics and Intellectual Disability: Newsletter of the Network on Ethics and Intellectual Disability, 10*(1), 1–2, 7–8.

TASH. (2007). Attenuating growth. . . .

Turnbull, R., Wehmeyer, M., Turnbull, A., & Stowe, M. (2007). *KU experts examine issues in surgery to halt girl's growth.* . . .

EXPLORING THE ISSUE

May Doctors Offer Medical Drugs and Surgery to Stop a Disabled Child from Maturing?

Critical Thinking and Reflection

1. What would be the best way, in your view, of helping a family care for a severely disabled child? Is the strategy chosen by Ashley's parents an acceptable strategy, in your view, given the help available to them?
2. Dignity is invoked in two different ways by Theresa Savage—as one of the possible reasons for offering the Ashley treatment, and as a reason for prohibiting the treatment. Explain these two uses, and explain which you find more persuasive, if you are drawn to one or the other side.
3. Are there policy options in between banning this kind of intervention and doing nothing to limit its use?

Is There Common Ground?

Ashley is now 14 years old and according to a blog her parents keep about her development and their family life (www.pillowangel.org/), she is happy and doing well. (An earlier blog at http://ashleytreatment.spaces.live.com/blog/ has been discontinued.) The blog contains pictures of Ashley, interviews with the family, and stories about children who have undergone versions of "the Ashley treatment."

Most of the commentaries on the "Ashley treatment" have acknowledged the parents' deep love for their child and their good intentions but have criticized the treatment on several grounds: unknown risks, the possibility of abuse in other cases; focus on the parent's convenience rather than benefit to Ashley; and failure to consider the rights of persons with disabilities.

Edwards, a British philosopher, develops a theme that was common in the initial reaction in 2007 to news about the Ashley treatment. He argues that the treatment sets a worrisome precedent that could be used to justify even more radical interventions. Another kind of reaction, however, is articulated by the bioethicist Erik Parens, who argues that parents' wishes—as well as those expressed by people with disabilities themselves, when they are able to express them—should be respected, as long as their assumptions can be discussed to ensure that they are truly informed.

Additional Resources

Daniel F. Gunther and Douglas A. Diekema, physicians involved in the case, describe their decision-making process in "Attenuating Growth in Children with Profound Developmental Disability: A New Approach to an Old Dilemma," *Archives of Pediatric and Adolescent Medicine* (October 2006).

S.D. Edwards discussion is in "The Ashley Treatment: A Step Too Far, or Not Far Enough?" *Journal of Medical Ethics* (May 2008).

Erik Parens's discussion of the Ashley treatment is "Respecting Children with Disabilities—and Their Parents," *Hastings Center Report* (January–February 2009). It is part of a set of essays on the use of medical technologies to alter children's bodies.

Heather T. Battles and Lenore Manderson emphasize the importance of medical anthropological research on the meanings of personhood and childhood disability, autonomy, and the ethics of body modification surgery ("The Ashley Treatment: Furthering the Anthropology of/on Disability," *Medical Anthropology* [vol. 27, no. 3, July 2008]).

N. Tan and I. Brassington look at the Ashley treatment from the viewpoint of professional responsibilities and find worrisome aspects ("Agency, Duties, and the 'Ashley Treatment,'" *Journal of Medical Ethics* [vol. 35, 2009]).

After weighing all the arguments, Peter A. Clark and Lauren Vasta conclude that "When solutions exist that allow individuals with severe brain impairments to be cared for without interfering with their natural developmental patterns, then these solutions should always take priority." They recommend a moratorium on the Ashley treatment ("The Ashley Treatment: An Ethical Analysis," *The Internet Journal of Law, Healthcare and Ethics* [vol. 5, no. 1, 2007]).

See also S. Matthew Liao, Julian Savulescu, and Mark Sheehan, "The Ashley Treatment: Best Interests, Convenience, and Parental Decision-Making," *Hastings Center Report* (March–April 2007).

ISSUE 15

Should Scientists Create Artificial Organisms?

YES: Mark A. Bedau, from "The Intrinsic Scientific Value of Reprogramming Life," *Hastings Center Report* (July/August 2011)

NO: Christopher J. Preston, from "Synthetic Biology: Drawing a Line in Darwin's Sand," *Environmental Values* (February 2008)

Learning Outcomes

After reading this issue, you should be able to:

- Briefly explain "synthetic biology" and discuss some of the ethical questions it raises.
- Explain the idea of "intrinsic value."
- Discuss whether the alteration of nature can be intrinsically morally troubling.

ISSUE SUMMARY

YES: Philosopher Mark A. Bedau argues that the effort to "create life"—the goal of the field known as synthetic biology—would be both socially useful and a huge step forward in the quest to understand what life is.

NO: Christopher J. Preston, an environmental ethicist, warns that synthetic biology is a threat to the concept of "natural" that has guided moral thinking about the environment in North America.

On May 20, 2010, the J. Craig Venter Institute (JCVI) announced that it had engineered the "first self-replicating synthetic bacterial cell." This achievement was described in some media reports as "creating life" or "playing God." Although the achievement was indeed significant, the self-replicating cell involved the complete replacement of genetic material, including more than one million base pairs of DNA and almost 1,000 genes. Most careful commentators held that JCVI had not created life; it had instead synthesized a cell's genome and inserted it into an existing cell. Possibly, however, researchers following in JCVI's footsteps will someday manage to do something that looks more like creating life.

JCVI's "synthetic cell" represents one of several lines of work in a field called "synthetic biology." JCVI is working on synthesizing whole cellular genomes. Others in synthetic biology are working on creating short, standardized genetic sequences that can be put together in various combinations and inserted into to do useful or interesting things. Others start with existing organisms such as *Escherichia coli* and modify their metabolisms. Still others are intent on creating living organisms using entirely new kinds of materials, rather than borrowing from existing life forms.

Much work in synthetic biology can also be viewed as essentially an extension of genetic engineering, that is, of the modification of biological systems by inserting genes from other sources and combining them in new ways. But if scientists succeed in creating new kinds of living organisms, it seems to bring biotechnological control over life to a whole new level. As Joachim Boldt and Oliver Müller from Freiburg University explain, "If we look at nature through the glasses of genetic engineering, we see a world filled with entities that are already useful to us in many respects and that just need some reshaping here and there to perfectly match our interests. In contrast, synthetic biology does not soften edges, but creates life-forms that are meant not to have any edges from the start. . . . Nature is a blank space to be filled with whatever we wish" (*Nature Biotechnology*, April 2008, p. 388).

These new microorganisms will be designed to serve a specific purpose, such as creating new biofuels or clean water. There are potential medical uses as well, such as developing new medications or destroying cancer cells. Synthetic biology has accelerated in recent years because of the increased sophistication and power of genetic sequencing technologies. At the same time, these technologies have become much cheaper. The basic components are readily available.

The introduction of a new technology raises both hopes and fears. While many scientists see enormous possibilities in synthetic biology, others worry about the risk that the engineered cell will escape the laboratory, cause environmental havoc, or be used by terrorists. Other worries are more philosophical—that the very enterprise will somehow imperil other important societal values, such as environmentalism and protection of nature.

This discussion has historical roots. In the early 1970s, when genetic engineering was introduced, the scientists who had developed the ability to splice and combine genes were themselves concerned about the implications, primarily risk to laboratory workers. They agreed on a voluntary moratorium on conducting the most dangerous experiments and convened a conference at Asilomar in Pacific Grove, California, in 1975 to discuss the potential hazards. They lifted the moratorium but established safety guidelines, including containment standards and a review system. Over the years, with the benefit of extensive experience, scientists and government agencies have modified the restrictions. One of the current questions is whether existing government oversight for genetic engineering is adequate for synbio.

The YES and NO selections provide two opposing views of this new technology. Mark A. Bedau, a philosopher, acknowledges the unknowns but concludes on balance that the potential benefits of synthetic biology outweigh the possible risks. Indeed, says Bedau, synthetic biology's capacity to challenge our philosophical assumptions about the place of humans in the cosmos is itself valuable. Christopher J. Preston, a philosopher and environmentalist, addresses the question of "natural" as it relates to the environment. He fears that the newly created forms depart so radically from the core principle of Darwinian natural selection—descent through modification—that there will be a direct negative impact on environmental ethics.

YES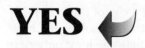

Mark A. Bedau

The Intrinsic Scientific Value of Reprogramming Life

The general public's attention to synthetic biology has been accelerated by the achievement a year ago of a so-called synthetic cell by a team of scientists at the J. Craig Venter Institute, and also by the helpful and timely report on the ethics of synthetic biology from the Presidential Commission for the Study of Bioethical Issues. Most attention has focused on synthetic biology's practical implications, such as the need for safeguards in the laboratory and the environment and security procedures to prevent malicious use. But we should give more attention to some of synthetic biology's less practical implications. In particular, I urge us not to overlook the intrinsic scientific value of making synthetic cells.

First, let us be clear about what the JCVI team actually accomplished. Although their achievement is often called a "synthetic cell," it is a *partly* synthetic cell. They were working with normal bacteria, the simplest known cellular forms of life. They first sequenced the entire genome of one natural bacterial species (*Mycoplasma mycoides*). They next synthesized copies of the entire *M. mycoides* genome—a technical tour de force that involved making new copies of the *mycoides* genome out of nonliving raw materials that can be ordered from chemical supply houses. Next, they inserted their synthetic genomes into bacteria from *Mycoplasma capricolum*, a closely related species, and got the *capricolum* bacteria to express the synthetic *mycoides* genome. This in effect changed the *capricolum* bacterium into a *mycoides* bacterium. However, 99 percent of the dry weight of the resulting bacterium is simply a normal living *M. capricolum* bacterium used as the genome-transplant recipient. So, the JCVI synthetic cell is only partly synthetic. Furthermore, the resulting construct is not a new *kind* of bacterium, but merely (a slightly modified version of) an old, familiar bacterium produced by artificial means.

Because the JCVI cell is only partly synthetic, and because the resulting cell is merely an artificially produced example of a natural life form, the commission's report can correctly deny that the JCVI has "created life." However, there is an active scientific research program aimed at making *fully* synthetic cells being carried out today by a number of different laboratory teams in the United States, Europe, and Japan. The commission report downplays these efforts, claiming that creating a fully synthetic cell "remains remote for the foreseeable future."[1] Yet many—including me—are convinced that fully synthetic cells might very well be created within our lifetimes, perhaps even within the next decade. The reason for this optimism is that most of the components of such cells have already been synthesized, and many of them have already been combined in the laboratory. Fully synthetic cells will in all likelihood be a form of life that is rather new and perhaps very unnatural. There is no reason why a fully synthetic cell must closely mimic any natural form of life; novel molecular mechanisms might make the project much more feasible. Furthermore, it will be easier to create fully synthetic cells if they are much simpler than any natural form of life. So making a fully synthetic cell would be creating genuinely new forms of life from wholly nonliving materials. (Of course, human scientists are needed to create the laboratory conditions in which nonliving materials will assemble into a synthetic cell. Nobody supposes that any synthetic cell will arise without the intentional efforts of intelligent, living beings.)

The commission report warns against using "sensationalist buzzwords" and phrases such as "creating life" because "ultimately such words impede ongoing understanding of both the scientific and ethical issues at the core of public debates on these topics."[2] I disagree. When synthetic biologists do create fully synthetic cells—and they will, at some point—then we *should* describe it as creating life, for that would be true. Similarly, those who are trying to make fully synthetic cells should be forthright about the fact that they aim to create life. This will encourage us all to face squarely the resulting social and ethical issues.

The main point of making synthetic cells is to make new kinds of cells—cells that perform useful and desired functions beyond the capability of any existing form of life. The JCVI achievement opens the door to this possibility. This is one of the reasons why the JCVI achievement is game changing. To make a synthetic genome, one needs a supply of the nucleotides out of which a genome is constructed, and one needs the information describing the entire genetic sequence of the genome. While the JCVI team used the sequence of *M. mycoides*, they could have started with a different genetic sequence. In fact, in principle they could have started with virtually *any* genetic sequence; they could have invented an entirely new sequence and created an entirely new genome. If you think of the genome as a kind of software that drives a cell's development and behavior, you could say that the JCVI team demonstrated they could *arbitrarily reprogram* simple forms of life. Fully synthetic cells will take full advantage of life's programmability. This point is often unappreciated, and it is largely ignored in the commission report. But it is precisely this arbitrary programmability that opens the door to synthetic biology's great intrinsic scientific value.

Arbitrarily reprogrammable synthetic cells are a fantastic new tool for illuminating the complex molecular mechanisms that can give rise to simple forms of life. Even the simplest forms of life are enormously complex biomolecular complexes, about which there are a multitude of unanswered questions. The ability to reprogram simple life forms however we wish enables us to make vast arrays of precise experimental modifications of the cells' molecular conditions. The JCVI achievement enables us to construct any new genome we want and observe what happens when we put them inside donor cells. The eventual achievement of fully synthetic cells will expand this reprogrammability to include modifications of every aspect of a cell's molecular constituents. A molecular biologist could hardly dream of a more powerful and flexible experimental methodology. For this reason, arbitrarily reprogrammable synthetic cells can propel a basic scientific research program to reveal all the molecular mechanisms underlying simple life forms.

In addition, efforts to make fully synthetic cells will also help us better understand exactly what it is for a simple molecular aggregate to be alive. At the time of his death, the blackboard of Nobel laureate Richard Feynman contained the sentence, "What I cannot create, I do not understand." Feynman's dictum succinctly captures why our ability to make synthetic cells has such great intrinsic scientific value. The nature of life remains one of the deepest fundamental mysteries about our world. Once we finally figure out how to make wholly new forms of life entirely from nonliving materials, we will be able to design research programs to probe what kinds of radically novel chemical systems deserve to be considered as alive. We can test radically different genetic programs, with new kinds of metabolic systems, new kinds of containers, and new kinds of interactions among them. Making just one kind of synthetic cell will not tell us very much about the nature of life. But experimenting with a great variety of different synthetic cells is exactly what will eventually enable us to learn what is and what is not required to turn a collection of inert molecules into a living organism.

Make no mistake. It is one thing to conduct a research program to unlock the remaining molecular secrets of life. It is quite another thing to program synthetic cells to do whatever we want. There is nothing stopping us from embarking on the research program. But today nobody has any idea how to program a partly or fully synthetic cell to do whatever we want—neither the JCVI team nor anybody else. If we could, then we already would have reprogrammed bacteria to produce inexpensive fuels, foods, building materials, pharmaceuticals, you name it. People are actively working on these tasks, and no doubt many will eventually succeed. But today we can program only pretty trivial traits, and only one synthetic biology reprogramming project has had notable commercial success (making cheaper malaria drugs). Synthetic biology has reprogrammed bacteria to do many things, but progress is painstaking and each achievement requires surmounting many challenges. Furthermore, the difficulty increases by leaps and bounds as we try to reprogram much more complex traits. The JCVI team unlocked the door to arbitrarily reprogramming simple life forms, but figuring out how to go through that door and end up where we want remains a largely unsolved scientific challenge.

Here is one way to get some sense of the difficulty. It has been estimated that it would take about 1080 hydrogen atoms to fill the entire known universe. The number 1080 can be written as a one followed by eighty zeros, and

YES / Mark A. Bedau **299**

typing this number on an ordinary piece of paper would take one to two lines of text. The genome that the JCVI team synthesized consists of a little over one million base pairs. Since there are four nucleotides, there are about $4^{1,000,000}$, or about $10^{600,000}$, different genomes of the same length that the JCVI team could have synthesized instead. To get a feel for the size of this number, bear in mind that written out, it would be a one followed by 600,000 zeros, which would fill about two hundred pages. In other words, the number of different genomes of the size of *M. mycoides*'s genome (which is uncommonly small, as genomes go) that could be synthesized is many, many, many times larger than the number of hydrogen atoms that would fill the entire known universe. So, choosing which genome will produce a specific kind of synthetic cell is like finding the proverbial needle in a haystack. Although the JCVI team has unlocked the door to reprogramming life, we need further research on programming different kinds of synthetic cells before we can take advantage of this new ability.

Of course, any such research program must be conducted in a socially responsible manner. Most of the public commentary on synthetic biology so far has focused on concerns about safety and security, and such concerns must be adequately met. Furthermore, addressing them can be difficult, because life forms can adapt and evolve in unanticipated and unintended directions. So there is good reason for synthetic biology to exercise all due caution—and the synthetic biology community should be commended for making serious and sensible efforts to do just that.

The awareness of life's arbitrary reprogrammability will no doubt shock and disturb some people. In particular, constructing synthetic cells entirely from nonliving materials will provide overwhelming evidence that simple life forms are nothing more than very complex molecular mechanisms. Overwhelming evidence is not absolutely conclusive proof; one could still consistently believe that simple life forms are more than complex molecular mechanisms, just as one could consistently hold the belief that everything in the universe, including everyone's memories and beliefs about past experiences, was created only five minutes ago. But both beliefs would be equally desperate attempts to deny the obvious. Now, if the simplest life forms are just complex molecular mechanisms, then there is good reason to conclude that the same holds for more complex life forms—even human beings. Humans are vastly more complex than bacteria, of course, and humans have conscious mental states and complex moral attitudes that are worlds beyond anything true of any bacterium. Nevertheless, since the simplest and original life forms are just complex chemical machinery, and since humans evolved from those simple life forms by a long series of evolutionary transitions and innovations, it stands to reason that something like the same conclusion will apply to human life, too. That is, synthetic biology drives us to acknowledge that we, too, are complex chemical mechanisms.

Rather than ignoring this conclusion, or being frightened or embarrassed by it, we should face it squarely. What consequences follow? Does it undermine respect for humans and other life forms? Does it debunk the pretensions of conventional morality? Does it imply that life is not a legitimate source of awe and wonder? All of these questions remain open. Debate on these issues will be provoked by, and should be informed by, the new scientific insights that result from our efforts to make and reprogram synthetic cells.

Notes

1. Presidential Commission for the Study of Bioethical Issues, *New Directions: The Ethics of Synthetic Biology and Emerging Technologies* (Washington, D.C.: Government Printing Office, 2010), 3.

2. Ibid., 15.

Christopher J. Preston   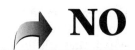 **NO**

Synthetic Biology: Drawing a Line in Darwin's Sand

Introduction

Two years shy of celebrating the 150 year anniversary of the publication *Origin of Species*—a book without which it is hard to imagine either modern biology or modern environmentalism existing in any recognisable form—synthetic biology and nanotechnology threaten to usurp the most important principle of Darwinian natural selection. These emerging technologies strike at the very heart of the distinction between biotic nature and artefact. They create organisms that lack significant connections to the historical evolutionary process. With the threat provided by these technologies looming, those for whom the ideas of 'nature' and the 'historical evolutionary process' comes with any kind of normative punch have some serious self-reflection to do. Many environmental ethicists are about to lose the ground from underneath one of their favourite philosophical ideas. . . .

At Stake for Environmental Ethics

A large number of positions in environmental ethics rest on a substantial normative commitment to the value of what is biologically natural over what is artefactual. In environmental philosophy the term the 'natural' generally prompts some form of moral approbation while objects classed as 'unnatural' or 'artefactual' are viewed more suspiciously. Aldo Leopold introduced his landmark Sand County Almanac with a request for a re-appraisal of things 'unnatural, tame, and confined' in terms of things 'wild, natural, and free' (Leopold, 1949: ix). Contemporary environmental ethicist Holmes Rolston, III, captured a similar sentiment in his statement that '[m]y concept of the good is not coextensive with the natural, but it does greatly overlap it', adding '[N]o one has learned the full scope of what it means to be moral until he has learned to respect the integrity and worth of those things we call wild' (Rolston, 1986: 49,46). Both theorists point to the fact that the *naturalness* of wild nature carries moral weight.

To sustain this line of thinking, the small matter of how to delimit the natural and mark it off from the non-natural (or artefactual) has always been central to environmental philosophy. Typically, environmental ethicists have

From *Environmental Values*, vol. 17, no. 1, February 2008. Copyright © 2008 by The White Horse Press. Reprinted by permission.

put great stock in the distinction tidily made by Aristotle more than two thousand years ago. Aristotle characterised a natural object in *The Physics* as one
which 'has within itself a principle of movement and of stationariness (in
respect of place, or of growth and decrease, or by way of alteration)' (192b8-11)
(Aristotle, 1941). Any change the object undergoes over time is determined
from wholly within that object's nature. Acorns grow into oaks, silverback
gorillas grow grey and arthritic, and mountains slowly erode. An artefact,
by contrast, lacks 'the source of its own production . . . that principle is in
something else external to the thing' (192b28). The external source to which
Aristotle refers is the intentional action of a human. Artefacts thus display the
presence of human intention. Natural objects do not. Keekok Lee, anchoring a
good deal of her work entirely on Aristotle's distinction, usefully summarised
the point this way:

> '[T]he natural' . . . refers to whatever exists which is not the result of
> deliberate human intervention, design, and creation in terms of its mate-
> rial efficient, formal, and final causes . . . The natural comes into exist-
> ence, continues to exist, and goes out of existence entirely independent
> of human volition and manipulation . . . [B]y contrast, 'the artefactual'
> embodies a human intentional structure. (Lee, 1999: 82) . . .

The apparent simplicity of Aristotle's distinction turns out, of course,
to be an illusion. The problems inherent in distinguishing the natural from
the artefactual have long been known to environmental philosophers. In his
1874 essay 'Nature', John Stuart Mill noticed immediately what appears to be
the most central paradox. On the one hand, all human actions are natural
because humans have a natural origin and none of their actions transcend
natural laws. Yet at the same time, Mill saw how everything a human does, by
Aristotle's definition, leaves nature in a non-natural state. . . .

Despite its problems, the idea of nature unmodified by human activity is
so central to environmentalism that it is almost impossible to imagine letting
it go. Certainly the history of the North American environmental movement
could hardly be so abruptly rewritten. The emotional connections run deep. As
a matter of political reality, the idea that wild nature is morally significant is
one that motivates millions. Images of polar bears prowling arctic ice-flows,
humpback whales breaching in front of snow-capped mountains, and lionesses
lounging with their young on the African savannah adorn the walls of bedrooms
and boardrooms across the world. Denying the moral significance of the biologically natural is almost inconceivable for environmentalists.

In addition to the politics of the matter, there are also important non-
pragmatic reasons to retain the Aristotelian idea of 'nature'. Nature unmodified by human intention may be increasingly hard to find today but, as a matter
of historical fact, there were close to 4.6 billion years of geological history on
Earth that preceded the arrival of our first, artefact-creating ancestor, *Homo habilis,*
approximately 2 million years ago. During these 4.598 billion years of earth's
history there were independent processes at work ultimately responsible for creating everything environmentalists find of value today. For 4.598 billion years,

there really did exist—as a matter of historical fact—something one could call 'nature' in an unproblematically Aristotelian sense.

For almost 80 per cent of that long reach of time, there was also something one could call the 'natural historical evolutionary process' slowly working its effects on living beings. As Charles Darwin explained in 1859, natural variations appearing in successive generations of biological organisms would tend to be preserved if those variations provided survival and breeding advantage. Over the millions of years of evolutionary history before the arrival of early hominids, Darwinian processes were responsible for creating great biological diversity and complexity, progenitors of the same diversity and complexity environmentalists seek to preserve today. It is for good reason that many environmental philosophers think this historical process morally important. Part of the reason we protect wildlands, claims Holmes Rolston, III, is that they provide 'the profoundest historical museum of all, a relic of the way the world was during 99.9% of past time' (Rolston, 1988: 14). Eugene Hargrove, pushing a quite different aesthetics-based approach to environmental protection, also suggests 'nature aesthetically is not simply what exists at this point in time; it is also the entire series of events and undertakings that have brought it to that point. When we admire nature, we also admire that history' (Hargrove, 1989: 195). This blending of historical fact and normative overlay is why the idea of non-humanised nature, despite the objections of Steven Vogel and the gloomy outlook of Bill McKibben, still serves a valuable purpose. The pertinent question to ask is how today's environmentalist might effectively use Aristotle's distinction between nature and artefact in the light of its numerous acknowledged problems. . . .

The Last Stand for Aristotle's Distinction

Synthetic biologists assemble short DNA sequences with known properties to create synthetic organisms that perform desirable functions. The self-appointed task of a synthetic biologist is to 'create living systems from the scratch and then endow these systems with new and novel functions' (Chopra and Kamma, 2006). The products of the technology potentially include drugs for medical applications, vehicles for targeted drug delivery, biosensors to detect and neutralise contamination in the environment, biotic components for information technology applications, new biodegradable materials, and the environmentally sensitive generation of methane or ethanol for energy projects. Due to the scale at which this work is carried out, some synthetic biologists call the technique 'natural nanotechnology'.

These are still relatively early days for the research. Nevertheless, Israeli scientists have engineered DNA to carry out basic mathematical functions that could theoretically be integrated into functioning computers. A Princeton University team has made an artificial organism within an *E. coli* bacterium that blinked predictably. Both teams in effect designed a biological machine to perform a chosen function, with the product of their efforts located entirely within a living cell. This form of engineering seems to successfully blur the line between a living biological organism and a purpose-built machine.

One of the major preliminary tasks for synthetic biologists is to isolate the properties of particular DNA sequences so that those sequences might be used as 'bio-bricks' to build future synthetic organisms. MIT has set up a Registry of Standard Biological Parts in order to catalogue these bio-bricks. This element of synthetic biology is sometimes characterised in terms of the bioscientific project of 'understanding life'. But the project of gaining more knowledge about living systems takes on a different hue when bio-bricks are used to engineer functional synthetic bio-systems. In these endeavours, synthetic biology is more appropriately characterised as the engineering of life (Endy, 2005). The goal of redesigning life using engineering principles is the true framework under which synthetic biology operates.

Environmental ethicists have long recognised that not all biological organisms are created equal. Most agree that there is a significant moral difference between wild genomes and genomes influenced by conscious human intention. Nineteenth century environmental advocate John Muir was one of the first to take up this point when he decried the artificially created stupidity of domestic sheep, famously calling them the 'hooved locusts' of the High Sierra. Contemporary environmental philosopher J. Baird Callicott, thinking along similar lines, categorises domestic animals as 'living artefacts' constituting 'yet another mode of extension of the works of man into the ecosystem' (Callicott, 1980: 330). Callicott's attack against biological organisms that are not 'wild, natural, and free' is even more vitriolic than Muir's. 'From the perspective of the land ethic', Callicott has insisted, 'a herd of cattle, sheep, or pigs is as much or more a ruinous blight on the landscape as a fleet of four-wheel drive off-road vehicles' (Callicott, 1980: 330). But however much both these theorists condemn domestic animals as 'biotic artefacts', the products of future synthetic biology will reach a whole new level of artificity.

One of Keekok Lee's main objections to molecular nanotechnology was its ability to 'construct *de novo* synthetic, abiotic kinds, from the design board' (Lee, 1999: 118). Synthetic biologists do exactly this but with biotic, rather than abiotic, kinds. The rhetoric used by synthetic biologists reveals just how ambitious are their construction projects. 'Think of it as Life, version 2.0' suggested the author of an article in *Scientific American* in 2004. The side-stepping manoeuvre synthetic biology makes around the historical evolutionary process is unique. Craig Venter, a synthetic biologist who earlier headed the consortium that mapped the human genome, is described as desiring to 'short-circuit millions of years of evolution and create his own version of a second genesis'. Other researchers share the goal of replacing evolution with something better. 'It will be a marvelous challenge to see if we can outdesign evolution' offered George Whitesides (2001).

Statements such as these bring out the difference between synthetic biology and traditional biotechnology. The relevant difference is that traditional biotechnology has always started with the genome of an existing organism and modified it by deleting or adding genes. The biologist has always taken a viable organism and made a selective change, hoping in the process not to modify the existing organism to such a degree that it is no longer able to survive. In every case of traditional biotechnology—even in the case of transgenic organisms—the genome on which the modification takes place is either the product of natural evolutionary processes or is the descendent of such a product. In every case in traditional biotechnology, there exists prior to the modification a viable organism on which the manipulation takes place.

This is not the case in synthetic biology. Synthetic biology does not start with a viable genome and modify it. It starts afresh with bio-bricks possessing known properties. There is no existing genome that undergoes modification. In the current state of the technology, the synthetically engineered DNA sequences have all been inserted into existing single-celled organisms. The idea, however, is not to preserve properties of the existing bacteria with modified behaviour. It is to create an entirely new organism with DNA constructed in its entirety according to human plan. The products of synthetic biology do not borrow any genetic function from genomes produced by the historical evolutionary process. To the contrary, synthetic biology is guided by the idea of leaving evolution and existing genomes behind in order to do a better job of creation with human goals in mind.

There are a number of familiar prudential worries that immediately arise with synthetic biology. Environmentalists might be concerned about risks that range from bioterrorism to the havoc such synthetic organisms might potentially wreak on the natural world. Synthetic biologists themselves already recognise this latter worry. The Venter Institute in California states on its website that '[T]he group has long been committed to fully exploring and educating the public about the ethical issues surrounding synthetic life. As such the team is dedicated to developing only synthetic organisms that completely lack the ability to survive outside the lab.' Steve Benner, a synthetic biology pioneer at the University of Florida, tries to create similar reassurance with his claim that the more different an artificial system is from a natural biological system, the less likely it is to survive in the wild. But in addition to the important prudential arguments, it seems there is also a clear basis for a deontological argument against synthetic biology.

In a famous article against the coupling of nanotechnology with biotechnology in *Wired Magazine* in 2000, Bill Joy, founder of Sun Microsystems, came close to articulating the problem. Joy claimed that future bio-nano technologies will cross a fundamental line when they allow the 'replicating and evolving processes that have been confined to the natural world . . . to become realms of human endeavor' (Joy, 2000). Joy's worry can be refined to apply to synthetic biology. Arteficity is again the problem. But the reason that the arteficity in synthetic biology is particularly worrisome is that it is a kind of arteficity that departs from the fundamental principle of Darwinian evolution, namely, descent through modification.

Charles Darwin himself, when searching for clues as to how the transmutation of species occurred in nature, spent many hours amongst dog and pigeon breeders admiring what these breeders had created using selective breeding techniques. His comfort level in this company is revealing. Darwin appreciated that when an experimenter modifies an existing genome through selective breeding he or she is doing much the same thing as natural selection has been doing continuously for over 3 billion years. In fact, it was because these breeders were doing something so similar to natural selection that Darwin was able to gain important insights he incorporated into his emerging theory.

Since natural selection works by taking an existing viable genome and modifying it incrementally, it seems plausible to characterise many previous types of biotechnology the same way. We might accept selective breeding, hybridisation and genetic technologies on the basis that they, like natural selection, work with the fundamental principle of descent through modification. They take existing genomes and modify them, even though they do it intentionally rather than randomly. All late twentieth century molecular biotechnology, including (perhaps rather surprisingly) the creation of transgenic organisms, follows this basic pattern. Viable genomes are modified with humans in laboratories now playing an integral role in making it happen. Clearly the modifications are not as incremental as they were in the case of pigeon breeding. Many of today's modifications would likely never have happened through natural selection or selective breeding. Nevertheless the biotechnology of the late twentieth century might charitably be recognised to retain the essence of Darwinian descent through modification.

As a result of retaining this Darwinian essence, genetically modified organisms possess a continuous causal chain between the genome currently being manipulated and the historical evolutionary process. At every point in this chain, there has existed a viable organism. This is true even if the organism being modified is itself the product or selective breeding or is transgenic. No product of twentieth century biotechnology has ever lacked this causal connection to the historical evolutionary past. Before synthetic biology, every organism had ancestors connecting it to the historical processes environmentalists value.

When a synthetic biologist creates a genome from scratch, by contrast, building organisms *de novo* from bio-bricks, causal continuity with the historical evolutionary past has been severed. With synthetic biology, all trace of descent from naturally selected ancestors has been eliminated. Though they still contain the nucleic acids, the biotic artefacts created by synthetic biology borrow none of their genetic sequencing from viable products of the historical evolutionary process. A genome built from bio-bricks is as complete an artefact as any biological organism can be. This makes it possible to offer an argument that accepts hybridisation, selective breeding and late twentieth century genetic biotechnology but rejects synthetic biology. The argument hinges on the fact that synthetic biology creates a more fundamental type of biotic artefact.

The heart of this argument against synthetic biology is consistent with the worries articulated by Keekok Lee but finds them realised in a different place. Lee argued, correctly it seems, that 'the supercession of natural evolution' (Lee, 2003: 190-3) is a serious worry for environmentalists. But the supercession of natural evolution does not occur, as Lee had suggested, when humans take a genome created through natural processes and modify it. Nor does it occur when humans take a modified genome and modify *that*. It occurs when humans create new genomes from scratch. In the former cases, there remains in place a chain of viable organisms connecting the latest modification to the 3.6 billion years of the natural evolutionary process. This causal connection remains even when the last few steps in the chain have involved the active manipulation of the genome by humans. Lee was right about unnaturalness being the problem, but she drew the line in the wrong place. Contra Lee, humans do not usurp the historical evolutionary process when they simply modify an existing genome. In certain senses, by doing this humans are doing to biological organisms exactly what evolution has 'done' to them over natural history, namely, descent through modification.

But in the case of a bacterium with its DNA created through synthetic biology, there is no causal chain of viable organisms connecting the synthetic organism with the historical evolutionary process. As Lee suggested was the problem with molecular nanotechnology, synthetic biologists create biotic kinds *de novo*. It is this creation of organisms *de novo* that makes synthetic biology different from previous biotechnologies. . . .

References

Aristotle. [1941]. *Physics,* trans. R.P. Hardie and R.K. Gaye. New York: Random House.

Callicott, J. Baird. 1980. 'Animal liberation: A triangular affair'. *Environmental Ethics* 2: 311–338.

Chopra, Paras and Akhil Kamma. 2006. 'Engineering life through Synthetic Biology'. *In Silico Biology* 6, 0038.

Darwin, Charles, 1898. *The Origin of Species, By Means of Natural Selection,* Vol. 1. New York: Appleton and Company.

Endy, D. 2005. 'Foundations of engineering biology'. *Nature* **438**: 449–453, doi: 10.1038/nature04342.

Hargrove, Eugene. 1989. *The Foundations of Environmental Ethics.* Englewood Cliffs, NJ: Prentice Hall.

Joy, Bill. 200. 'Why the future does not need us'. *Wired Magazine* 8(4). http://www.wired.com/wired/archive/8.04/joy.html (accessed 30 Aug 2007).

Lee, Keekok. 1999. *The Natural and the Artifactual: The Implications of Deep Science and Deep Technology for Environmental Philosophy.* New York: Lexington Books.

Lee, Keekok. 2003. *Philosophy and Revolutions in Genetics: Deep Science and Deep Technology.* Basingstoke: Palgrave MacMillan.

Leopold, Aldo. 1949. *A Sand County Almanac.* New York: Oxford University Press.

Rolston, Holmes, III. 1986. 'Can we and ought we to follow nature?' in Holmes Rolston, III, *Philosophy Gone Wild* (Buffalo, NY: Prometheus), pp. 30–52.

Rolston, Holmes, III. 1988. *Environmental Ethics: Duties to and Values in the Natural World.* Philadelphia, PA: Temple University Press.

Whitesides, George. 2001. 'The once and future nanomachine'. *Scientific American* (Sept).

EXPLORING THE ISSUE

Should Scientists Create Artificial Organisms?

Critical Thinking and Reflection

1. What would "creating life" really mean? In what way would the creation of life be valuable?
2. Preston argues that nature has intrinsic value; explain and evaluate that idea. Are concerns about protecting animals, species, or wild places best explained with this idea?
3. If part of the reason that naturally occurring species are valuable (and should be protected) is that they are natural phenomena, would a living thing that was not natural lack intrinsic value?
4. In the NO selection, Preston argues that the creation of artificial organisms is an attack on evolution. Evaluate that claim.

Is There Common Ground?

The ethical issues around synthetic biology were the subject of the first report that President Obama requested from his bioethics advisory body, the President's Commission for the Study of Bioethical Issues. The commission held three public meetings, featuring presentations from invited experts and discussion, and in December 2010 issued a report titled "New Directions: The Ethics of Synthetic Biology and Emerging Technologies." The overall recommendation from the commission was that development and use of the technology be allowed to proceed but that a stance of "prudent vigilance" be maintained toward the technology: Potential benefits and risks should be carefully weighed and assessed so that appropriate steps can be taken to ensure that the risks do not outweigh the potential benefits.

In 2012, a group of advocacy organizations led by Friends of the Earth published a contrasting document titled "Principles for the Oversight of Synthetic Biology," which calls for adherence to a more cautious approach to balancing risks and benefits, known as the "precautionary principle." The precautionary principle has been formulated in different ways, some stronger and some weaker, but the core idea in them is that risks can be hard to anticipate, and development of a new technology should be held back until the evidence suggests that the benefits outweigh the risks.

The commission concluded that concerns about how synthetic biology may alter the natural world do not constitute a decisive reason to call for a moratorium on it, although the commission also encouraged further public discussion of such moral and religious concerns.

Additional Resources

New directions and transcripts from the Presidential Commission's meetings are available at www.bioethics.gov/.

The Woodrow Wilson International Center for Scholars offers a variety of resources on synthetic biology at the following Web site, www.synbioproject.org/.

Bedau's selection is one of a set of essays on synthetic biology that appeared in the *Hastings Center Report* (July–August 2011).

"Principles for the Oversight of Synthetic Biology" can be accessed at www.foe.org/publications/reports. For criticism of the document, see Gregory E. Kaebnick, "Carefully Precautionary about Synthetic Biology?" *Bioethics Forum* (March 22, 2012); www.thehastingscenter.org/Bioethicsforum/Post.aspx?id=5781&blogid=140.

The Boldt and Müller article cited in the Introduction is titled "Newtons of the Leaves of Grass," *Nature Biotechnology* (April 2008).

Jonathan B. Tucker and Raymon A. Zilinskas, "The Promise and Perils of Synthetic Biology," *The New Atlantis,* offers a summary and also a reading list. It is available at www.thenewatlantis.com/publications/the-promise-and-perils-of-synthetic-biology.

Jonathan D. Moreno offers an optimistic view of synthetic biology in "Synthetic Biology Grows Up," *Science Progress* (May 20, 2010), which is available at www.scienceprogress.org/2010/05/synthetic-biology-grows-up.

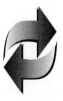

Internet References . . .

Organ Donation

This site provides current statistics and background information on the allocation of transplantable organs in the United States.

www.organdonor.gov

Kaiser Family Foundation

This research organization's Web site has reports and data about health care coverage in the United States, including state data.

www.kff.org/

Undocumented Patients

This Web site, created in a research project at The Hastings Center, offers information about undocumented immigrants and access to health care.

www.undocumentedpatients.org/

National Conference of State Legislatures

This organization keeps track of state legislation on a wide range of policy issues, including access to health care.

www.ncsl.org/

Access to Health Care

*I*n its modern infancy, biomedical ethics was almost exclusively concerned with issues relating to individual doctor–patient relationships.
Questions of resource allocation and public policy did occur, but mostly
within the context of whether or not a patient could pay for certain kinds
of care. In the past several decades, as medical care costs have skyrocke-
ted, the issues concerning equitable distribution of scarce resources have
become paramount. As medical care became more costly, it became less
accessible to the uninsured and to the underinsured (people who have
some employment-based health insurance but not enough to cover their
own illnesses or those of their families). In this new world of market-
driven health care, some old problems of resource allocation and public
policy take on new urgency. How far should commercialism extend? The
threat of war and bioterrorism has created new dilemmas for military
doctors and policymakers as they struggle to define a balance between
protecting the public's health in case of an attack and preserving the basic
liberties that Americans prize so highly. This unit takes up these issues.

- Is an Individual Mandate to Purchase Health Insurance Fair?
- Is There an Ethical Duty to Provide Health Care for All Immigrants to the United States?
- Should New Drugs Be Given to Patients Outside Clinical Trials?
- Should Vaccination for HPV Be Mandated for Teenage Girls?
- Should There Be a Market in Human Organs?

ISSUE 16

Is an Individual Mandate to Purchase Health Insurance Fair?

YES: Karen Davenport, from "Should Everyone Be Required to Have Health Insurance? Yes: It's the Key to Reform," *The Wall Street Journal* (January 23, 2012)

NO: Michael F. Cannon, from "Should Everyone Be Required to Have Health Insurance? No: Premiums Will Rise," *The Wall Street Journal* (January 23, 2012)

Learning Outcomes

After reading this issue, you should be able to:

- Identify core issues in recent health care reform initiatives.
- Discuss moral and policy arguments for and against mandating that individuals purchase health insurance.

ISSUE SUMMARY

YES: Karen Davenport, a health policy analyst, argues that an individual mandate to purchase health insurance emphasizes conservative ideals of personal responsibility and is necessary to ensure that health care is available and affordable for all citizens.

NO: Michael F. Cannon, also a health policy analyst, argues that it will promote irresponsibility, restrict personal freedom, increase the cost of health care, and lead ultimately to government rationing.

On March 23, 2010, President Obama signed into law the Patient Protection and Affordable Care Act (often cited as ACA), a major change in the way health care is financed and delivered in the United States. The United States has long been the only industrialized country without a national health care system, despite the efforts over the past 50 years of Republican and Democratic presidents to introduce change. The ACA is intended to address two major health care problems: lack of access and high costs.

Most of the people who have health insurance today obtain it through their employers. It was not always the case, however. Employer-based insurance was introduced in World War II as an incentive to recruit and retain workers because wartime regulations prevented them from offering higher wages.

Even though there is no national health care system, government programs have long played a major role. Medicare, a federal program, was enacted in 1965 to cover people over the age of 65 and those with end-stage kidney disease. Medicaid, introduced at the same time, is a joint federal–state program that covers people below the poverty line. There are other government-sponsored programs—TRICARE (formerly CHAMPUS) for uniformed service members, retirees, and their families; federal employees' insurance; and the Children's Health Insurance Program (CHIP) for poor children. These government-sponsored programs are administered by private insurance companies.

Even with these programs aimed at special populations, around 50 million people lack health insurance in the United States. According to the Commonwealth Fund, a private foundation that addresses health reform, data from the U.S. Census Bureau shows that provisions of the ACA that have already gone into effect have lowered the number of young adults who lack insurance. Because of the weak job market, however, the overall number of uninsured still increased by about 5 million between 2007 and 2009. Many employers also dropped or limited coverage or raised employee contributions.

Most of the adults without health insurance are in working families but have low incomes. Twenty-seven percent of people whose families have incomes under $25,000 were without health insurance in 2010, according to the Commonwealth Fund, and nearly 22 percent of those in families with incomes between $25,000 and $50,000 were uninsured. About 80 percent of the uninsured are U.S. citizens.

Hospitals with emergency departments are required by law to treat patients whether they have insurance or not. "Treatment," however, is limited to stabilizing the patient, not providing follow-up care. And hospitals can still bill for the care, at a rate that is often higher than the one negotiated with health insurance plans.

The ACA addresses the lack of access by expanding Medicaid to cover nearly all of the nonelderly lowest income adults. To spread this cost over the greatest number, beginning in 2014 almost every American (with a few exemptions) will be required to have health insurance or pay a penalty. An individual can choose to enroll in an employer-based plan as long as it meets certain standards. Insurance will be available through new state-based insurance marketplaces called exchanges, with subsidies for low-income people. People younger than 30 will be able to satisfy the mandate by buying low-cost, high-deductible plans. In 2006, Massachusetts expanded access through a similar plan with an individual mandate provision.

The public has been deeply divided about the ACA, and the "individual tax mandate" is one of the most controversial aspects of the health reform law. The ACA was challenged by several states, but in June 2012, the U.S. Supreme Court ruled that the mandate was constitutional. The Court's opinion concluded that the mandate would be unconstitutional if it were considered a "penalty" but that it could be considered a tax and as such fell within the U.S. federal government's power to levy taxes.

The YES and NO selections discuss the merits of individual mandates. Karen Davenport argues that an individual mandate is tailored to appeal to conservatives because it emphasizes conservative ideals of personal responsibility. She also claims that any reform that keeps private health insurance but tries to make health care affordable for all citizens depends on making sure that everybody actually purchases health insurance. Michael F. Cannon, a libertarian health policy analyst, argues that the mandate will promote irresponsibility, restrict personal freedom, and increase the cost of health care. Ultimately, he concludes, it will lead to government rationing.

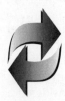

YES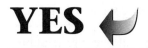

Should Everyone Be Required to Have Health Insurance? Yes: It's the Key to Reform

All Americans should be responsible for holding insurance coverage. It's the key to making health care more available, more affordable and more reliable for everybody.

It's instructive to remember where the idea for an individual mandate began. In the late 1980s and early 1990s, a group of conservative health-policy experts began looking for an alternative to the employer-mandate proposal that ultimately became a central pillar of Bill Clinton's health-care reform effort. The conservatives landed on an approach that called for individual responsibility, maintained a significant role for the private health-insurance market, and dealt with the "free-rider" problem of individuals who choose not to purchase health insurance and so pass their health-care bills on to those who do.

Sound familiar?

Three Premises

The Affordable Care Act is built on three premises: Health insurance must be more accessible, particularly to people with pre-existing conditions; more affordable, including for people with very low incomes; and always there, including for people with very high health-care costs.

To that end, the law makes important changes to the non-group insurance market, where most individuals and small businesses seek coverage. These changes include: requiring insurers to offer coverage to all applicants, regardless of health status; requiring insurers to renew coverage, regardless of the policyholder's claims history; requiring insurers to price premiums without regard to health status; and prohibiting insurers from using exclusions for pre-existing condition and lifetime or annual limits to restrict coverage.

Like in a masonry arch, the keystone of the individual mandate enables all the other pieces of reform to lock into place. Without it, the arch crumbles.

Think about it. People could wait until they were seriously ill to buy coverage, knowing that insurance companies could not turn them down. Insurers, because they would be covering mostly sick people, would need to raise premiums to stay afloat.

Davenport, Karen. From *The Wall Street Journal,* January 23, 2012. Copyright © 2012 by Dow Jones & Company, Inc. Reprinted by permission.

Some opponents of the mandate argue that making coverage mandatory will drive up overall premiums, and that requiring some to pay for others' health-care costs is unfair. Certainly, some individuals will pay higher premiums than they currently do—for example, someone who is young and healthy, or who has bare-bones coverage today, will likely pay more. But the young and healthy person will not stay young, and might not stay healthy, while the person with bare-bones coverage may end up needing far more care than the policy will cover. We therefore share risk through insurance—paying for sicker people's health-care costs when we are healthy, with the promise that if we need expensive care, others will cover the costs.

It's not the mandate that will drive up premiums. Quite the opposite. The mandate is meant to help keep a lid on premiums by ensuring that the risk pool includes enough healthy people to spread the costs. At the same time, payment and delivery system changes that reward high-quality, efficient care will produce systemwide savings that also reduce premiums. In a 2010 report by the Commonwealth Fund, a private foundation supporting health-care reform, experts predict that by 2019, these changes will save each family almost $2,000 a year in premiums.

Opponents tend to see the mandate as federal interference in a private decision of whether to buy insurance or accept the financial risks of being uninsured.

But let's be clear. Uninsured individuals who need care, particularly catastrophically expensive care, generally receive these services anyway. A decision not to pay for insurance—to become a free rider—leads hospitals and other providers to charge other patients more to make up the difference. People shouldn't have the freedom to shift the burden to everybody else.

And it's a real burden. Yes, uncompensated care in 2008 as measured by the Urban Institute was a modest proportion of total health spending in the U.S. But when you're talking about health care, "modest" is still a lot of money. In 2008, 2.2% of total spending equaled $56 billion.

A Lot of Care

To put this amount in context, the Affordable Care Act is expected to spend $56 billion on expanding coverage to 15 million people via the Medicaid program in 2015. So you can buy a lot of health coverage and care for $56 billion. To be sure, reducing unnecessary care would realize even more significant savings—and the law promotes reforms to address that issue as well.

Opponents also charge that the individual mandate in Massachusetts has led to rationing. On the contrary, data show that access to care has improved on a variety of measures, including reduced levels of unmet health-care needs. In some cases, the critics suggest that payment changes under consideration in Massachusetts—aimed at reducing the growth in health-care costs—will, if implemented, lead to rationing. This charge ignores the fact that global payment approaches and other payment changes are designed to improve care for patients with chronic illnesses. Under these approaches, physicians and health-care systems would coordinate with each other and more carefully manage their patients to ensure that patients receive needed care and enjoy better health. They would likely provide less unnecessary care and generally reduce overtreatment—thereby reducing potential risks to patients and reclaiming some of the 30% of health-care spending currently dedicated to unnecessary care.

Michael F. Cannon 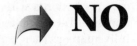 **NO**

Should Everyone Be Required to Have Health Insurance? No: Premiums Will Rise

When Washington begins penalizing people for not purchasing health insurance in 2014, it will mark the first time in history the federal government has required nearly all Americans to buy a private product as a condition of lawful residence in the U.S. No part of the health-care law is less popular, or more essential to preventing it from crumbling like a house of cards, than this individual mandate.

Even if the mandate were popular and constitutional, it would still be a bad idea. It will increase premiums, cost shifting and government rationing, while promoting irresponsibility. Indeed, its entire purpose is to enable supporters to avoid responsibility for their decisions.

Let's start with premiums. The mandate will increase premiums for households who currently do not purchase coverage, and tens of millions more (including at least half of employer-sponsored plans) who will have to purchase additional coverage to satisfy the mandate. A study issued by the left-leaning Commonwealth Fund estimates the law has already increased premiums 1.8% on average. That will rise as the mandate takes full effect. Some of the increase will reflect the cost of additional coverage—but if consumers valued that coverage, they would have bought it already.

Magnified Effects

True, the law will force insurers to reduce premiums for the sick, and the mandate will magnify that effect. But those same government price controls will increase premiums for healthier customers—and the mandate will magnify that effect, too. (Economist Jonathan Gruber, one of the law's biggest proponents, projects that for some who buy policies in the individual market, premiums will more than double.) At best, those two effects cancel each other out. But these provisions also create incentives for healthy people to drop coverage, driving average premiums higher still.

Then there's how a mandate leads to government rationing. Like President Obama, ex-Massachusetts Gov. Mitt Romney tied a mandate to subsidies that help people buy the mandatory coverage. The higher-than-projected cost[s] of those subsidies, plus the premium increases caused by the mandate, are leading desperate state officials to reduce those costs by rationing care.

Officials have imposed price controls on premiums, which force insurers to limit services. They are pushing price controls on providers, which could exacerbate Massachusetts' already long waits for care. And they hope to impose Canadian-style "payment reforms" that would financially reward providers for limiting services. (An early experiment has delivered zero savings and in some cases increased spending, yet it may still be denying care to people.)

Though supporters claim the mandate will reduce cost shifting from uninsured free riders to the insured, the latter will see no savings. Researchers at the left-leaning Urban Institute estimate that in 2008, such cost shifting amounted to just $56 billion, or 2% of total health spending, and increased premiums by "at most 1.7 percent." For comparison, the Dartmouth Institute for Health Policy and Clinical Practice estimates we waste more than 14 times that amount on unnecessary care. More important, the Commonwealth Fund study shows the federal law has already increased premiums by more than the mandate could reduce them by eliminating free riding.

The federal law actually promotes free riding and cost shifting. My colleague Victoria Payne and I calculated that individuals could save up to $3,000 a year—and families of four could save as much as $8,000—by dropping their health insurance, paying the penalty, and waiting until they are sick to purchase coverage. Massachusetts reported a nearly fivefold increase in such free riding after its mandate took effect. The federal law also offers $1 trillion in subsidies to tens of millions of Americans—shifting $1 trillion of the cost of their health care to taxpayers.

Personal Responsibility

The mandate's greatest pretense is the idea that it promotes personal responsibility. If that were the goal, Congress need only have enhanced the courts' ability to collect medical debts. Supporters instead demanded a mandate precisely because it lets them avoid responsibility for their decisions.

Here's how. The federal law promotes irresponsibility by allowing healthy people to wait until they get sick to buy coverage. It creates that free-rider problem, which has been known to make insurance markets collapse. Supporters of the law could have taken personal responsibility for this instability they introduced into the market—say, by volunteering to pay the free riders' premiums. Instead, they imposed a mandate, which attempts to stabilize the market by depriving others of their money and freedom.

Forcing others to bear the costs of your decisions is the opposite of personal responsibility. It is selfishness, not altruism.

The mandate is not a conservative or free-market idea. Some Republicans who were for it are now against it, just as some Democrats once against it are now for it. A majority of conservatives and the overwhelming majority of libertarians always opposed it. It's snake oil, no matter who prescribes it.

Free markets—which no living American has seen in health care—would make health care better, more affordable, and more secure. The mandate makes such progress impossible.

If the public understood the rest of the health-care overhaul as well as it does the mandate, the law would already be history.

EXPLORING THE ISSUE

Is an Individual Mandate to Purchase Health Insurance Fair?

Critical Thinking and Reflection

1. The YES and NO selections describe the balance between individual liberty and the social good in different ways; what is the most compelling account of this balance, in your view, and why?
2. Communitarians (who may be liberal or conservative on many social issues) argue that an individual's identity, life prospects, and personal triumphs are deeply influenced by the individual's relationship to the community, whereas libertarians see the individual's identity, life prospects, and personal triumphs as belonging solely to the individual. Where do you fall on this debate? Could there be a spectrum of views in it? How does it relate to the debate about access to health care? How does it relate to the debate about the individual mandate?
3. These selections also make competing claims about how an individual mandate will affect the cost of health-care insurance; explain these connections in your own words.

Is There Common Ground?

The divisive political debate since 2009 over the Patient Protection and Affordable Care Act would seem to leave little hope of finding common ground on this issue. During the 2012 presidential election, both candidates held that the law illustrated the gap between the competing visions or philosophies endorsed by Republicans and Democrats. Nonetheless, maybe turning to the underlying values offers some hope of discovering some common ground beneath the political infighting.

Philosopher Paul Menzel is one commentator on health-care reform who has made this kind of case. Menzel points out, for example, that conservatives in most of the rest of the world have health-care reform efforts that aim to achieve broader access to health care because that goal promotes conservative goals such as personal responsibility, individual opportunity, and the strong and stable social foundation that allows for prosperity. The problem, then, is to identify the particular reform strategies that both liberals and conservatives can recognize as advancing their underlying values.

Additional Resources

To find out more about health reform and its implementation, go to the Kaiser Family Foundation website www.kff.org/ or Health Reform GPS www.healthreformgps.org/. Both sites are updated frequently.

For discussion of the Supreme Court's 2012 ruling about the constitutionality of the individual mandate and the implications of its ruling for the philosophical debate about the values inherent in the individual mandate, see a set of essays in the September–October 2012 issue of the *Hastings Center Report*. See also Paul Menzel and Donald W. Light, "A Conservative Case for Universal Access to Health Care," *Hastings Center Report* (July–August 2006).

A discussion of what the individual mandate actually requires of people can be found at Politico: Joanne Kenen, "5 Myths of the Individual Mandate," June 28, 2012; www.politico.com/news/stories/0612/77997.html

For an older but still helpful overview of the contrasting positions on the mandate, see Sara Rosenbaum and Jonathan Gruber, "Buying Health Care, the Individual Mandate, and the Constitution," *The New England Journal of Medicine* (July 29, 2010), and Glen Whitman, "Hazards of the Individual Health Care Mandate," *Cato Policy Report* (September–October 2007); www.cato.org/pubs/policy_report/v29n5/cpr29n5-1.html.

ISSUE 17

Is There an Ethical Duty to Provide Health Care for All Immigrants to the United States?

YES: **Rajeev Raghavan and Ricardo Nuila**, from "Survivors—Dialysis, Immigration, and U.S. Law," *The New England Journal of Medicine* (June 9, 2011)

NO: **James Dwyer**, from "When the Discharge Plan Is Deportation: Hospitals, Immigrants, and Social Responsibility," *Bioethics* (vol. 23, no. 3, 2009)

Learning Outcomes

After reading this issue, you should be able to:

- Explain the societal challenge of extending health insurance to undocumented immigrants.
- Discuss arguments for and against extending health insurance to undocumented immigrants.

ISSUE SUMMARY

YES: Rajeev Raghavan and Ricardo Nuila, physicians who work with end-stage renal disease patients, argue that standardized coverage for dialysis treatments would alleviate the burden on taxpayers where the most undocumented residents live and would improve these patients' health, allowing them to return to work.

NO: James Dwyer, a philosopher and bioethicist, looks at another response to treatments for immigrants—deporting them. While he opposes deportation, he asserts that placing the financial responsibility on individual hospitals or regions is unfair.

In October 2009, Grady Memorial Hospital in Atlanta, a "safety-net" public hospital, announced it was closing its free dialysis center because it was losing too much money. Fifty patients, many of them undocumented immigrants who had no insurance coverage, had until January 2010 to find alternative dialysis providers in the United States or in their home countries. Without regular dialysis treatment for their kidney disease, they would die. Yet, other dialysis providers would not accept the patients without payment. In December 2009, a federal judge dismissed a lawsuit challenging the center closing, and it closed as planned. Grady paid for 3 months' treatment for the 13 patients who agreed to be repatriated. And it contracted with a large for-profit provider to cover the other patients' treatment until September 2010.

At different points in American history, immigrants have been welcomed as cheap, unskilled labor; at others, immigrants have been excluded as potential revolutionaries or threats to social order. An immigrant's health status was considered crucial in the massive waves of immigration from Eastern and Southern Europe in the nineteenth and early twentieth centuries. Public health officials examined immigrants at Ellis Island in New York harbor and marked with chalk the coats of those suspected of having a "loathsome or dangerous contagious disease." They might be sent to a hospital on site or sent back home. In fact, immigration officials were really worried about accepting people whose conditions were likely to make them "public charges." In 1924, legal immigration was sharply curtailed.

Even so, immigration to the United States increased dramatically in the 1990s and thereafter (but has recently slowed somewhat), as waves of people from Mexico, other Latin American countries, and Asia, as well as other countries, came seeking work. Again health status is an issue, but this time the questions are not about people seeking legal entry (although they still have to answer medical questions) but about people who have crossed the border without the required permission. Are these undocumented immigrants entitled to health care? And if so, who should pay if they are uninsured?

In 2005, there were an estimated 36 million foreign-born residents in the United States, about 35 percent of them naturalized citizens, 33 percent documented immigrants, and 31 percent (about 12 million) undocumented immigrants. Many of these families include children. In 1995, the Personal Responsibility and Work Opportunity Reconciliation Act made recent immigrants ineligible for Medicaid and other public benefits for 5 years. Although one goal of the Affordable Care Act is to increase access to health insurance to the 45 million Americans without it, the act specifically excludes undocumented immigrants from all its programs aimed at this goal. This ban also applied to the State Children's Health Insurance Program (SCHIP) of 1997.

Undocumented immigrants are likely to be poor, work at low-wage jobs without health insurance, and avoid going to doctors until an emergency because they fear being deported. Under the Emergency Medical Treatment and Active Labor Act (EMTALA), they are entitled to emergency treatment but not follow-up care. There is no evidence that undocumented immigrants use emergency rooms more than any other group of uninsured people. In fact, most people who come to emergency rooms for treatment have insurance.

While undocumented immigrants are moving into states that have previously not been known for foreign-born residents, certain areas of the country and even certain hospitals are more likely to treat them for emergency conditions. A major financial problem arises when the patient cannot safely be discharged, requires further rehabilitation or chronic treatment, or lacks family to provide needed care.

The YES and NO selections address this dilemma. Neither selection advocates a drastic solution such as deportation but each brings a different perspective. Physicians Rajeev Raghavan and Ricardo Nuila believe that a better and cheaper solution to the needs of undocumented dialysis patients would be to provide standardized coverage so that patients would not come to treatment as a last resort. Philosopher James Dwyer argues for a national solution to the problem so that individual hospitals and areas are not financially or technically overburdened.

YES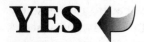

**Rajeev Raghavan and
Ricardo Nuila**

Survivors—Dialysis, Immigration, and U.S. Law

Santiago is in the ER again. He sits in a special row of 20 patients, all of whom are waiting for one result: the potassium. Is it high enough today? Two days ago he was here, and it was only 6 meq per liter. We discharged him. Right now his chest hurts, and he is short of breath. Nothing new, and Santiago knows that if he's to be dialyzed today, these symptoms don't matter. Only the potassium matters.

One of us is the nephrologist on service, and the other is the hospitalist taking admissions. We both trained here as medical students and have continued to work in the county hospital system as faculty members. Some of these patients remember us as residents. Now they recognize us as the gatekeepers, the people deciding which patients go home and which sit in the chair. We know them, too. There's Juan, who is 67 years old and lives 50 miles away in Hempstead. His children take turns bringing him in. There's Maria; she's 38, a mother of three. She began dialysis 5 years ago, initially just once a month; now it's twice every week. Hugo is back. He was admitted for line sepsis last month and spent 2 weeks in-house receiving antibiotics and a new catheter. He was referred for an arteriovenous fistula 6 months ago, but the waiting list is more than a year long. Hugo was brought to the United States at the age of 5; he works in an upscale restaurant and speaks perfect English. Some of the patients appear miserable, but most are like Santiago—they are just waiting patiently for a doctor to quantify their malaise.

Santiago emigrated from Mexico at the age of 20. He had no papers and no job, but he had a family to support, so he hired a smuggler to help him cross the border. He worked in construction from his first day here and helped to build Houston's highways, until one day he became inexplicably ill. He presented to our county hospital, where on his first encounter with a doctor, he was found to have a serum creatinine concentration of 15 mg per deciliter. An ultrasound and laboratory tests confirmed the diagnosis: irreversible kidney failure. A tunneled hemodialysis catheter was inserted into his right internal jugular vein, and the demands of his new life were explained: you are to come to the emergency room every time you feel sick. And every fourth day for 5 years now, Santiago has come to our ER.

More than 11 million undocumented residents live in the United States, and 6000 of them have end-stage renal disease (ESRD).[1] This number seems small in the context of the 400,000-plus Americans currently undergoing dialysis,[2] but the direct and indirect costs are not small. The annual cost of hemodialysis is approximately $72,000 per patient.[2] Through the End Stage Renal Disease program, passed by Congress in 1973, all U.S. citizens with advanced kidney failure qualify for Medicare or Medicaid to defray these high costs.[1] The Consolidated Omnibus Budget Reconciliation Act (COBRA) passed in 1986 explicitly prohibits the use of federal funds for covering undocumented residents for nonemergency services such as dialysis.[3] Some states such as California and Massachusetts use state-allocated Medicaid or county taxes to pay for thrice-weekly hemodialysis for undocumented residents. Most states—including ours, Texas—do not. Here, undocumented residents with ESRD depend on public safety-net hospitals for emergency dialysis. That is to say, even though we know when these patients become ill, we must wait until their lives are at risk before we provide dialysis.

Nephrology guidelines recommend initiating dialysis when the estimated glomerular filtration rate (GFR) falls below 15 ml per minute in patients with diabetes or 10 ml per minute in patients without diabetes. Because of a lack of resources, we often delay initiation of dialysis in undocumented residents until the GFR is much lower or a patient requires emergency treatment. Our inpatient dialysis unit has 12 chairs, and priority is given to admitted patients. The line in the ER begins to swell by 6 a.m. Over the years, we've had some small victories—a special row of chairs, blood for laboratory tests drawn at triage, EKGs performed in assembly-line fashion—which have helped us maximize the provision of hemodialysis. Still, our capacity is grossly insufficient to meet the demands of the more than 180 undocumented residents (and counting) who depend on emergency dialysis in our city.[3]

Emergency dialysis is good for nobody. It places patients' lives at risk, and it results in more ER visits, more hospitalizations, and more blood transfusions than does scheduled dialysis. In total, these excesses result in costs of more than $200,000 per emergency-dialysis patient annually.[4] Furthermore, the community loses these patients' labor, and they lose out on wages, because of their irregular dialysis schedules and poor health. These effects are apparent in our population of patients, the majority of whom immigrated to the United States to work. In our experience, very few patients immigrate to this country because of their illness. Most are like Santiago: they are survivors.

This issue lies at the intersection of debates over the soaring cost of health care and the need for immigration reform. Do we have an ethical duty to provide the same standard of care for all sick patients within our borders? Or would mandating the provision of health care (and of maintenance-dialysis treatments) create an incentive for illegal immigration and worsen the current situation?

There is no easy solution. But with this particular disease, there are cheaper, more compassionate alternatives: dialyzing at home using peritoneal dialysis, kidney transplantation, or funding of maintenance hemodialysis. Resources in our city have allowed for 100 undocumented residents to receive thrice-weekly hemodialysis treatments in a county-funded clinic.[3] Patients undergoing dialysis in this clinic are healthier and happier than those who must receive emergency treatment, and many of them have returned to work.[3] Like the undocumented residents cared for in other centers, our patients are young, with an average age of 43 years.[3] These patients are excellent candidates for transplantation, and many have potential donors. However, the out-of-pocket costs for transplantation and immunosuppressive medications make this option untenable, despite the potential savings for taxpayers.[5]

In order for any of these options to work, dialysis coverage for this patient population must be standardized throughout the country. Standardization would alleviate the burden that is unfairly placed on taxpayers in areas where the most undocumented residents live, such as California and Texas.[3] In states like ours, standardization of care would improve these patients' health and allow them to return to work.

Santiago would love to work, but he can't work like this—not with his body so weak. On the days he qualifies for dialysis, he arrives here by bus at 5 a.m. and leaves in the evening, exhausted. When he doesn't qualify, he comes back the very next day. Today he waits. It's July in Houston—the heat index is 110°F—and Santiago is wearing his blue hoodie. He's cold. By any moral or medical standard, he should already be upstairs, but he "looks stable," and so we wait for the potassium. There are mouths to feed and bills to pay, but though Santiago would like nothing more than to work, his body tells him he can't, and so he rests. And in 2 days, he will begin the process again.

References

1. Campbell GA, Sanoff S, Rosner MH. Care of the undocumented immigrant in the United States with ESRD. Am J Kidney Dis 2010;55:181–91.

2. USRDS. 2008 Annual data report: atlas of chronic kidney disease and end-stage renal disease in the United States. Bethesda, MD: National Institutes of Health, National Institute of Diabetes and Digestive and Kidney Diseases; 2008.

3. Raghavan R, Sheikh-Hamad D. Descriptive analysis of undocumented residents with ESRD in a public hospital system. Dial Transplant 2011;2:78–81.

4. Sheikh-Hamad D, Paiuk E, Wright AJ, Kleinmann C, Khosla U, Shandera WX. Care for immigrants with end-stage renal disease in Houston: a comparison of two practices. Tex Med 2007;103:54–8.

5. Goldberg MJ, Simmerling M, Frader JE. Why nondocumented residents should have access to kidney transplantation: arguments for lifting the federal ban on reimbursement. Transplantation 2007;83:17–20.

James Dwyer

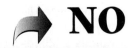

When the Discharge Plan Is Deportation: Hospitals, Immigrants, and Social Responsibility

Some hospitals in the United States have taken to deporting illegal immigrants.[1] Consider a typical case. A man from Guatemala was not able to support his family with the work he could find in his village. So he decided to go north. He agreed to pay a guide to smuggle him into the United States. After he arrived, he made contact with a relative in Florida and found work as a gardener. Although the work was hard and the pay was low, he was able to save some money every month. He dreamed of saving enough money to return home, build a house, and start a small business. But one day, after several years in the US, he was in a serious automobile accident. An ambulance took him to the nearest hospital. There he received blood transfusions, extensive surgery, and medical treatment. After a long period of treatment, his condition stabilized, but he was left with severe brain injury from the trauma.

At this point the usual discharge plan would have been to transfer the patient from the acute-care hospital to a long-term care facility that provided rehabilitation for patients with brain injuries. But no long-term care facility would take the patient because he lacked insurance. Most public insurance programs in the US do not cover long-term care for immigrants, legal or illegal, until they can establish that they've been residents for at least five years. And most private charities are overburdened. So the acute-care hospital kept the patient for over one year, at a cost of over one million dollars. Then, with no other solution in sight, the hospital arranged to place the patient in a public rehabilitation hospital in Guatemala. The patient lacked the decisional capacity to consent to this plan, and his guardian objected, but the hospital went ahead. It hired a private air ambulance and flew the patient, accompanied by a nurse, to the placement in Guatemala. In this case, the discharge that the hospital arranged was a form of deportation or repatriation.

How widespread is this practice? No one knows for sure; but some facts suggest that it is fairly common. Each year, hospitals contact consulates from many countries to arrange repatriations. In one year, a hospital in Florida repatriated about 7 patients and a hospital in Arizona repatriated almost 100 patients. The practice is now common enough that at least one company specializes in finding placements in and transporting patients back to Latin America.

Although deporting patients may seem shocking, the practice is under-standable within a given legal and economic context. US law requires that hospitals evaluate all patients and provide them with emergency care until their condition is stable. Thus hospitals are required to treat patients even if they lack insurance and funds to pay. The federal government reimburses hos-pitals for part of this emergency treatment. After the patients are stable, the hospitals are required to arrange a safe discharge. Depending on the case, a safe discharge might be letting the patient walk out the door, sending the patient home for care by the family, or placing the patient in a rehabilitation facility. The problem is that many patients lack insurance that covers long-term reha-bilitation. Because lawmakers wanted to save money and encourage individual responsibility, most forms of public assistance do not cover immigrants. So hospitals are in a bind. After they have treated and stabilized uninsured immi-grants, they have nowhere to send these patients.

Acute-care hospitals are inappropriate places for long-term rehabilita-tion. They are not designed and staffed for rehabilitation, and they are often short of beds. Furthermore, few hospitals can afford to house patients indefi-nitely. Even not-for-profit hospitals need to make enough money to stay in business. Without some margin, they will not be able to sustain their mission of caring for the sick. When faced with this bind, even some Catholic hospitals have repatriated patients they could not place in local long-term care.

In order to evaluate this practice from an ethical perspective, I want to view it within a wider context.[2] Although the health care system and immi-gration policy in the US are particularly bureaucratic and inhumane, very few societies have responded in a morally adequate way to the problems faced by immigrants, refugees, migrant workers, and undocumented workers. When people picture undocumented workers, they imagine Mexicans working in the United States or Africans working in France. But people without visas are liv-ing and working all over the world. There are undocumented workers from Indonesia in Malaysia, from Burma in Thailand, from Haiti in the Dominican Republic, from Zimbabwe in South Africa, and so on. Although China has very few foreign migrants, over 100 million Chinese have left the rural areas to seek work in the cities. Many of these Chinese workers face problems similar to those faced by undocumented workers in other countries: dangerous jobs, poor pay, social exclusion, and inadequate health care.

What is pushing people out of the source countries? Poverty, unemploy-ment, structural adjustment policies, war, and environmental degradation. What is pulling them into the destination countries? The desire to earn more money, provide better support for their families, and construct better lives. To do this, they are willing to work wherever they can. In most societies, undocu-mented workers do the most disagreeable work, in the most difficult condi-tions. They sew apparel, wash dishes, clean toilets, harvest crops, and slaughter animals. Many women immigrants are employed, and often exploited, in serv-ice jobs as maids, health care aides, and sex workers.

Do societies have an ethical obligation to provide healthy conditions, acute health care, and long-term care for these workers? I want to sketch three responses to this question. The first response appeals to a narrow account of desert. It begins with the assertion that people who have no right to be in a country have no right to benefits in that country. There is no denying that undocumented workers have violated a law by entering or staying in a country, but it does not follow that they have no ethical right or claim to health care services. Many citizens have violated a law by working off the books to avoid taxes—a practice we might call undocumented work. But it does not follow that these citizens forfeit all claims to health care. To deal with this objection, the first response adds a related assertion: given that health care resources are limited, governments should prioritize needy citizens over illegal immigrants. With this assertion, a narrow account of desert tends to pit the interests of poor citizens against the interests of undocumented workers. Of course, resources will always be somewhat limited and trade-offs will sometimes be necessary, but pitting these disadvantaged groups against one another is not an inevitable tragedy. It is a social choice that needs to be evaluated, based in part on the alternatives.

The second response to the question appeals to an expansive account of human rights. Since national borders are rather arbitrary, and the disparities in health and wealth between countries are quite shocking, this response focuses on what people are entitled to not as citizens, but as human beings. The International Covenant on Economic, Social and Cultural Rights recognizes 'the right of everyone to the enjoyment of the highest attainable standard of physical and mental health.'[3] Although this claim embodies many worthy sentiments, it is problematic in two ways. First, it is too easy, and not very enlightening, to claim a relatively limitless right. This claim doesn't shed much light on the relative responsibilities that people have and the relative priorities that institutions should set. Second, since a claim based on a human right is a claim based on people's common humanity, it tends to collapse distinctions between cases. But doesn't the Guatemalan man who lived and worked for years in the US have a different kind of ethical claim from a man who stayed and worked in Guatemala? And don't US citizens have different responsibilities in the two cases? In general, we should recognize a basic core of human rights, but we shouldn't try to couch all our moral concerns in the discourse of human rights.

The response in terms of human rights is too broad and fails to account for important distinctions, while the response in terms of desert is too narrow and makes invidious distinctions. To focus on either the human status or the legal status of undocumented workers leaves out many morally salient points: background conditions, employment patterns in society, structural relationships between undocumented workers and other social members, and the whole idea of taking responsibility for conditions and practices. Societies have often used marginalized and vulnerable people—slaves, indentured servants, minorities, and migrants—to do the most disagreeable and difficult labour. The use of illegal immigrants is a contemporary form of this old pattern. Although some laws proscribe the use of undocumented workers, the economic system encourages and relies on it. This employment pattern is not a natural phenomenon beyond human control but a social construction based on laws, norms, institutions, conditions, and ideas. We need to take some responsibility for it because, by our actions, most of us participate in or contribute to the conditions and structures that support it.[4] The strawberries that I eat connect me, in complex and indirect ways, to the lives of many undocumented workers.

Although all the people involved need to take some responsibility for changing unjust patterns, individual persons and individual hospitals cannot take full financial responsibility for all the undocumented workers to whom they are connected in myriad and indirect ways. Most individuals would be overwhelmed; many hospitals would go out of business. So societies need to devise fair ways to apportion this responsibility. That probably can't be done in a fragmented health care system where hospitals flourish by shifting costs. It will require political discussion and collective action. Repatriating patients who lack insurance mutes the discussion that we need to have and avoids the action that we need to take. It takes both the patients and us in the wrong direction.

References

1. D. Sontag. 2008. Immigrants Facing Deportation by US Hospitals. *New York Times* 3 August; D. Sontag. 2008. Deported in a Coma, Saved Back in US. *New York Times* 9 November. The case that follows is based on these articles, and so are the facts about the practice.

2. J. Dwyer. Illegal Immigrants, Health Care, and Social Responsibility. *Hastings Cent Rep* 2004;34(5):34–41.

3. United Nations Office of the High Commissioner for Human Rights. 1976. *International Covenant on Economic, Social and Cultural Rights.* New York: United Nations: Article 12.

4. I.M. Young. Responsibility and Global Justice: A Social Connection Model. *Soc Philos Policy* 2006;23(1):102–130.

EXPLORING THE ISSUE

Is There an Ethical Duty to Provide Health Care for All Immigrants to the United States?

Critical Thinking and Reflection

1. There are two contrasting ways to frame the question of whether health insurance should be extended to undocumented immigrants: We might ask whether they have a right to it, or we might ask whether our society is the kind of society that accepts an obligation to address their needs. Which would you find more persuasive? How do Raghavan and Nuila argue for extending insurance?
2. What kind of response to the problem of undocumented workers does Dwyer propose? Do you think Dwyer is addressing the problem more honestly, or sidestepping the problem?

Is There Common Ground?

Extending health insurance to undocumented immigrants remains controversial. Although the Affordable Care Act (ACA) excludes undocumented immigrants from the state-run health-care exchanges through which, starting in 2014, citizens without employer-provided insurance should be able to buy health insurance, the ACA does include increased funding for constructing and staffing Federally Qualified Health Centers, which provide primary care for medically underserved populations, including seasonal and migrant workers.

In August 2010, Grady Memorial Hospital and several Atlanta dialysis providers reached an agreement to provide dialysis for 38 end-stage renal disease patients, most of them undocumented immigrants. The hospital agreed to help pay for continuing dialysis for most of the immigrants, while the rest would be distributed among the local providers as charity cases. There is no plan for managing the care of newly diagnosed patients, except for emergency room care when they become desperately ill.

Additional Resources

A selection of resources are available at a Web site developed by The Hastings Center, "Undocumented Patients: Undocumented Immigrants & Access to Health Care," www.undocumentedpatients.org/.

For further reading, see Stephen Zukerman, Timothy A. Waldman, and Emily Lawton, "Undocumented Immigrants, Left Out of Health Reform, Likely to Continue to Grow as Share of the Uninsured," *Health Affairs* (pp. 1997–2007, October 2011). Also, Susan Okie, "Immigrants and Health Care—At the Intersection of Two Broken Systems," *The New England Journal of Medicine* (pp. 525–529, August 9, 2007).

Elizabeth R. Chesler argues that denying undocumented immigrants' access to Medicaid under the 1996 Personal Responsibility and Work Opportunity Reconciliation Act violates their right to equal protection (www.bu.edu/law/central/jd/organizations/journals/pilj/vol17no2/documents/17-2CheslerNote.pdf).

"Immigrants in the U.S. Health Care System: Five Myths That Misinform the American Public" (2007), by Meredith L. King, is available on the website of the Center for American Progress (www.americanprogress.org/projects/healthprogress/articles.html). Among the beliefs she cites as erroneous is "Restricting immigrants' access to the health care system will not affect American citizens."

For a different view, see James R. Edwards Jr., "The Medicaid Costs of Legalizing Illegal Aliens," a July 2010 memorandum from the Center for Immigration Studies, an organization opposed to expanding immigration.

The National Conference of State Legislatures has an immigration policy project that provides updates on activities in state legislatures. The most recent report covers the period from January 1, 2011 to December 7, 2011; www.ncsl.org/?tabid=19897.

The Kaiser Commission on Medicaid and the Uninsured has data on immigrants' health care coverage and access; www.kff.org/medicaid/upload/Connecting-Eligible-Immigrant-Families-to-Health-Coverage-and-Care-Key-Lessons-from-Outreach-and-Enrollment-Workers-pdf.pdf

ISSUE 18

Should New Drugs Be Given to Patients Outside Clinical Trials?

YES: Emil J. Freireich, from "Should Terminally Ill Patients Have the Right to Take Drugs that Pass Phase I Testing?" *British Medical Journal* (September 8, 2007)

NO: George J. Annas, from "Cancer and the Constitution—Choice at Life's End," *The New England Journal of Medicine* (July 26, 2007)

Learning Outcomes

After reading this issue, you should be able to:

- Discuss the ethical and policy issues that arise in the development and marketing of new drugs.
- Explore critically the individual right to make one's own risk–benefit decisions and society's reasons for limiting that right.

ISSUE SUMMARY

YES: Physician Emil J. Freireich believes that patients with advanced cancer and limited life expectancy should have the same privilege as all individuals in a free society.

NO: Law professor George J. Annas argues that there is no constitutional right to demand experimental interventions, and that fully open access would undermine the FDA's ability to protect the public from unsafe drugs.

$\mathbf{A}$t the beginning of the twentieth century, any American could manufacture a medication and sell it to the public. The era of "patent medicines" led at best to harmless but useless "cure-alls," and at worst, to illness and death. Alarmed by this practice, in 1906 the U.S. Congress enacted the Food and Drug Act, prohibiting the sale of misbranded, mislabeled, and adulterated foods and drugs in interstate commerce. In 1938, more than 100 people died as a result of taking elixir sulfanilamide, a powder that had been made into a liquid form by adding diethylene glycol, a poison used in antifreeze. In response, Congress created the Food and Drug Administration (FDA) to prevent future tragedies.

Under the current rules, drug manufacturers must submit "investigational new drug" applications to the agency and provide evidence of their safety and effectiveness before they can bring new drugs to the market. In general, drug trials involve stages of testing and data are collected from small, carefully selected groups, analyzed, and then tested in wider populations. Phase I includes a small number of patients and is designed to determine levels of toxicity (bad reactions). This process is costly and can take considerable time.

Over the years, the FDA has been criticized on grounds that it allows unsafe drugs to be marketed to the public, and in recent years several drugs have been taken off the market. It has also been criticized for its slow review process because of which promising new drugs are unavailable to people who desperately need them. In the 1980s and 1990s, HIV/AIDS activists in particular lobbied for faster access to drugs, and the FDA responded with a plan to allow access to some experimental drugs for patients with serious diseases and no other therapeutic options.

But for many people facing death, the FDA does not go far enough. They want to be able to take drugs that are in early stages of development and without being enrolled in a clinical trial, for which they may not be eligible. The Abigail Alliance, founded in 2001 by Frank Burroughs, is one of the most prominent advocates of this position. Mr. Burroughs' daughter Abigail died that year from cancer of the head and neck. He had tried unsuccessfully to obtain two drugs that were then in clinical trials, although not for her type of cancer. (One of the drugs has since been approved for that indication.) Abigail was not eligible for the clinical trials because as Mr. Burroughs said, "She had the right cells in the wrong place."

In 2003, the Alliance sued the FDA in federal district court, claiming that the agency's failure to permit the sale of investigational new drugs to terminally ill patients violated the patients' rights to privacy and due process under the Fifth Amendment of the U.S. Constitution. The three-judge panel on the first court to hear the case agreed that there was a constitutional right to such access, but 15 months later this decision was reversed by the District of Columbia Circuit Court of Appeals. In January 2008, the U.S. Supreme Court declined to hear the case.

The YES and NO selections take different views of the basic issue. Physician Emil J. Freireich asserts that dying individuals for whom all approved medications have failed should have the right to take drugs still in the investigational stage. Law professor George J. Annas believes that access to unproven drugs has to be limited to protect the public.

YES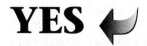

Emil J. Freireich

Should Terminally Ill Patients Have the Right to Take Drugs That Pass Phase I Testing?

Around half a million people will die from cancer-related causes in the United States this year. In the US, as in much of the Western world, patients know their diagnosis and are often given a hopeless prognosis. For most, the option of participating in phase I and phase II clinical trials of new drugs that offer some promise helps them remain optimistic. Clearly, they should have the right to take drugs that have passed phase I testing.

The problem is that most cancer patients cannot participate in phase II trials because they are either ineligible or they are unable to fulfil the financial and social requirements for participating in such trials, such as staying in the centres conducting these trials, sometimes for many weeks or months. The problem is clearly not one of safety because these drugs have completed phase I clinical trials and there is sufficient information about them to justify a phase II trial to determine efficacy.

Phase II trials are designed to give the highest probability of a positive outcome. Thus, they have patient eligibility requirements which assure that only the healthiest patients at the earliest point in their disease are entered. These decisions are not based on any reasonable evidence that patients who are ineligible would not benefit, but are strictly designed to fulfil the regulatory requirements established by bodies such as the Food and Drug Administration (FDA) and the regulatory components of industry and academia that govern these clinical trials.

Compassionate Prescribing

In the modern electronic era, most of the patients with hopeless cancer diagnoses have access through the media and the internet to information about promising new drugs that are in phase II clinical trials. These patients would like very much to receive these drugs to offer them some hope, but for the reasons mentioned above are unable to participate in those trials. So why not offer these drugs to these patients on a compassionate basis?

The first reason given is usually the safety concerns. Without knowledge about how renal function, cardiac function, age, etc. affect the action of the

From *British Medical Journal*, September 8, 2007, vol. 335, pp. 335. Copyright © 2007 by BMJ Publishing Group. Reprinted by permission via Rightslink.

phase I drug, side effects might occur that could be harmful to the patient or, perhaps more importantly, the continued development of the drug. I think this objection is relatively minor since it simply states the benefit:risk ratio problem—that is, these patients are prepared to volunteer to expose themselves to increased risk because of their hopeless prognosis and because of the promise of the new drug.

The second objection is that it will interfere with the development of the drug. However, in the past, the FDA and the National Cancer Institute have allowed compassionate use of drugs and have found that it actually accelerates development. This is because when patients are offered compassionate use of an experimental drug, their doctors have to collect information as systematically as in the research protocol and submit it to the sponsor. Information is therefore available about use of the drug outside trial conditions. For example, if patients with impaired renal function not only tolerate the drug but respond, it will assist in drug development to have that knowledge collected systematically.

Drug Industry Profits

Another objection is that the drug industry might use this device to profit from investigation of a phase I drug. I believe this is a trivial objection because the usual strategy for compassionate use is that the drug is provided at cost. The last, and perhaps the most serious, objection is that expanded access would interfere with the clinical trial process. This certainly should not be the case. The clinical trial process is governed by the regulatory bodies in government, in industry, and in academic institutions. The unfortunate consequence of this is that physician scientists, who have the most experience, the most training, the most knowledge, the most productivity, and the most creativity, are completely excluded from this process. Because of the relationship between the regulatory organisations of government, industry, and academia, the academic physician scientist can only implement protocols that have been developed by the drug developer with direction from the regulatory agencies. Expanded access would bring the doctors back into the drug development process and, rather than damage the clinical trial system, would greatly expand its effectiveness and value.

In summary, patients with advanced cancer and limited life expectancy should have the same privilege as all individuals in a free society—that is, to decide their own benefit:risk ratio. It is tragic that regulatory bodies have created a circumstance where people have to live in an aura of hopelessness even though they have the will, the resources, and the ability to expose themselves to the risk of participating in investigational studies and to enjoy the potential for benefit. The solution is legislation or judicial action to permit expanded access to experimental treatments for patients with limited life expectancy.

George J. Annas

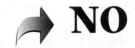

Cancer and the Constitution—
Choice at Life's End

J.M. Coetzee's violent, anti-apartheid *Age of Iron,* a novel the *Wall Street Journal* termed "a fierce pageant of modern South Africa," is written as a letter by a retired classics professor, Mrs. Curren, to her daughter, who lives in the United States. Mrs. Curren is dying of cancer, and her daughter advises her to come to the United States for treatment. She replies, "I can't afford to die in America. . . . No one can, except Americans."[1] Dying of cancer has been considered a "hard death" for at least a century, unproven and even quack remedies have been common, and price has been a secondary consideration. Efforts sponsored by the federal government to find cures for cancer date from the establishment of the National Cancer Institute (NCI) in 1937. Cancer research was intensified after President Richard Nixon's declaration of a "war on cancer" and passage of the National Cancer Act of 1971.[2] Most recently, calls for more cancer research have followed the announcement by Elizabeth Edwards, wife of presidential candidate John Edwards, that her cancer is no longer considered curable.

Frustration with the methods and slow progress of mainstream medical research has helped fuel a resistance movement that distrusts both conventional medicine and government and that has called for the recognition of a right for terminally ill patients with cancer to have access to any drugs they want to take. Prominent examples include the popularity of Krebiozen in the 1950s and of laetrile in the 1970s. As an NCI spokesperson put it more than 20 years ago, when thousands of people were calling the NCI hotline pleading for access to interleukin-2, "What the callers are saying is, 'Our mother, our brother, our sister is dying at this very moment. We have nothing to lose.'"[2] Today, families search the Internet for clinical trials, and even untested chemicals such as dichloroacetate, that seem to offer them some hope. In addition, basing advocacy on their personal experiences with cancer, many families have focused their frustrations on the Food and Drug Administration (FDA), which they see as a government agency denying them access to treatments they need.

In May 2006 these families won an apparent major victory when the Court of Appeals for the District of Columbia, in the case of *Abigail Alliance v. Von Eschenbach* (hereafter referred to as *Abigail Alliance*),[3] agreed with their argument that patients with cancer have a constitutional right of access to

Annas, George J. From *The New England Journal of Medicine,* July 26, 2007. Copyright © 2007 by Massachusetts Medical Society. All rights reserved. Reprinted by permission via Rightslink.

investigational cancer drugs. In reaction, the FDA began the process of rewriting its own regulations to make it easier for terminally ill patients not enrolled in clinical trials to have access to investigational drugs.[4] In November 2006, the full bench of the Court of Appeals vacated the May 2006 opinion, and the case was reheard in March 2007.[5] The decision of the full bench, expected by the fall, will hinge on the answer to a central question: Do terminally ill adult patients with cancer for whom there are no effective treatments have a constitutional right of access to investigational drugs their physicians think might be beneficial?

The Constitutional Controversy

The Abigail Alliance for Better Access to Developmental Drugs (hereafter called the Abigail Alliance) sued the FDA to prevent it from enforcing its policy of prohibiting the sale of drugs that had not been proved safe and effective to competent adult patients who are terminally ill and have no alternative treatment options. The Abigail Alliance is named after Abigail Burroughs, whose squamous-cell carcinoma of the head and neck was diagnosed when she was only 19 years old. Two years later, in 2001, she died. Before her death she had tried unsuccessfully to obtain investigational drugs on a compassionate use basis from ImClone and AstraZeneca and was accepted for a clinical trial only shortly before her death. Her father founded the Abigail Alliance in her memory.[6]

The district court dismissed the Abigail Alliance lawsuit. The appeals court, in a two-to-one opinion written by Judge Judith Rogers, who was joined by Judge Douglas Ginsburg, reversed the decision. It concluded that competent, terminally ill adult patients have a constitutional "right to access to potentially life-saving post-Phase I investigational new drugs, upon a doctor's advice, even where that medicine carries risks for the patient," and remanded the case to the district court to determine whether the FDA's current policy violated that right.[3]

The Right to Life

The appeals court found that the relevant constitutional right was determined by the due-process clause of the Fifth Amendment: "no person shall be . . . deprived of life, liberty, or property without due process of law." In the court's words, the narrow question presented by *Abigail Alliance* is whether the due-process clause "protects the right of terminally ill patients to make an informed decision that may prolong life, specifically by use of potentially life-saving new drugs that the FDA has yet to approve for commercial marketing but that the FDA has determined, after Phase I clinical human trials, are safe enough for further testing on a substantial number of human beings."[3]

The court answered yes, finding that this right has deep legal roots in the right to self-defense, and that "Barring a terminally ill patient from the use of a potentially life-saving treatment impinges on this right of self-preservation."[3] In a footnote, the court restated this proposition: "The fundamental right to take action, even risky action, free from government interference, in order to save one's own life undergirds the court's decision."[3] The court relied primarily on the *Cruzan* case,[7] in which the Supreme Court recognized the right of a competent adult to refuse life-sustaining treatment, including a feeding tube:

> The logical corollary is that an individual must also be free to decide for herself whether to assume any known or unknown risks of taking a medication that might prolong her life. Like the right claimed in *Cruzan,* the right claimed by the [Abigail] Alliance to be free of FDA imposition does not involve treatment by the government or a government subsidy. Rather, much as the guardians of the comatose [sic] patient in Cruzan did, the Alliance seeks to have the government step aside by changing its policy so the individual right of self-determination is not violated.[3]

The appeals court concluded that the Supreme Court's 1979 unanimous decision on laetrile,[8] in which the Court concluded that Congress had made no exceptions in the FDA law for terminally ill cancer patients, was not relevant because laetrile had never been studied in a phase 1 trial and because the Court did not address the question of whether terminally ill cancer patients have a constitutional right to take whatever drugs their physicians prescribe.

The Dissent

Judge Thomas Griffith, the dissenting judge, argued that the suggested constitutional right simply does not exist. He noted, for example, that the self-defense cases relied on are examples of "abstract concepts of personal autonomy," and cannot be used to craft new rights. As to the nation's history and traditions, he concluded that the FDA's drug-regulatory efforts have been reasonable responses "to new risks as they are presented."[3] Accepting his argument leaves the majority resting squarely on *Cruzan* and the laetrile case. As to *Cruzan,* the dissent argued that "A tradition of protecting individual *freedom* from life-saving, but forced, medical treatment does not evidence a constitutional tradition of providing affirmative *access* to a potentially harmful, even fatal, commercial good."[3] As to the laetrile case, the judge noted simply that the Court had agreed with the FDA that, "For the terminally ill, as for anyone else, a drug is unsafe if its potential for inflicting death or physical injury is not offset by the possibility of therapeutic benefit."[3, 8]

Finally, the dissenting judge argued that if the new constitutional right were accepted, it was too vague to be applied only to terminally ill patients seeking drugs that had been tested in phase 1 trials. Specifically, the judge asked, must the right also apply to patients with "serious medical conditions," to patients who "cannot afford potentially life-saving treatment," or to patients whose physicians believe "marijuana for medicinal purposes . . . is potentially life saving?"[3] In other words, there is no principled reason to restrict the constitutional right the majority created to either terminally ill patients or to post–phase 1 drugs.

Discussion

The facts as illustrated by stories of patients dying of cancer while trying unsuccessfully to enroll in clinical trials are compelling, and our current system of ad hoc exceptions is deeply flawed. The central constitutional issue, however, rests primarily on determining whether this case is or is not like the right-to-refuse-treatment case of Nancy Cruzan, a woman in a permanent vegetative state whose family wanted tube feeding discontinued because they believed that discontinuation was what she would have wanted. I do not think *Abigail Alliance* is like *Cruzan*. Rather, it is substantially identical to cases involving physician-assisted suicide, in which a terminally ill patient claims a constitutional right of access to physician-prescribed drugs to commit suicide.

The Supreme Court has decided, unanimously, that no right to physician-prescribed drugs for suicide exists.[9, 10] There is no historical tradition of support for this right. And although the right seems to be narrowly defined, it is unclear to whom it should apply—why only to terminally ill patients? Don't patients in chronic pain have even a stronger interest in suicide? Why is the physician necessary, and why are physician-prescribed drugs the only acceptable method of suicide? None of these questions can be answered by examining the Constitution.[11]

Similarly, in *Abigail Alliance,* the new constitutional right proposed has no tradition in the United States, and it cannot be narrowly applied. For example, why should a constitutional right apply only to people who have a particular medical status? And why should a physician be involved at all? If patients have a right to autonomy, why isn't the requirement of a government-licensed physician's recommendation at least as burdensome as the requirement of the FDA's approval of the investigational drug? And why would the Constitution apply only to investigational drugs for which phase 1 trials have been completed? Why not include access to investigational medical devices, like the artificial heart, or even to Schedule I controlled substances, like marijuana or lysergic acid diethylamide (LSD)? If it is a constitutional right, these should be available too, at least unless the state can demonstrate a "compelling interest" in regulating them.

My prediction is that after rehearing this case en banc, the full Circuit Court will reject the position of the Abigail Alliance for the same reasons that the Supreme Court rejected the "right" of terminally ill patients to have access to physician-prescribed drugs they could use to end their lives.[9, 11] To decide otherwise would entirely undermine the legitimacy of the FDA. Patients in the United States have always had a right to refuse any medical treatment, but we have never had a right to demand mistreatment, inappropriate treatment, or even investigational or experimental interventions. This will not, however, be the end of the matter. After the physician-assisted–suicide cases, the fight appropriately shifted to the states, although so far only one, Oregon, has provided its physicians with immunity for prescribing life-ending drugs to their competent, terminally ill patients.[12] In the Abigail Alliance case, the debate will continue in the forum in which it began—the FDA—and in Congress.

Congress

Congressional action also had its birth with the story of one patient with cancer and was also heavily influenced by another individual patient involved in a controversy over removal of a feeding tube. "Terri's Law" was enacted in Florida in 2003 to try to prevent the removal of a feeding tube from Terri Schiavo; the case was substantially similar to *Cruzan.* Terri's case gained national attention 2 years later.[13] In the midst of it, in March 2005, the *Wall Street Journal* asserted, in an editorial titled "How About a 'Kianna's Law'?," "If Terri Schiavo deserves emergency federal intervention to save her life, people like Kianna Karnes deserve it even more."[14] At the time, Kianna Karnes was a 44-year-old mother of four who was dying of kidney cancer. Her only hope of survival, according to the editorial, was to gain access to one of two experimental drugs in clinical trials, but neither of the two companies running the trials (Bayer and Pfizer) would make the drugs available to her on a compassionate-use basis. This was because, according to the *Wall Street Journal,* the FDA "makes it all but impossible" for the manufacturers "to provide [drugs] to terminal patients on a 'compassionate use' basis."[14]

Almost immediately after the editorial was published, both drug manufacturers contacted Kianna's physicians to discuss releasing the drugs to her. But within 2 days after publication, she was dead. The *Wall Street Journal* editorialized, "Isn't it a national scandal that cancer sufferers should have to be written about in the *Wall Street Journal* to be offered legal access to emerging therapies once they've run out of other options?"[15] It noted that Mrs. Karnes' father, John Rowe—himself a survivor of leukemia—was working with the Abigail Alliance on a "Kianna's Law." That law, formally titled the "Access, Compassion, Care, and Ethics for Seriously Ill Patients Act" or the "ACCESS Act," was introduced in November 2005 and is an attempt to make it much easier for seriously ill patients to gain access to experimental drugs.[16, 17]

The act begins with a series of congressional findings, including that "Seriously ill patients have a right to access available investigational drugs, biological products, and devices." The act permits the sponsor to apply for approval to make an investigational drug, biologic product, or device available on the basis of data from a completed phase 1 trial, "preliminary evidence that the product may be effective against a serious or life-threatening condition or disease," and an assurance that the clinical trial will continue.[17] The patient, who must have exhausted all approved treatments, must provide written informed consent and must also sign "a written waiver of the right to sue the manufacturer or sponsor of the drug, biological product, or device, or the physicians who prescribed the product or the institution where it was administered, for an adverse event caused by the product, which shall be binding in every State and Federal court."[17]

Although Congress is the proper forum to address this issue, this initial attempt has some of the same problems as the *Abigail Alliance* decision: the patients to whom it applies are ambiguously classified, and clinical research seems to be equated with clinical care. Also troubling is that the patients (and would-be subjects) are asked to assume all of the risks of the uncontrolled experiments, and current rules of research—which protect subjects by prohibiting mandatory waivers of rights—are jettisoned, with the requirement of such waivers becoming the price of obtaining the investigational agent from an otherwise reluctant drug company.

FDA Proposal

In direct response to *Abigail Alliance,* the FDA proposed amending its rules to encourage more drug companies to offer their investigational drugs through compassionate-use programs.[4] These programs first came into prominence during the early days of infection with the human immunodeficiency virus (HIV) and AIDS, when there were no effective treatments and AIDS activists insisted that they have early access to investigational drugs because, in the words of their inaccurate slogan, "A Research Trial Is Treatment Too."[18] Because the FDA could not stand the political pressure generated by the activists, the compassionate-use program was developed as a kind of political safety valve to provide enough exceptions to save their basic research rules. In early December 2006, the FDA continued this political-safety-valve approach by issuing new proposed regulations with a title that could have been taken directly from the AIDS Coalition to Unleash Power (ACT-UP): "Expanded Access to Investigational Drugs for Treatment Use."[19]

The FDA's expanded-access proposal applies to "seriously ill patients when there is no comparable or satisfactory alternative therapy to diagnose, monitor, or treat the patient's disease or condition."[4] Manufacturers are required to file an "expanded access submission," and the product must be administered or dispensed by a licensed physician who will be considered an "investigator," with all the reporting requirements that role entails.[3]

Whether or not the proposal is adopted, it will do little to increase access, since the major bottleneck in the compassionate-use program has never been the FDA. The manufacturers have no incentives to make their investigational products available outside clinical trials. This is because direct access to investigational drugs by individuals may make it more difficult to recruit research subjects, and thus to conduct the clinical trials necessary for drug approval, and could also subject the drug manufacturer to liability for serious adverse reactions. Even without a lawsuit, a serious reaction to a drug outside a trial could adversely affect the trial itself.[4, 16, 20] The drug companies are right to worry that the approaches of the judiciary, Congress, and the FDA will probably make clinical trials more difficult to conduct, because few seriously ill patients who have exhausted conventional treatments would rather be randomly assigned to an investigational drug than have a guarantee that they will receive the investigational drug their physician recommends for them. This could result in significant delays in the approval and overall availability of drugs that demonstrate effectiveness—a result no one favors. Even if patients with cancer are willing buyers, drug manufacturers are not willing sellers.

Physicians and Patients

The cover story for all the proposed changes is patients' choice. But without scientific evidence of the risks and benefits of a drug, choice cannot be informed, and for seriously ill patients, fear of death will predictably overcome fear of unknown risks. This is understandable. As psychiatrist Jay Katz, the leading scholar on informed consent, has noted, when medical science seems impotent to fight nature, "all kinds of senseless interventions are tried in an unconscious effort to cure the incurable magically through a 'wonder drug,' a novel surgical procedure, or a penetrating psychological interpretation."[21] Another *Wall Street Journal* article, entitled "Saying No to Penelope,"[22] illustrates the impossibility of limiting access to unproven cancer drugs to competent adults. The article tells the story of 4-year-old Penelope, who is dying from neuroblastoma that has proved resistant to all conventional treatments. Her parents seek "anything [that] has a prayer of saving her." In her father's words, "The chance of anything bringing her back from the abyss now is very low. But the only thing I know for sure is if we don't treat her, she will die." With Penelope hospitalized and in pain, her parents continue "searching Penelope's big brown eyes for clues as to how long she wants to continue to battle for life."

It is suggested that the requirement of a physician's recommendation can safeguard against "magical thinking" and help make informed consent real.[23] But as Katz has noted, although physicians (and, he could have added, drug companies) often justify such last-ditch interventions as simply being responsive to patient needs, the interventions "may turn out to be a projection of their own needs onto patients."[21]

Government and the Market

Another recurrent theme is the belief that government regulation is evil, a central tenet of the laetrile litigation of the 1970s. The court hearing *Abigail Alliance* was correct to note that laetrile never underwent a phase 1 trial, but every indication was that the drug, also known as vitamin B_{17}, was harmless, albeit also ineffective against cancer. Laetrile became a legal cause celebre in 1972, when California physician John A. Richardson was prosecuted for promoting laetrile. Richardson was a member of the John Birch Society, which quickly formed the Committee for Freedom of Choice in Cancer Therapy, with more than 100 committees nationwide.[24] It took another 7 years before the FDA prevailed in its case against laetrile before the Supreme Court.[8] The basic arguments against FDA regulation remain the same today: the FDA follows a "paternalistic public policy that prevents individuals from exercising their own judgment about risks and benefits. If the FDA must err, it should be on the side of patients' freedom to choose."[25]

Public Policy

The FDA will prevail again today, not only because there is no constitutional right of access to unapproved drugs but also because even if there were, the state has the same compelling interest in approving drugs as it has in licensing physicians. From a public policy view, the *Abigail Alliance* court, the Congress, and the FDA all seem to be suffering from the "therapeutic illusion" in which research, designed to test a hypothesis for society, is confused with treatment, administered in the best interests of individual patients.[21, 26, 27] Of course there is a continuum, and it is perfectly understandable that many patients with cancer, told that there is nothing conventional medicine can do for them, will want access to whatever is available in or outside the context of clinical trials. But this is a problem for patients, physicians, the FDA, and drug manufacturers. First, because terminally ill patients can be harmed and exploited, there are better and worse ways to die.[21, 26] Second, it is only through research, not "treatment," that cancer may become a chronic illness that is treated with a complex array of drugs, given either together or in a progression.[28, 29] The right to choose in medicine is a central right of patients, but the choices can and should be limited to reasonable medical alternatives, which themselves are based on evidence.

This is, I believe, good public policy. But it is also much easier said than done.[30] Death is feared and even dreaded in our culture, and few Americans are able to die at home, at peace, with our loved ones in attendance, without seeking the "latest new treatment." There always seems to be something new to try, and there is almost always anecdotal evidence that it could help. This is one reason that even extremely high prices do not affect demand for cancer drugs, even ones that add little or no survival time.[31, 32] When does caring for the patient demand primary attention to palliation rather than to long-shot, high-risk, investigational interventions? Coetzee's Mrs. Curren, who rejected new medical treatment for her cancer and insisted on dying at home, told her physician, whom she saw as "withdrawing" from her after giving her a terminal prognosis—"His allegiance to the living, not the dying"—"I have no illusions about my condition, doctor. It is not [experimental] care I need, just help with the pain."[1]

References

No potential conflict of interest relevant to this article was reported.

From the Department of Health Law, Bioethics, and Human Rights, Boston University School of Public Health, Boston.

1. Coetzee JM. Age of iron. London: Seeker & Warburg, 1990.
2. Patterson JT. The dread disease: cancer and modern American culture. Cambridge, MA: Harvard University Press, 1987.
3. Abigail Alliance v. Von Eschenbach, 445 F.3d 470 (DC Cir 2006). Vacated 469 F.3d 129 (DC Cir 2006).
4. Proposed rules for charging for investigational drugs and expanded access to investigational drugs for treatment use. Rockville, MD: Food and Drug Administration, 2006. (Accessed July 6, 2007, at http://www.fda.gov/cder /regulatory/applications/IND_PR.htm.)
5. Abigail Alliance v. Von Eschenbach, 429 F.3d 129 (DC Cir 2006).
6. Jacobson PD, Parmet WE. A new era of unapproved drugs: the case of Abigail Alliance v Von Eschenbach. JAMA 2007;297:205–8.
7. Cruzan v. Director, Missouri Dept. of Health, 497 U.S. 261 (1990).
8. United States v. Rutherford, 442 U.S. 544 (1979).
9. Washington v. Glucksberg, 521 U.S. 702 (1997).
10. Vacco v. Quill, 521 U.S. 793 (1997).
11. Annas GJ. The bell tolls for a constitutional right to assisted suicide. N Engl J Med 1997;337:1098–103.

12. Gonzales v. Oregon, 546 U.S. 243 (2006).

13. Annas GJ. "I want to live": medicine betrayed by ideology in the political debate over Terri Schiavo. Stetson Law Rev 2005;35:49–80.

14. How about a "Kianna's Law"? Wall Street Journal. March 24, 2005:A14.

15. Kianna's legacy. Wall Street Journal. March 29, 2005:Al4.

16. Groopman J. The right to a trial: should dying patients have access to experimental drugs? The New Yorker. December 18, 2006:40–7.

17. ACCESS Act (Access, Compassion, Care, and Ethics for Seriously Ill Patients), S. 1956, 109th Cong (2005).

18. Annas GJ. Faith (healing), hope and charity at the FDA: the politics of AIDS drug trials. Villanova Law Rev 1989;34:771–97.

19. FDA proposes rules overhaul to expand availability of experimental drugs: the agency also clarifies permissible charges to patients. Rockville, MD: Food and Drug Administration, December 11, 2006. (Accessed July 6, 2007, at http://www.fda.gov/bbs/topics/NEWS/2006/NEW01520.html.)

20. Prud'homme A. The cell game: Sam Waksal's fast money and false promises—and the fate of ImClone's cancer drug. New York: Harper Business, 2004.

21. Katz J. The silent world of doctor and patient. New Haven, CT: Yale University Press, 1984:151.

22. Anand G. Saying no to Penelope: father seeks experimental cancer drug, but a biotech firm says risk is too high. Wall Street Journal. May 1, 2007:A1.

23. Robertson J. Controversial medical treatment and the right to health care. Hastings Cent Rep 2006;36:15–20.

24. Culbert ML. Vitamin B17: Forbidden weapon against cancer. New Rochelle, NY: Arlington House, 1974.

25. Miller HI. Paternalism costs lives. Wall Street Journal. March 2, 2006:A15.

26. Annas GJ. The changing landscape of human experimentation: Nuremberg, Helsinki, and beyond. Health Matrix J Law Med 1992;2:119–40.

27. Appelbaum PS, Lidz CW. Re-evaluating the therapeutic misconception: response to Miller and Joffe. Kennedy Inst Ethics J 2006;16:367–73.

28. Nathan D. The cancer treatment revolution: how smart drugs and other therapies are renewing our hope and changing the face of medicine. New York: John Wiley, 2007.

29. Brugarolas J. Renal-cell carcinoma—molecular pathways and therapies. N Engl J Med 2007;356:185–6.

30. Callahan D. False hopes: why America's quest for perfect health is a recipe for failure. New York: Simon and Schuster, 1998.

31. Berenson A. Hope, at $4,200 a dose: why a cancer drug's cost doesn't hurt demand. New York Times. October 1, 2006:BU1.

32. Anand G. From Wall Street, a warning about cancer drug prices. Wall Street Journal. March 15, 2007:A1.

EXPLORING THE ISSUE

Should New Drugs Be Given to Patients Outside Clinical Trials?

Critical Thinking and Reflection

1. What other kinds of risk–benefit decisions does society allow individuals to make for themselves? What are some examples of risk–benefit decisions that society attempts to impose on individuals?
2. How do the examples above compare to the proposed right to make decisions about experimental drugs? How far does the right to make one's own decisions about risks extend, in your view—are there risks one could not claim a right to accept?
3. In recent years, some libertarians have called for eliminating the FDA altogether. In your view, on the basis of the YES and NO selections, would that improve or worsen access to drugs?

Is There Common Ground?

In August 2008, another case involving access to experimental treatment reached the courts. While the appeals court in the Abigail Alliance case determined that there was no constitutional right to experimental drugs, Judge William J. Martini of the United States District Court in Newark ruled that 16-year-old Jacob Gunvalson, suffering from a rare and fatal form of Duchenne muscular dystrophy, should be allowed to use an experimental drug for that condition. Jacob did not meet the criteria for a clinical trial organized by the manufacturer. Jacob's mother claimed that drug company officials had led her to believe that her son would be allowed to take part in a clinical trial, but then refused to accept him. In December 2008, the U.S. Court of Appeals reversed Judge Martini's decision and ruled that PTC therapeutics did not have to provide the experimental drug to Jacob Gunvalson.

The Access, Compassion, Care, and Ethics for Seriously Ill Patients Act, known as the Compassionate Access Act, were introduced in the Senate in 2008 and in the House in 2010. The act would require the Secretary of Health and Human Services to permit a still-experimental drug or device to be made available to sick people under certain circumstances. The law has not been passed.

An alternative approach is simply to speed the review of drugs. In 2012, the Food and Drug Administration announced that it had developed several different mechanisms to accelerate the approval of drugs and make them available to patients faster.

Additional Resources

Additional information about the Abigail Alliance's activities can be found at www.Abigail-Alliance.org. The Alliance supports the Compassionate Access Act of 2010 (H.R. 4732), introduced in March 2010, to create a new conditional approval process for drugs, biologics, and devices for seriously ill patients.

Jerome Groopman addresses the issue and its background in "The Right to a Trial: Should Dying Patients Have Access to Experimental Drugs?" *The New Yorker* (December 18, 2006). This article is available online at www.newyorker.com/archives.

See also Susan Okie, "Access before Approval—A Right to Take Experimental Drugs?" *The New England Journal of Medicine* (August 3, 2006); and Peter D. Jacobson and Wendy E. Parmet, "A New Era of Unapproved Drugs: The Case of Abigail Alliance v. Von Eschenbach," *Journal of the American Medical Association* (January 10, 2007). These articles express concerns about unregulated access to experimental drugs.

For opposing views, see Roger Pilon, "New Right to Life," *Wall Street Journal* (August 13, 2007); and A. Puckett, "The Proper Focus for FDA Regulations: Why the Fundamental Right to Self-Preservation Should Allow Terminally Ill Patients with No Treatment Options to Attempt to Save Their Lives," *SMU Law Review* (Spring 2007).

The FDA's accelerated review policies are described in "Fast Track, Accelerated Approval and Priority Review: Accelerating Availability of New Drugs for Patients with Serious Diseases," www.fda.gov/forconsumers /byaudience/forpatientadvocates/speedingaccesstoimportantnewtherapies /ucm128291.htm.

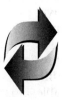

ISSUE 19

Should Vaccination for HPV Be Mandated for Teenage Girls?

YES: **R. Alta Charo**, from "Politics, Parents, and Prophylaxis—Mandating HPV Vaccination in the United States," *New England Journal of Medicine* (May 10, 2007)

NO: **Gail Javitt, Deena Berkowitz, and Lawrence O. Gostin**, from "Assessing Mandatory HPV Vaccination: Who Should Call the Shots?" *The Journal of Law, Medicine and Ethics* (Summer 2008)

Learning Outcomes

After reading this issue, you should be able to:

- Identify and discuss the ethical issues raised by public health policies that attempt to influence or compel individuals' behavior.
- Explain the public health problem posed by the human papillomavirus (HPV) and how the HPV vaccine can be used to address it.

ISSUE SUMMARY

YES: Law professor R. Alta Charo argues that vaccination against the human papillomavirus, which causes most cases of cervical cancer, should be mandatory except in cases of medical, religious, or philosophical objection.

NO: Law professors Gail Javitt and Lawrence O. Gostin and physician Deena Berkowitz believe that, given the limited data and experience, and the fact that HPV does not pose imminent and significant risk to others, mandating HPV vaccine is premature.

Human papillomavirus (HPV) is the most common sexually transmitted infection in the United States, with about 6.2 million individuals newly infected every year. Over a quarter (26.8 percent) of females aged 14–24 have an HPV infection, and among the age group 20–24, almost half (44.8 percent) are infected. There is no treatment, but the vast majority (90 percent) of the women clear the virus within 2 years.

HPV is the cause of nearly all cases of cancer of the cervix (the narrow end of the uterus, or womb), which the National Institutes of Health lists as the third most common cancer among women globally. Each year around the world, a little less than half a million new cases of cervical cancer are diagnosed, and up to 300,000 deaths from this disease are reported. Most of these cases are among young women in their child-bearing and child-rearing years. More than 80 percent of the cases occur in developing countries, and this percentage is rising. In the United States, the incidence of cervical cancer is low, but still significant; about 11,000 new cases occur every year, and about 4,000 women die of the disease. The risk of death in the United States is much lower because of the widespread use of the Papanicolaou (Pap) test, which detects cervical cancer at an early and usually treatable stage.

But for those whose infection does not go away, the consequences are serious, especially if the infection comes from the high-risk strain of HPV. The high-risk strain is present in nearly all (99 percent) of cervical cancers. If a young woman is infected with the lower-risk variation, the association with cervical cancer is relatively low.

Clearly, cervical cancer related to HPV infection in the developing world is a major public health problem. But what about the United States? The chances of becoming infected with HPV are quite high, but the chances of this infection leading to cervical cancer are relatively low.

This issue was moved from the theoretical to the real world in June 2006 when the Food and Drug Administration (FDA), which must approve the safety and effectiveness of a medication or vaccine before it is introduced to the general public, licensed a prophylactic (preventive) vaccine against four strains of HPV. The vaccine protects against 70 percent of cervical cancers linked to HPV, but not against all cancer-causing types of HPV. The vaccine was approved for females aged 9–26. Commonly known as Gardasil, its trade name, the vaccine is manufactured and marketed by Merck. In October 2009, the FDA approved a second HPV vaccine, Cervarix, which targets a different HPV strain and is manufactured by GlaxoSmithKline.

The Advisory Committee on Immunization Practices of the Centers for Disease Control and Prevention (CDC) recommends routine vaccination of 11- and 12-year-old girls with three doses of the vaccine as well as vaccination of 13- to 26-year-olds who had no opportunity to receive the vaccine when they were younger. The three-dose vaccination costs about $375, making it one of the most costly vaccines available.

The CDC's recommendations were just that—recommendations. The controversy began when Merck officials lobbied state legislatures to require the vaccine as a condition of school entry for girls entering the sixth grade. By executive order from the governor, in 2007 Texas became the first state to mandate this use of the vaccine, but the state legislature passed legislation to override the executive order and the governor did not veto it. As a result of the controversy, Merck withdrew its lobbying campaign.

The following selections explore this controversy from different perspectives. Law professor R. Alta Charo argues that states are justified in promoting HPV vaccination and even in making it mandatory unless parents object. Gail Javitt and Lawrence O. Gostin, law professors, and Deena Berkowitz, a physician, based their objections on the lack of long-term data on safety and effectiveness and on the lack of imminent risk to others posed by HPV. They believe that mandates would undermine trust in the vaccine and contribute to the widespread fear of vaccination in general.

YES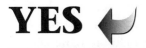

R. Alta Charo

Politics, Parents, and Prophylaxis—Mandating HPV Vaccination in the United States

Cancer prevention has fallen victim to the culture wars. Throughout the United States, state legislatures are scrambling to respond to the availability of Merck's human papillomavirus (HPV) vaccine, Gardasil, and to the likely introduction of GlaxoSmithKline's not-yet-approved HPV vaccine, Cervarix, which have been shown to be effective in preventing infection with HPV strains that cause about 70% of cases of cervical cancer. At the Centers for Disease Control and Prevention (CDC), the Advisory Committee on Immunization Practices (ACIP) has voted unanimously to recommend that girls 11 and 12 years of age receive the vaccine, and the CDC has added Gardasil to its Vaccines for Children Program, which provides free immunizations to impoverished or underserved children.

Yet despite this federal imprimatur, access to these vaccines has already become more a political than a public health question. Though the more important focus might be on the high cost of the vaccines—a cost that poses a genuine obstacle to patients, physicians, and insurers—concern has focused instead on a purported interference in family life and sexual mores. This concern has resulted in a variety of political efforts to forestall the creation of a mandated vaccination program. In Florida and Georgia, for example, efforts to increase adoption of the vaccine have been stalled by legislative maneuvering. The Democratic governor of New Mexico has announced that he will veto a bill that mandates vaccinations. And the Republican governor of Texas came under fire (and under legal attack from his own attorney general) when he issued an executive order to the same effect, mandating that all girls entering the sixth grade receive the vaccine; the policy was attacked as an intrusion on parental discretion and an invitation to teenage promiscuity. But all these measures included a parental right to opt out, whether on religious or secular grounds. The opposition seemed more about acknowledging the realities of teenage sexuality than about the privacy and autonomy of the nuclear family.

For more than a century, it has been settled law that states may require people to be vaccinated, and both federal and state court decisions have consistently upheld vaccination mandates for children, even to the extent of denying unvaccinated children access to the public schools. State

From *The New England Journal of Medicine*, vol. 356, no. 19, May 10, 2007, pp. 1905–1907. Copyright © 2007 by Massachusetts Medical Society. All rights reserved. Reprinted by permission.

requirements vary as to the range of communicable diseases but are often based on ACIP recommendations. School-based immunization requirements represent a key impetus for widespread vaccination of children and adolescents[1] and are enforceable even when they allegedly conflict with personal or religious beliefs.[2] In practice, however, these requirements usually feature exceptions that include individual medical, religious, and philosophical objections.

HPV-vaccination mandates, which are aimed more at protecting the vaccinee than at achieving herd immunity, have been attacked as an unwarranted intrusion on individual and parental rights. The constitutionality of vaccination mandates is premised on the reasonableness of the risk–benefit balance, the degree of intrusion on personal autonomy, and, most crucial, the presence of a public health necessity. On the one hand, to the extent that required HPV vaccination is an example of state paternalism rather than community protection, mandatory programs lose some of their justification. On the other hand, the parental option to refuse vaccination without interfering in the child's right to attend school alters this balance. Here the mandates act less as state imperatives and more as subtle tools to encourage vaccination. Whereas an opt-in program requires an affirmative effort by a parent, and thus misses many children whose parents forget to opt in, an opt-out approach increases vaccination rates among children whose parents have no real objection to the program while perfectly preserving parental autonomy.

Opposition to HPV vaccination represents another chapter in the history of resistance to vaccination and, on some levels, reflects a growing trend toward parental refusal of a variety of vaccines based on the (erroneous) perception that many vaccines are more risky than the diseases they prevent. In most cases, pediatricians have largely restricted themselves to educating and counseling objecting families, since it is rare that the risks posed by going unvaccinated are so substantial that refusal is tantamount to medical neglect. In the case of HPV vaccine, parents' beliefs that their children will remain abstinent (and therefore uninfected) until marriage render it even more difficult to make the case for mandating a medical form of prevention. Even with an opt-out program, critics may argue that the availability of a simple and safe alternative—that is, abstinence—undermines the argument for a state initiative that encourages vaccination through mandates coupled with an option for parental refusal.

But experience shows that abstinence-only approaches to sex education do not delay the age of sexual initiation, nor do they decrease the number of sexual encounters.[3] According to the CDC, though only 13% of American girls are sexually experienced by 15 years of age, by 17 the proportion grows to 43%, and by 19 to 70%.[4] School-based programs are crucial for reaching those at highest risk of contracting sexually transmitted diseases, and despite the relatively low rate of sexual activity before age 15, the programs need to begin with children as young as 12 years: the rates at which adolescents drop out of school begin to increase at 13 years of age,[1] and younger dropouts have been shown to be especially likely to engage in earlier or riskier sexual activity.

Another fear among those who oppose mandatory HPV vaccination is that it will have a disinhibiting effect and thus encourage sexual activity among teens who might otherwise have remained abstinent. This outcome, however, seems quite unlikely. The threat of pregnancy or even AIDS is far more immediate than the threat of cancer, but sex education and distribution of condoms have not been shown to increase sexual activity. Indeed, according to a study conducted by researchers at the University of Pennsylvania, it is the comprehensive sex-education approaches that include contraceptive training that "delay initiation of sexual intercourse, reduce frequency of sex, reduce frequency of unprotected sex, and reduce the number of sexual partners."[5] Opposition to the HPV-vaccination mandates, then, would seem to be based more on an inchoate concern: that to recognize the reality of teenage sexual activity is implicitly to endorse it.

Public health officials may have legitimate questions about the merits of HPV vaccine mandates, in light of the financial and logistic burdens these may impose on families and schools, and also may be uncertain about adverse-event rates in mass-scale programs. But given that the moral objections to requiring HPV vaccination are largely emotional, this source of resistance to mandates is difficult to justify. Since, without exception, the proposed laws permit parents to refuse to have their daughters vaccinated, the only valid objection is that parents must actively manifest such refusal. Such a slight burden on parents can hardly justify backing away from the most effective means of protecting a generation of women, and in particular, poor and disadvantaged women, from the scourge of cervical cancer. To lighten that burden even further, the governor of Virginia has proposed that refusals need not even be put in writing. Perhaps it is time for parents who object to HPV vaccinations to take a lesson from their children and heed the words of Nancy Reagan: Just say no.

References

1. Adolescent vaccination: bridging from a strong childhood foundation to a healthy adulthood. Bethesda, MD: National Foundation for Infectious Diseases, 2005....

2. Hodges J, Gostin L. School vaccination requirements: historical, social, and legal perspectives. Ky Law J 2001–2002;90:831–90.

3. Trenholm C, Devaney B, Fortson K, Quay L, Wheeler J, Clark M. Impacts of four Title V, Section 510 abstinence education programs: final report. Princeton, NJ: Mathematica Policy Research, April 2007....

4. Dailard C. Legislating against arousal: the growing divide between federal policy and teenage sexual behavior. Guttmacher Policy Rev 2006;9:12–6.

5. Bleakley A, Hennessy M, Fishbein M. Public opinion on sex education in US schools. Arch Pediatr Adolesc Med 2006;160:1151–6.

Gail Javitt, Deena Berkowitz, and Lowrence O. Gostin

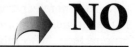 **NO**

Assessing Mandatory HPV Vaccination: Who Should Call the Shots?

Why Mandating HPV Is Premature

The approval of a vaccine against cancer-causing HPV strains is a significant public health advance. Particularly in developing countries, which lack the health care resources for routine cervical cancer screening, preventing HPV infection has the potential to save millions of lives. In the face of such a dramatic advance, opposing government-mandated HPV vaccination may seem foolhardy, if not heretical. Yet strong legal, ethical, and policy arguments underlie our position that state-mandated HPV vaccination of minor females is premature.

A. Long-Term Safety and Effectiveness of the Vaccine Is Unknown

Although the aim of clinical trials is to generate safety and effectiveness data that can be extrapolated to the general population, it is widely understood that such trials cannot reveal all possible adverse events related to a product. For this reason, post-market adverse event reporting is required for all manufacturers of FDA-approved products, and post-market surveillance (also called "phase IV studies") may be required in certain circumstances. There have been numerous examples in recent years in which unforeseen adverse reactions following product approval led manufacturers to withdraw their product from the market. . . .

In the case of HPV vaccine, short-term clinical trials in thousands of young women did not reveal serious adverse effects. However, the adverse events reported since the vaccine's approval are, at the very least, a sobering reminder that rare adverse events may surface as the vaccine is administered to millions of girls and young women. Concerns have also been raised that other carcinogenic HPV types not contained in the vaccines will replace HPV types 16 and 18 in the pathological niche.

The duration of HPV vaccine-induced immunity is unclear. The average follow-up period for Gardasil during clinical trials was 15 months after the third dose of the vaccine. Determining long-term efficacy is complicated by the fact that even during naturally occurring HPV infection, HPV antibodies

From *The Journal of Law, Medicine and Ethics*, Summer 2008, pp. 384–395 (excerpts). Copyright © 2008 by American Society of Law, Medicine & Ethics. Reprinted by permission of Wiley-Blackwell via Rightslink.

are not detected in many women. Thus, long-term, follow-up post-licensure studies cannot rely solely upon serologic measurement of HPV-induced antibody titers. . . .

The current ACIP recommendation is based on assumptions about duration of immunity and age of sexual debut, among other factors. As the vaccine is used for a longer time period, it may turn out that a different vaccine schedule is more effective. In addition, the effect on co-administration of other vaccines with regard to safety is unknown, as is the vaccines' efficacy with varying dose intervals. Some have also raised concerns about a negative impact of vaccination on cervical cancer screening programs, which are highly effective at reducing cervical cancer mortality. These unknowns must be studied as the vaccine is introduced in the broader population.

At present, therefore, questions remain about the vaccine's safety and the duration of its immunity, which call into question the wisdom of mandated vaccination. Girls receiving the vaccine face some risk of potential adverse events as well as risk that the vaccine will not be completely protective. These risks must be weighed against the state's interest in protecting the public from the harms associated with HPV. As discussed in the next section, the state's interest in protecting the public health does not support mandating HPV vaccination.

B. Historical Justifications for Mandated Vaccination Are Not Met

HPV is different in several respects from the vaccines that first led to state-mandated vaccination. Compulsory vaccination laws originated in the early 1800s and were driven by fears of the centuries-old scourge of smallpox and the advent of the vaccine developed by Edward Jenner in 1796. By the 1900s, the vast majority of states had enacted compulsory smallpox vaccination laws.[1] While such laws were not initially tied to school attendance, the coincidental rise of smallpox outbreaks, growth in the number of public schools, and compulsory school attendance laws provided a rationale for compulsory vaccination to prevent the spread of smallpox among school children as well as a means to enforce the requirement by barring unvaccinated children from school.[2] In 1827, Boston became the first city to require all children entering public school to provide evidence of vaccination.[3] Similar laws were enacted by several states during the latter half of the 19th century.[4]

The theory of herd immunity, in which the protective effect of vaccines extends beyond the vaccinated individual to others in the population, is the driving force behind mass immunization programs. Herd immunity theory proposes that, in diseases passed from person to person, it is difficult to maintain a chain of infection when large numbers of a population are immune. With the increase in number of immune individuals present in a population, the lower the likelihood that a susceptible person will come into contact with an infected individual. There is no threshold value above which herd immunity exists, but as vaccination rates increase, indirect protection also increases until the infection is eliminated. . . .

The smallpox laws of the 19th century, which were almost without exception upheld by the courts, helped lay the foundation for modern immunization statutes. Many modern-era laws were enacted in response to the transmission of measles in schools in the 1960s and 1970s. In 1977, the federal government launched the Childhood Immunization Initiative, which stressed the importance of strict enforcement of school immunization laws.[5] Currently, all states mandate vaccination as a condition for school entry, and in deciding whether to mandate vaccines, are guided by ACIP recommendations. At present, ACIP recommends vaccination for diphtheria, tetanus, and acellular pertussis (DTaP), Hepatitis B, polio, measles, mumps, and rubella (MMR), varicella (chicken pox), influenza, rotavirus, haemophilus Influenza B (HiB), pneumococcus, Hepatitis A, meningococcus, and, most recently HPV. State mandates differ; for example, whereas all states require DTaP, polio, and measles in order to enter kindergarten, most do not require Hepatitis A.[6]

HPV is different from the vaccines that have previously been mandated by the states. With the exception of tetanus, all of these vaccines fit comfortably within the "public health necessity" principle articulated in *Jacobson* [v. *Massachusetts* (1905)], in that the diseases they prevent are highly contagious and are associated with significant morbidity and mortality occurring shortly after exposure. And, while tetanus is not contagious, exposure to *Clostridium tetani* is both virtually unavoidable (particularly by children, given their propensity to both play in the dirt and get scratches), life threatening, and fully preventable only through vaccination. Thus, the public health necessity argument plausibly extends to tetanus, albeit for different reasons.

Jacobson's "reasonable relationship" principle is also clearly met by vaccine mandates for the other ACIP recommended vaccines. School-aged children are most at risk while in school because they are more likely to be in close proximity to each other in that setting. All children who attend school are equally at risk of both transmitting and contracting the diseases. Thus, a clear relationship exists between conditioning school attendance on vaccination and the avoidance of the spread of infectious disease within the school environment. Tetanus, a non-contagious disease, is somewhat different, but school-based vaccination can nevertheless be justified in that children will foreseeably be exposed within the school environment (e.g., on the playground) and, if exposed, face a high risk of mortality.

HPV vaccination, in contrast, does not satisfy these two principles. HPV infection presents no public health necessity, as that term was used in the context of *Jacobson*. While non-sexual transmission routes are theoretically possible, they have not been demonstrated. Like other sexually transmitted diseases which primarily affect adults, it is not immediately life threatening; as such, cervical cancer, if developed, will not manifest for years if not decades. Many women will never be exposed to the cancer-causing strains of HPV; indeed the prevalence of these strains in the U.S. is quite low. Furthermore, many who are exposed will not go on to develop cervical cancer. Thus, conditioning school attendance on HPV vaccination serves only to coerce compliance in the absence of a public health emergency.[7]

The relationship between the government's objective of preventing cervical cancer in women and the means used to achieve it—that is, vaccination of all girls as a condition of school attendance—lacks sufficient rationality. First, given that HPV is transmitted through sexual activity, exposure to HPV is not directly related to school attendance.[8] Second, not all children who attend school are at equal risk of exposure to or transmission of the virus. Those who abstain from sexual conduct are not at risk for transmitting or contracting HPV. Moreover, because HPV screening tests are available, the risk to those who choose to engage in sexual activity is significantly minimized. Because it is questionable how many school-aged children are actually at risk—and for those who are at risk, the risk is not linked to school attendance—there is not a sufficiently rational reason to tie mandatory vaccination to school attendance.

To be sure, the public health objective that proponents of mandatory HPV vaccination seek to achieve is compelling. Vaccinating girls before sexual debut provides an opportunity to provide protection against an adult onset disease. This opportunity is lost once sexual activity begins and exposure to HPV occurs. However, that HPV vaccination may be both medically justified and a prudent public health measure is an insufficient basis for the state to compel children to receive the vaccine as a condition of school attendance.

C. In the Absence of Historical Justification, the Government Risks Public Backlash by Mandating HPV Vaccination

Childhood vaccination rates in the United States are very high; more than half of the states report meeting the Department of Health and Human Services (HHS) Healthy People 2010 initiative's goal of ≥95 percent vaccination coverage for childhood vaccination.[9] However, from its inception, state mandated vaccination has been accompanied by a small but vocal anti-vaccination movement. Opposition has historically been "fueled by general distrust of government, a rugged sense of individualism, and concerns about the efficacy and safety of vaccines."[10] In recent years, vaccination programs also have been a "victim of their tremendous success,"[11] as dreaded diseases such as measles and polio have largely disappeared in the United States, taking with them the fear that motivated past generations. Some have noted with alarm the rise in the number of parents opting out of vaccination and of resurgence in anti-vaccination rhetoric making scientifically unsupported allegations that vaccination causes adverse events such as autism.[12]

The rash of state legislation to mandate HPV has led to significant public concern that the government is overreaching its police powers authority. As one conservative columnist has written, "[F]or the government to mandate the expensive vaccine for children would be for Big Brother to reach past the parents and into the home."[13] While some dismiss sentiments such as this one as simply motivated by right wing moral politics, trivializing these concerns is both inappropriate and unwise as a policy matter. Because sexual behavior is involved in transmission, not all children are equally at risk. Thus, it is a reasonable exercise of a parent's judgment to consider his or her child's specific risk and weigh that against the risk of vaccination.

To remove parental autonomy in this case is not warranted and also risks parental rejection of the vaccine because it is perceived as coercive. In contrast, educating the public about the value of the vaccine may be highly effective without risking public backlash. According to one poll, 61 percent of parents with daughters under 18 prefer vaccination, 72 percent would support the inclusion of information about the vaccine in school health classes, and just 45 percent agreed that the vaccine should be included as part of the vaccination routine for all children and adolescents.[14]

Additionally, Merck's aggressive role in lobbying for the passage of state laws mandating HPV has led to some skepticism about whether profit rather than public health has driven the push for state mandates.[15] Even one proponent of state-mandated HPV vaccination acknowledges that Merck "overplayed its hand" by pushing hard for legislation mandating the vaccine.[16] In the face of such criticisms, the company thus ceased its lobbying efforts but indicated it would continue to educate health officials and legislators about the vaccine.[17]

Some argue that liberal opt-out provisions will take care of the coercion and distrust issues. Whether this is true will depend in part on the reasons for which a parent may opt out and the ease of opting out. For example, a parent may not have a religious objection to vaccination in general, but nevertheless may not feel her 11-year-old daughter is at sufficient risk for HPV to warrant vaccination. This sentiment may or may not be captured in a "religious or philosophical" opt-out provision.

Even if opt-out provisions do reduce public distrust issues for HPV, however, liberal opt outs for one vaccine may have a negative impact on other vaccine programs. Currently, with the exception of those who opt out of all vaccines on religious or philosophical grounds, parents must accept all mandated vaccines because no vaccine-by-vaccine selection process exists, which leads to a high rate of vaccine coverage. Switching to an "a la carte" approach, in which parents can consider the risks and benefits of vaccines on a vaccine-by-vaccine basis, would set a dangerous precedent and may lead them to opt out of other vaccines, causing a rise in the transmission of these diseases. In contrast, an "opt in" approach to HPV vaccine would not require a change in the existing paradigm and would still likely lead to a high coverage rate.

Conclusion

Based on the current scientific evidence, vaccinating girls against HPV before they are sexually active appears to provide significant protection against cervical cancer. The vaccine thus represents a significant public health advance. Nevertheless, mandating HPV vaccination at the present time would be premature and ill-advised. The vaccine is relatively new, and long-term safety and effectiveness in the general population is unknown. Vaccination outcomes of those voluntarily vaccinated should be followed for several years before mandates are imposed. Additionally, the HPV vaccine does not represent a public health necessity of the type that has justified previous vaccine mandates. State mandates could therefore lead to a public backlash that will undermine both

HPV vaccination efforts and existing vaccination programs. Finally, the economic consequences of mandating HPV are significant and could have a negative impact on financial support for other vaccines as well as other public health programs. These consequences should be considered before HPV is mandated.

The success of childhood vaccination programs makes them a tempting target for the addition of new vaccines that, while beneficial to public health, exceed the original justifications for the development of such programs and impose new financial burdens on both the government, private physicians, and, ultimately, the public. HPV will not be the last disease that state legislatures will attempt to prevent through mandatory vaccination. Thus, legislatures and public health advocates should consider carefully the consequences of altering the current paradigm for mandatory childhood vaccination and should not mandate HPV vaccination in the absence of a new paradigm to justify such an expansion.

Note

The views expressed in this article are those of the author and do not reflect those of the Genetics and Public Policy Center or its staff.

References

1. J. G. Hodge and L. O. Gostin, "School Vaccination Requirements: Historical, Social, and Legal Perspectives," *Kentucky Law Journal* 90, no. 4 (2001–2002): 831–890.

2. J. Duffy, "School Vaccination: The Precursor to School Medical Inspection," *Journal of the History of Medicine and Allied Sciences* 33, no. 3 (1978): 344–355.

3. See Hodge and Gostin, *supra* note 1.

4. *Id.*

5. A. R. Hinman et al., "Childhood Immunization: Laws that Work," *Journal of Law, Medicine & Ethics* 30, no. 3 (2002): 122–127; K. M. Malone and A. R. Hinman, "Vaccination Mandates: The Public Health Imperative and Individual Rights," in R. A. Goodman et al., *Law in Public Health Practice* (New York: Oxford University Press, 2006).

6. Centers for Disease Control and Prevention, *Childcare and School Immunization Requirements, 2005–2006,* August 2006, *available at* <http://www.immunize.org/laws/2005-06_izrequirements.pdf> (last visited March 5, 2008).

7. B. Lo, "HPV Vaccine and Adolescents' Sexual Activity: It Would Be a Shame If Unresolved Ethical Dilemmas Hampered This Breakthrough," *BMJ* 332, no. 7550 (2006): 1106–1107.

8. R. K. Zimmerman, "Ethical Analysis of HPV Vaccine Policy Options," *Vaccine* 24, no. 22 (2006): 4812–4820.

9. C. Stanwyck et al., "Vaccination Coverage Among Children Entering School—United States, 2005–06 School Year," *JAMA* 296, no. 21 (2006): 2544–2547.

10. See Hodge and Gostin, *supra* note 1.

11. S. P. Calandrillo, "Vanishing Vaccinations: Why Are So Many Americans Opting Out of Vaccinating Their Children?" *University of Michigan Journal of Legal Reform* 37 (2004): 353–440.

12. *Id.*

13. B. Hart, "My Daughter Won't Get HPV Vaccine," *Chicago Sun Times,* February 25, 2007, at B6.

14. J. Cummings, "Seventy Percent of U.S. Adults Support Use of the Human Papillomavirus (HPV) Vaccine: Majority of Parents of Girls under 18 Would Want Daughters to Receive It," *Wall Street Journal Online* 5, no. 13 (2006). . . .

15. J. Marbella, "Sense of Rush Infects Plan to Require HPV Shots," *Baltimore Sun*, January 30, 2007. . . .

16. S. Reimer, "Readers Worry About HPV Vaccine: Doctors Say It's Safe," *Baltimore Sun*, April 3, 2007.

17. A. Pollack and S. Saul, "Lobbying for Vaccine to Be Halted," *New York Times,* February 21, 2007. . . .

EXPLORING THE ISSUE

Should Vaccination for HPV Be Mandated for Teenage Girls?

Critical Thinking and Reflection

1. How great must a vaccine's public benefit be in order to justify that the vaccine be mandated? How would you apply your thinking to other public health measures, such as campaigns to promote healthy eating or limit the consumption of sugary drinks?
2. Is an opt-out approach sufficient to ensure that individual liberty is respected? Would there be different ways of making the opt-out known and available to patients that you would find either acceptable or unacceptable?

Is There Common Ground?

As of July 2012, according to the National Conference of State Legislatures, at least 41 states and the District of Columbia have introduced legislation to require the vaccine or to fund or educate the public about the vaccine, and at least 21 states have enacted legislation.

In October 2009, Gardasil also was licensed for use in males aged 9–26 years. It works better in younger males, however, and the CDC now recommends routine vaccination of boys aged 11 or 12 years with three doses of Gardasil. On August 1, 2008, Gardasil became one of the required vaccinations for young immigrant females. A 1996 immigration law requires applicants for a green card (legal entry into the United States) have all the vaccinations recommended (not required) by the CDC. This action has been criticized by immigration advocates and even members of the original CDC panel that recommended the use of the vaccine, as well as Merck representatives. Even though only one dose is required, this adds about $120 to an already expensive list of requirements.

The trend in public policy toward greater use of HPV vaccines is occurring against a backdrop of widespread public resistance toward vaccines in general. In October 2008, the CDC announced that one in four girls aged 13–17 have been vaccinated with Gardasil since its introduction. This is a lower percentage than vaccine advocates had anticipated.

Additional Resources

J. L. Schwartz, A. L. Caplan, R. R. Faden, and J. Sugarman review the "unexpectedly early" activity in state legislatures from an ethical perspective ("Lessons from the Failure of Human Papillomavirus Vaccine State Requirements," *Clinical Pharmacological Therapy* [December 2007]).

R. I. Field and A. L. Caplan see the controversy as one between autonomy (in this case freedom from government intrusion) and beneficence, utilitarianism, and justice, all of which lend support to intervention. They would support a mandate based on utilitarianism if certain conditions are met and if "herd immunity" (protecting the community by vaccinating the few) is a realistic objective ("A Proposed Ethical Framework for Vaccine Mandates: Competing Values and the Case of HPV," *Kennedy Institute of Ethical Journal* [June 2008]).

For a complete list of state legislation from the National Conference of State Legislatures, go to www.ncsl.org/programs/health/HPVVaccine.htm.

For additional commentary on the HPV vaccine, see these articles in the May 10, 2007, issue of *The New England Journal of Medicine*: George F. Sawaya and Karen Smith-McCune, "HPV Vaccination—More Answers, More Questions"; Lindsey R. Baden, Gregory D. Curfman, Stephen Morrissey, and Jeffry M. Drazen, "Human Papillomavirus Vaccine—Opportunity and Challenge"; Jan M. Agosti and Sue J. Goldie, "Introducing HPV Vaccine in Developing Countries—Key Challenges and Issues." The scientific report that inspired these commentaries, also in this issue, is "Quadrivalent Vaccine against Human Papillomavirus to Prevent High-Grade Cervical Lesions," by The FUTURE II Study Group.

ISSUE 20

Should There Be a Market in Human Organs?

YES: **Sally Satel**, from "Kidney for Sale: Let's Legally Reward the Donor," *Globe and Mail* (March 10, 2010)

NO: **The Institute of Medicine Committee on Increasing Rates of Organ Donation**, from *Organ Donation: Opportunities for Action* (2006)

Learning Outcomes

After reading this issue, you should be able to:

- Discuss the use of markets to allocate vital scarce resources, and explain the kinds of ethical claims offered for and against using markets to solve allocation problems.
- Discuss the concept of commodification and the relevance of that concept to topics such as organ transplantation.

ISSUE SUMMARY

YES: Psychiatrist Sally Satel contends that a regulated and legal system of rewarding organ donors will not only save lives but also stop the illegal trafficking that offers no protections for poor people around the world.

NO: The Institute of Medicine Committee on Increasing Rates of Organ Donation argues that a free market in organs is problematic because in live organ donation, both buyers and sellers may not have complete or accurate information, and selling organs of dead people raises concerns about commodification of human bodies.

Human organ transplantation, unachievable at mid-twentieth century and still experimental a few decades ago, has now become routine. Dr. Joseph E. Murray of Brigham and Women's Hospital in Boston performed the first successful kidney transplant in 1954. By the 1980s, livers, hearts, pancreases, lungs, and heart–lungs had also been successfully transplanted. Surgical techniques, as well as methods for preserving and transporting organs, had improved over the years. But the most significant advance came from a single drug, cyclosporine, discovered by Jean Borel in the mid-1970s and approved by the Food and Drug Administration in 1983. Cyclosporine suppresses the immune system so that the organ recipient's body does not reject the transplanted organ. However, the drug does not suppress the body's ability to fight infection from other sources.

This achievement has its darker side in that there is a shortage of transplantable organs and many seriously ill people wait for months to receive one. Some die before one becomes available. In 2009 almost 7,000 people on waiting lists died while waiting to receive an organ. According to the United Network of Organ Sharing (UNOS), the national agency responsible for allocating organs, on October 11, 2010, 108,952 people were waiting for organs. Over 86,000 of these patients were waiting for kidney transplants, and over 16,000 for liver transplants. Heart transplants were the next highest category, with over 3,000 patients on the waiting list.

By contrast, the UNOS data show that in 2009 only 28,463 transplants were performed, with kidney-alone transplants leading the list at 16,829. Of the total transplants, 21,854 came from deceased donors, and 6609 from living donors. Living donors are almost always relatives of the recipient, although there have been several highly publicized cases in which the donor was not related. Like any surgery, transplantation presents risks to the donor but these are usually not grave. A person can live with one kidney, although should that kidney fail, the donor would require regular dialysis (cleansing the blood of toxic substances through a machine) or a transplant.

The shortage of transplantable organs in the United States is attributed to many factors: the reluctance of families to approve donation after death, even if the donor has indicated the desire to do so; the reluctance of medical personnel to approach families at a time of crisis; religious objections; and mistrust of the medical system. Despite many educational programs and publicity about donation, Americans seem unwilling either to move to a system of required request (mandated in a few states) or to presume that potential donors would agree to having their organs used for transplantation, unless they had explicitly consented in advance.

The shortage of organs is even more acute in other parts of the world, where cultural or religious objections to removing organs from the deceased remain strong. Organ transplantation is one area in which "technology transfer"—the export of the science and training for the procedure—has been particularly strong. Organ transplant centers have grown rapidly in areas of the world that lack even basic public health measures. However, although some countries have the technology for transplantation, they do not have enough organs to meet the demand.

In the United States, the National Organ Transplant Act (Public Law 98-507), passed in 1984, made it illegal to buy and sell organs. Violators are subject to fines and imprisonment. Congress passed this law because it was concerned that traffic in organs might lead to inequitable access to donor organs with the wealthy having an unfair advantage. (Even with the ban, the wealthy have an advantage in being able to pay for the transplant and the necessary post-transplant supportive services, and thus are more likely to be accepted for a waiting list.)

Although many countries and international medical organizations officially ban the sale of organs as well, the practice goes on. The YES and NO selections present opposing views on whether the ban should be reexamined or more aggressively implemented. Sally Satel, a psychiatrist and recipient of a kidney donated by a friend, maintains that the ban on selling organs is unfair and should be replaced by a legal system of rewarding donors with in-kind rewards, such as lifetime health insurance. The Institute of Medicine's Committee on Transplantable Organs argues that selling organs of either living or dead people raises serious questions about the commodification of human bodies.

YES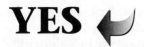

Sally Satel

Kidney for Sale: Let's Legally Reward the Donor

World Kidney Day [held every March] is part of a global health campaign meant to alert us to the impact of kidney disease. Sadly, there is little to celebrate.

According to the International Society of Nephrology, kidney disease affects more than 500 million people worldwide, or 10 per cent of the adult population. With more people developing high blood pressure and diabetes (key risks for kidney disease), the picture will only worsen.

There are nearly two million new cases of the most serious form of kidney disease—renal failure—each year. Unless patients with renal failure receive a kidney transplant or undergo dialysis—an expensive, lifelong procedure that cleanses the blood of toxins—death is guaranteed within a few weeks.

[In 2008], Australian nephrologist Gavin Carney held a press conference in Canberra to urge that people be allowed to sell their kidneys. "The current system isn't working," The Sydney Morning Herald quoted him as saying. "We've tried everything to drum up support" for organ donation, but "people just don't seem willing to give their organs away for free."

Dr. Carney wants to keep patients from purchasing kidneys on the black market and in overseas organ bazaars. As an American recipient of a kidney who was once desperate enough to consider doing that myself (fortunately, a friend ended up donating to me), I agree wholeheartedly that we should offer well-informed individuals a reward if they are willing to save a stranger's life.

If not, we will continue to face a dual tragedy: on one side, the thousands of patients who die each year for want of a kidney; on the other, a human-rights disaster in which corrupt brokers deceive indigent donors about the nature of surgery, cheat them out of payment and ignore their postsurgical needs.

The World Health Organization estimates that 5 per cent to 10 per cent of all transplants performed annually—perhaps 63,000 in all—take place in the clinical netherworlds of China, Pakistan, Egypt, Colombia and Eastern Europe.

Unfortunately, much of the world transplant establishment—including the WHO, the international Transplantation Society, and the World Medical Association—advocates only a partial remedy. They focus on ending organ trafficking but ignore the time-tested truth that trying to stamp out illicit markets either drives them further underground or causes corruption to reappear elsewhere.

For example, after China, India and Pakistan began cracking down on illicit organ markets, many patients turned to the Philippines. Last spring, after the Philippines banned the sale of kidneys to foreigners, a headline in *The Jerusalem Post* read: "Kidney transplant candidates in limbo after Philippines closes gates." (Israel has one of the lowest donation rates in the world, so the government pays for transplant surgery performed outside the country.) Similarly, patients from Qatar who travelled to Manila are "looking for alternative solutions," according to the Qatari daily *The Peninsula.*

True, more countries must develop efficient systems for posthumous donation, a very important source of organs. But even in Spain, which is famously successful at retrieving organs from the newly deceased, people die while waiting for a kidney.

The truth is that trafficking will stop only when the need for organs disappears.

Opponents allege that a legal system of exchange will inevitably replicate the sins of the black market. This is utterly backward. The remedy to this corrupt and unregulated system of exchange is a regulated and transparent regime devoted to donor protection.

My colleagues and I suggest a system in which compensation is provided by a third party (government, a charity or insurance) with public oversight. Because bidding and private buying would not be permitted, available organs would be distributed to the next in line—not just to the wealthy. Donors would be carefully screened for physical and psychological problems, as is currently done for all volunteer living kidney donors. Moreover, they would be guaranteed follow-up care for any complications.

Many people are uneasy about offering lump-sum cash payments. A solution is to provide in-kind rewards—such as a down payment on a house, a contribution to a retirement fund, or lifetime health insurance—so the program would not be attractive to people who might otherwise rush to donate on the promise of a large sum of instant cash.

The only way to stop illicit markets is to create legal ones. Indeed, there is no better justification for testing legal modes of exchange than the very depredations of the underground market.

Momentum is growing. In the *British Medical Journal,* a leading British transplant surgeon called for a controlled donor compensation program for unrelated live donors. [In 2008] the Israeli, Saudi and Indian governments have decided to offer incentives ranging from lifelong health insurance for the donor to a cash benefit. In the United States, the American Medical Association has endorsed a draft bill that would make it easier for states to offer noncash incentives for donation.

Until countries create legal means of rewarding donors, the fates of Third World donors and the patients who need their organs to survive will remain morbidly entwined. What better way to mark World Kidney Day than for global health leaders to take a bold step and urge countries to experiment with donor rewards?

The Institute of Medicine Committee on Increasing Rates of Organ Donation

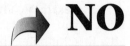 **NO**

Organ Donation: Opportunities for Action

Why a Free Market in Organs Is Problematic

Many economists begin from the position that a market is almost always the best way to allocate a scarce resource. In the standard model of a competitive market economy, markets use prices to allocate scarce resources in an automatic, decentralized fashion. In each market, the price of the good adjusts until the amount that suppliers are willing to sell at the prevailing price equals the amount that consumers are willing to pay. A higher price coaxes out more supply by making it worthwhile for producers to produce more of the good or, if the total amount of the good is fixed, by encouraging the current owners to put more of the good up for sale. On the demand side, a higher price chokes off demand, as some buyers decide that the good is not worth the new price to them.

In this model, the market outcome can be considered both efficient and equitable, provided the distribution of income and assets meets a community standard of fairness. On the demand side, price rations the good to the people who value it the most, that is, those who need it the most, where need is assessed by the people concerned rather than by a regulatory body. On the supply side, the supplier is compensated for the cost of production, including a reasonable profit, and in general, resources are directed to the most productive uses. If all markets are perfectly competitive, the resulting distribution of goods is efficient, and because it is the result of voluntary trades from a fair initial distribution of income and assets, it can be argued that it is also equitable.

On the basis of this model, permitting a market in organs could be an equitable and efficient way to achieve an increase in supply that would reduce the number of people on organ transplant waiting lists. However, this conclusion is dependent on the accuracy of the strong assumptions that underlie the theoretical model. When the assumptions do not hold, the normative arguments for the desirability of markets do not hold either. A market process might still be preferable to the available alternatives as an instrument for increasing the organ supply, but the case for it must be built, brick by brick, in light of the actual circumstances. Because the application of the market model raises different issues on the supply side and the demand side, the chapter will address them separately.

The Supply Side of an Organ Market

The market model's assumptions about supply seem most plausible for living donors. In living donation, a mentally competent adult has an organ (or organ part) that can be supplied to the market at some risk and financial cost. When the person donates the organ or organ part, that is, supplies it at a zero market price, he or she suffers a loss as a result of the discomfort of the operation, the opportunity cost of the time involved, and the long-term health risks. The donor's expectation of a benefit to the recipient is some compensation for this loss, which is why some organs are supplied at a zero price. Reducing the donor's loss by making a financial payment for the organ seems fair, however, and it seems likely that more people would be willing to provide organs as a result. In an efficient market, the additional organs would come from those who require the least financial compensation for the organ and for enduring the donation process.

In evaluating a policy of allowing payment for organs from living donors, two issues that are not assumed in the standard market model become important: distributional inequity and imperfect information. Many people would agree that large, unjust disparities in income and assets exist among Americans. Poor people value extra money more highly because they need it for basic necessities, so the additional organs are likely to come from the poor, a result many find morally troubling. A common economist's response to this concern is, "True, the distribution of income and assets is not fair. But if society cannot (or will not) do anything about it, is it fair to deprive people of an opportunity that they believe would improve their situations? Competent adults should be free to make their own decisions about the medical procedures that they will undergo and the risks that they will take."

This argument is compelling superficially, but it assumes that the organ suppliers have the information and the capacity that they need to make the decision. Information about the long-term risks of donation may not be complete, and the buyers of organs have an incentive to understate the risks. In an unregulated market, organs are likely to come from people who do not fully appreciate the risks that they are taking. Avoiding this result would require the development of complete information for potential living donors and other efforts to ensure that the decisions made by living donors are fully informed, which would require planning and substantial resources. Concerns about inadequate information arise, however, even under the gift model now in place. . . .

The living-donor case is mentioned here mainly to contrast it with the far less straightforward case of obtaining organs from deceased donors. In the latter case, the organs become available only when the person dies. There is no risk to the donor at that point, but a financial payment would not provide any direct benefit to the donor either—the benefit to the donor arises from the interest that the donor had while alive in providing for the well-being of his or her family after death. In practice, the family of the donor often makes the donation decision, and market advocates usually assume that the payment would be made to the family. Essentially, this means that the family is selling a relative's body parts, which raises the issue of cultural norms surrounding the treatment of dead bodies.

Commodification of Dead Bodies

Most societies hold that it is degrading to human dignity to view dead bodies as property that can be bought and sold. . . . [B]odies are supposed to be treated with respect—with funeral rites and burial or cremation—and not simply discarded like worn out household furniture and certainly not sold by the relatives (or anyone else) to the highest bidder. These norms are very powerful. Illicit markets for bodies have existed throughout history; for example, in the 19th century, England had an illicit market in which bodies were dug up in the night by body snatchers and sold for dissection, arguably a socially useful purpose (Richardson, 2000). Buying and selling bodies for dissection was considered a despicable business, however, and even desperately poor people did not willingly sell their relatives' bodies for whatever they could get.

Organ transplantation has provided a compelling justification for using the body parts of deceased individuals, namely, the opportunity to restore life and health to someone on the brink of death. Many people see donating a person's organs for this purpose as a highly meritorious act that honors the sacredness of the body rather than degrades it. At the same time, however, many people regard the act of donating the organs for this purpose as being conceptually and morally distinct from the act of selling the organs (even when the organs are to be used for the same purpose). Currently, the sale of solid organs is prohibited, but the prohibition reflects preexisting and widely accepted cultural norms. In the context of these norms, and the attitudes underlying them, it is not at all clear that the supply of organs from deceased donors would actually increase if sales were made legal. It is possible that the reasons people have for not donating cannot be overcome by money, or that offering money induces some to provide organs while leading an equal or greater number of people who would have provided organs to decide not to. For example, family members may wish to avoid appearing to be profiting from a deceased relative's body, especially if there is any chance of appearing to have participated in a treatment decision that might have hastened death. . . .

Barriers to a Futures Market

Traditionally, the relatives of deceased individuals had the final word about whether organs would be donated, but this has been changing. Because society supports the right of individuals to control what happens to their bodies when they are alive, it is a natural extension to assume that they should also decide what happens to their bodies after death. This adds more intricacy to the application of the market model. Because money is of no use to a corpse, for financial payments to influence the donor's decision, one must introduce a futures market or a bequest motive into the picture.

A futures market is a market in which the commodity bought and sold is the right to sell organs at a future time in the event that a person dies in circumstances that permit organs to be recovered and transplanted. The person receives payment for these contingent organ sale rights while he or she is still alive. Futures markets are inherently complex. In this case, the chances of dying in the appropriate circumstances are low, death may occur far into the future, and it may not be easy to execute the right to the organ at the appropriate moment; therefore, the right to a potential organ is not worth nearly as much as an actual organ at the time of death. What if sellers want to change their minds? Can they rescind their contracts and, if so, on what terms? Also, once the rights to an individual's organs have been sold, the buyer (who would probably be an organ broker) has a financial interest in the seller's death. Some people already worry about receiving suboptimal treatment at the end of life if they are registered organ donors and adding financial interests resulting from the selling of organ rights might add to those concerns. Further, it seems unlikely that there would be enough interested investors to allow a private futures market in organ rights to develop, given the long time horizon required and the uncertainty about the size of the profits.

Alternatively, one can assume that people get satisfaction in life from the knowledge that their heirs will receive inheritances when they die. If this is so, a person could be allowed to spell out his or her wishes for the disposition of his or her body in advance (in a will or in a special organ donor registry) stating whether his or her body should be buried or cremated intact, donated all or in part to a specific organization for a specific purpose, or sold whole or in part with the proceeds forming part of the estate. To the extent that more people would agree to organ removal if they had this option, the supply of organs would increase. This is an empirical question, and as before, there is no certainty of a positive effect. Again, implementation would be complex. For example, a registry would be better than a will, because one cannot wait until the will is probated to determine whether the organs can be sold. . . .

Other Complexities

It has been assumed thus far in the discussion that paying people or their families for organs would increase the supply of organs for transplantation. However, some other complexities of the organ procurement process suggest that the creation of financial incentives for organ donation may be less important for donors and their families than it is for healthcare organizations and the participating healthcare professionals. A family does not simply make the decision to donate (or to honor the decedent's wish to donate) and then it happens automatically. First, the potential donor must be in the process of dying under the right circumstances to be eligible to donate his or her organs. Second, the medical staff must make the family aware of the possibility of organ donation. Only then does the opportunity to say yes or no to donation arise. Many people have not thought much about organ donation before the issue arises, and in any case, they are in an extremely stressful situation. How and when they are told about the opportunity for organ donation and the way in which the request is made can make a significant difference to the relatives' response. Finally, the organs must be removed, the recipients must be identified, and the organs must be transported to their final destinations. These are complex tasks that must be carried out under extreme time pressure.

Many factors—including the structure of financial incentives to the healthcare workers and organizations that carry out these organ transplant-related activities—influence the way in which the process of notification, request, removal, and conveyance to a recipient occurs. If this process is the problem, the introduction of financial payments for organs may simply raise the cost of the transplantation process without having any effect on the number of organs recovered. The efforts and successes of the Organ Donation Breakthrough Collaboratives of the Health Resources and Services Administration suggest that the process is part of the problem and, indeed, is perhaps most of it. . . . The collaboratives have demonstrated that the application of quality improvement methods to the steps in this process can significantly increase the percentage of potential organ donations that are converted into actual donations. There is also potential to increase the organ supply through medical practice changes that make more decedents medically eligible to be organ donors . . . , that is, to give more people the opportunity to consent.

The Demand Side of an Organ Market

The demand side of an organ market is also complicated. The simple market model assumes that those who benefit from the use of the good pay for the good, and this is an important element in the normative theory in favor of markets. In the case of organs, advocates for payments for organs from deceased donors generally do not expect the recipients to make the payments. Most people believe that health care is a special kind of commodity that should not be allocated strictly according to an ability to pay because of the unusual importance of health care to the well-being of all people and the uneven distribution of illness among the population. The distribution of health care, especially life-saving health care, should be determined separately from the distribution of other goods and in accord with special ethical principles. This is a major departure from the standard market model and means that even if a fair distribution of income and assets could be arranged, letting health care be determined by voluntary market trades would not yield equitable outcomes, even under the highly unrealistic assumption of the existence of a perfectly competitive market.

In the United States, the result of this societal value judgment is a complex array of private and public policies that are implicitly or explicitly intended to provide people with care that they would not receive if all health care were distributed through unregulated private markets. Unfortunately, there is no general, transparent consensus on the nature and extent of healthcare services that people should be able to receive without regard to the ability to pay and how the cost of that care should be distributed across the population. The unfortunate result is a financing system that distributes both care and cost arbitrarily in a manner that meets no rational standard of efficiency or equity.

The U.S. healthcare system does not guarantee access to life-saving treatments such as organ transplantations, and the ability to pay does play a role in the distribution of this important good. Few people pay directly for organ transplantation, which is expensive even without payment for the organs.

People in need of organs rely on public or private insurance to pay the cost of acquiring the organs and transplanting them, and a transplant is not received unless insurance coverage or access to charity care is available (the so-called green screen).

Given this system of healthcare financing (or any system that might replace it), what would the demand side of a market for organs look like? Presumably, most of the actual buyers would be the healthcare organizations that perform transplantations. They would compete with one another for the available organs, the price would settle down at the market-clearing price, and the cost of organs would become part of the total charge to a third-party payer for an organ transplant. This market would inevitably be very complex.

So far the chapter has referred to "the price" of an organ, but an actual market would have multiple prices for organs because organs are highly differentiated products. For example, hearts differ from kidneys and kidneys differ from one another along many medically significant dimensions. Organ recipients also differ from one another, and matching an organ with the right recipient is important in achieving the benefits of transplantation. This means that the kidney market or the heart market would actually be a whole set of interconnected markets for goods that are close substitutes for each other (e.g., kidneys or hearts from people of different ages, with different blood types, or different human leukocyte antigen factors). The price of a kidney would therefore actually be a price structure for all the different kinds of kidneys. This price structure would result from the interaction of the array of kidneys available with the variety of patients in need of a kidney at any point in time and the trade-offs among kidney characteristics that are medically possible for transplantation into various patients.

Of course, the original suppliers and the end users of the organs do not have the medical knowledge to make sophisticated sales and purchase decisions, and even if they did, they are hardly in the best physical condition to apply their knowledge at the time of donation or transplantation. Like the rest of the healthcare market, this market would be characterized by complicated agency relationships (situations in which decisions are made by an expert on someone else's behalf). The various potential agents here would include the transplant recipient's physician, the organ donor's physician, the healthcare organizations in which the organ recovery and the transplantation occur, a specialized organ "broker" such as the United Network for Organ Sharing (UNOS), the private and public third-party payers that pay for the transplantation-related care, and so on.

Real-world markets in which differentiated products are sold under circumstances of imperfect information and intricate agency relationships do exist, and such markets can be superior to other methods of allocation. In the case of organs, however, it is interesting to note that a nonmarket process for allocating organs to recipients and managing waiting lists has been in place since the beginning of the transplantation era. The Organ Procurement and Transplantation Network system grew up in response to a perceived need to manage the organ allocation process within the transplantation community, although it has come to have substantial government involvement. There is ongoing pressure to adjust the process to make it more efficient and equitable, with the usual difficulties in defining exactly what efficiency and equity mean in such a complicated context. There is also recognition that financial and other incentives should be aligned with ultimate goals, but little enthusiasm for relying completely on an unregulated market process exists.

In summary, in a hypothesized market for organs, the good to be sold is highly differentiated and must be matched to the final user in many ways. The process of making an organ available requires skilled labor and technology. The good is highly perishable, and recovery and transfer to the final user must be accomplished under extreme time pressure. The good has unique cultural significance that would powerfully influence the response of suppliers to market incentives, even in the absence of the existing legal constraints on their behavior. Imperfect information issues are significant, and the end user is not in a position to act as an informed buyer. The need for information, skilled labor and technology, and third-party payment means that the market transactions involve complex agency relationships. With all of these departures from the standard assumptions of the market model, organ transplantation occurs in a world of imperfect markets when it comes to evaluating efficiency. A perfectly functioning market and a fair distribution of income and assets would not likely produce equity in the current healthcare system. As a society, it is not clear what an equitable distribution of health care and its cost would look like, but it is generally agreed that the distribution of organ transplants should not be totally determined by the ability to pay.

Given all of these factors, the committee doubts that it would even be possible to have a well-functioning free market in organs from deceased donors. If such a market existed, there is no certainty that it would produce a greater supply of organs. Moreover, a free market in organs would deviate substantially from prevailing norms in the United States regarding the nature of health care and the fair distribution of organs for transplantation, norms that have been developed within various communities of stakeholders and that are now well entrenched.

EXPLORING THE ISSUE

Should There Be a Market in Human Organs?

Critical Thinking and Reflection

1. Is the idea of treating human organs or bodies as commodities morally troubling to you? Are there some things that simply should not be bought or sold? If so, how do organs compare to them?
2. Do you think that the opportunity to sell a loved one's organ would generate an incentive for you to offer it for transplantation?
3. The Institute of Medicine committee argues that a market for organs would not function well. Explain and evaluate the committee's thinking.
4. Satel argues that a market for organs could be set up in such a way that organs would not go disproportionately to the rich: Are you persuaded that this would be possible? Do you agree that it would be problem?

Is There Common Ground?

Most scholars in the United States still hold that much can be done to improve the current organ donation system and that these measures should be tried before financial incentives or sales are permitted. These measures include continually refining the process of asking families of potential donors whether they would like to have their loved one's organs donated and improving the system by which organs are allocated to potential recipients.

A particularly controversial aspect of the allocation of transplantable organs in the United States is whether the organs should be allocated nationally or locally. The Department of Health and Human Services (DHHS) proposed in March 1998 that current geographic disparities in the allocation of scarce organs should be addressed by creating national uniform criteria for determining a patient's medical status and eligibility for placement on a waiting list. Under the current system, local centers have first chance at organs in their region, even though patients in other areas may have greater medical need or have been on the waiting list longer.

The proposal was received enthusiastically by the large transplant centers, which attract the most ill and most affluent recipients, who can travel to the center and remain for months. However, it was criticized by smaller transplant centers, which rely on local recipients and the value of being able to tell potential donors or their families that the organs will be given to a local resident. Congress asked the Institute of Medicine to study the impact of the rule. The IOM's report, issued in July 1999, titled "Organ Procurement and Transplantation: Assessing Current Policies and the Potential Impact of the DHHS Final Rule," agreed that organs should be allocated on the basis of medical need across wider geographical areas.

Additional Resources

The various reports on transplantation issued by the Institute of Medicine are available at www.nap.edu.

In *When Altruism Isn't Enough: The Case for Compensating Kidney Donors* (2009), Sally Satel and other authors expand the argument for abandoning the current ban on sale of organs.

Steve Farber, who received a kidney donated by his son, and Harlan Abraham describe their experience as well as another patient's in *On the List: Fixing America's Failing Organ Transplant System* (2009).

An approach that combines monetary compensation with donation is described in "Compensated Kidney Donation: An Ethical Review of the Iranian Model" by Alireza Bagheri (*Kennedy Institute of Ethics Journal* [vol. 16, no. 3, 2006]). In this program, donors receive compensation for their time taken from work, travel, and other expenses. While supporting this concept, the author warns that it does not have secure enough measures to prevent a direct monetary relationship between donors and recipients.

As alternatives to paid organ donations, Francis Delmonico and colleagues proposed donor medals of honor, reimbursement for funeral expenses, organ exchanges, medical leaves for organ donation, and other mechanisms, in "Ethical Incentives—Not Payment—for Organ Donation," *The New England Journal of Medicine* (June 20, 2002).

From a United Kingdom perspective, Charles Erin and John Harris have proposed an "ethical market" in organs. In their proposal, the market would be confined to a specific area, and only citizens from that area could buy and sell organs. One purchaser, probably a government agency, would buy all organs and distribute them according to some order of medical priority. Individuals would not be allowed to enter the market directly. See "An Ethical Market in Human Organs," *British Medical Journal* (July 20, 2002).

In the fall 2004 issue of the *American Journal of Bioethics,* David Steinberg proposes a new method for allocating organs for transplantation ("An 'Opting In' Paradigm for Kidney Transplantation"). His proposal would reward people who agree to donate their kidneys after they die by giving them preferences for a kidney should they need one while alive. Twenty-one commentaries follow the article.

UNOS policies prohibit designating donated organs for a group—that is, limiting a donation to patients who are white, black, Catholic, male, or any other category. In "Members First: The Ethics of Donating Organs and Tissues to Groups," Timothy F. Murphy and Robert M. Veatch raise questions about the implications of the activities of LifeSharers, a voluntary organization whose members agree that their organs will be donated first to other members (*Cambridge Quarterly of Healthcare Ethics* [vol. 15, 2006]). In the same issue, Barbro Bjorkman argues against selling of organs and calls instead for a "virtue ethics" approach in his article, "Why We Are Not Allowed to Sell That Which We Are Encouraged to Donate."

Contributors to This Volume

EDITOR

GREGORY E. KAEBNICK is a scholar at The Hastings Center and, since 2001, editor of the *Hastings Center Report*. He is currently leading the research project at Hastings titled "The Ethics of Synthetic Biology: An Examination of Four Case Studies" and participating in a project on the use of animals in research. Past Center research projects in which he has participated include work on the human relationship to nature, genetic paternity testing, agricultural biotechnology, end-of-life care, and behavioral genetics. He is the editor of *The Ideal of Nature: Debates about Biotechnology and the Environment* (Johns Hopkins, 2011), co-editor with Lori Knowles of *Shaping Our Future: Law, Policy, and Ethics in an Era of Reproductive Genetics* (Johns Hopkins Press, 2007), and co-editor with Mark O. Rothstein, Thomas H. Murray, and Mary Anderlik Majumder of *Genetic Ties and the Family: The Impact of Paternity Testing on Parents and Children* (Johns Hopkins Press, 2005). He received his PhD (1998) and MS (1994) in philosophy from the University of Minnesota and his BA in religion from Swarthmore College (1986).

AUTHORS

MARCIA ANGELL is a senior lecturer in the department of social medicine at Harvard Medical School and the former editor-in-chief of *The New England Journal of Medicine*.

GEORGE J. ANNAS is the Edward R. Utley Professor of Health Law and chairman of the Health Law Department at the Boston University School of Public Health in Boston, Massachusetts. He is also the cofounder of Global Lawyers & Physicians and the Patients' Rights Project.

ROBERT M. ARNOLD is the director of the Palliative Care Service at the University of Pittsburgh's Medical Center.

MARGARET P. BATTIN is the distinguished professor of philosophy and adjunct professor of internal medicine, Division of Medical Ethics, at the University of Utah, Salt Lake City.

KEN BAUM is a physician and attorney at the firm of Wiggin and Dana, New Haven, Connecticut.

MARK A. BEDAU teaches philosophy at Reed College, Portland, OR.

DEENA BERKOWITZ is an assistant professor of pediatrics at Georgetown University School of Medicine and Health Sciences in Washington, DC.

LILES BURKE is a justice on the Alabama Court of Criminal Appeals.

MICHAEL F. CANNON is the director of health policy studies at the Cato Institute, Washington, DC.

JULIE CANTOR is an attorney at Yale University School of Medicine.

R. ALTA CHARO is the Warren P. Knowles Professor of Law and Bioethics at the University of Wisconsin at Madison.

MEGAN CLAYTON is a research associate at the Oxford Centre for Applied Ethics, Oxford University, England.

KAREN DAVENPORT is the director of health policy at the National Women's Law Center, Washington, DC. Before joining NWLC, she worked as a research project director in the George Washington University's Department of Health Policy and as director of health policy at the Center for American Progress.

JAMES DWYER is a faculty member at the Center for Bioethics and Humanities, SUNY Upstate Medical University, Syracuse, New York.

ANGELA FAGERLIN is an experimental psychologist and member of the Center for Bioethics and Social Sciences in Medicine at the University of Michigan Health System, Ann Arbor, Michigan.

BENNETT FODDY is a research associate at the Oxford Centre for Applied Ethics, Oxford University, England.

KATHLEEN M. FOLEY holds The Society of Memorial Sloan-Kettering Cancer Center chair in pain research. She is a professor of neurology and pharmacology at the Weill Medical College of Cornell University and attending neurologist in the Pain and Palliative Care Service at Memorial Sloan-Kettering, New York City.

EMIL J. FREIREICH is a professor of special medical education at the MD Anderson Cancer Center, Houston, Texas.

ATUL GAWANDE practices general and endocrine surgery at Brigham and Women's Hospital in Boston. He is also a professor of surgery at Harvard Medical School and a professor in the Department of Health Policy and Management at the Harvard School of Public Health.

ROBERT P. GEORGE is McCormick Professor of Jurisprudence at Princeton University and the director of the James Madison Program in American Ideals and Institutions.

LAWRENCE O. GOSTIN is a professor of law at Georgetown University, a professor of public health at the Johns Hopkins University, and the director of the Center for Law and the Public's Health at Johns Hopkins and George Town universities.

BERNARD J. HAMMES is the director of medical humanities at Gundersen Lutheran Medical Foundation and Medical Center, LaCrosse, Wisconsin.

DONALD W. HERBE is an attorney in Cleveland, Ohio.

SUSAN E. HICKMAN is an associate professor, Department of Environments for Health, Indiana University School of Nursing, Indianapolis.

GAIL JAVITT is the law and policy director at the Genetics and Public Policy Center in Washington, DC. She is also a research scientist at the Berman Institute of Bioethics at Johns Hopkins University in Baltimore, Maryland.

TOM KOCH is the director of Information Outreach, Ltd., based in Vancouver, BC, where he conducts research on issues in bioethics and journalism.

PATRICK LEE is an associate professor of philosophy at the Franciscan University in Steubenville, Ohio. He is the author of *Abortion and Unborn Life* (1996).

CHARLES W. LIDZ is a professor of psychiatry at the University of Pittsburgh. Currently, he is on leave from the University of Pittsburgh and works at the University of Massachusetts Medical School, where he is the director of the Center for Mental Health Services Research.

MARGARET OLIVIA LITTLE is a philosopher at the Kennedy Institute of Ethics, Georgetown University. Her research interests focus on the intersection of ethics, feminist theory, and public policy.

ALVIN H. MOSS is a professor of medicine and the director of the Center for Health Ethics and Law at the Robert C. Byrd Health Sciences Center of West Virginia University, Morgantown, West Virginia.

THOMAS H. MURRAY is the president emeritus and senior research scholar at The Hastings Center in Garrison, New York.

RICARDO NUILA is a staff member of the Department of Medicine, Department of Family and Community Medicine, Baylor College of Medicine, Houston, Texas.

ONORA O'NEILL is a professor of philosophy at the University of Cambridge, England.

DAVID ORENTLICHER is Samuel R. Rosen Professor of Law and codirector of the William S. and Christine S. Hall Center for Law and Health at Indiana University Robert H. McKinney School of Law.

LYNN M. PALTROW is an attorney and executive director of National Advocates for Pregnant Women, New York, New York.

CHARLES PETERS is an associate professor of clinical pediatrics in the division of hematology–oncology and blood and marrow transplantation at the University of Minnesota Medical School in Minneapolis, Minnesota.

CHRISTOPHER J. PRESTON is an environmental ethicist at the University of Montana Missoula, MT.

RAJEEV RAGHAVAN is a staff member of the Department of Medicine, Division of Nephrology, Baylor College of Medicine, Houston, Texas.

JOHN A. ROBERTSON is the Vinson and Elkins Chair at The University of Texas School of Law at Austin.

LAINIE FRIEDMAN ROSS is an assistant professor of pediatrics in the McLean Center for Clinical Medical Ethics, Department of Medicine, at the University of Chicago in Chicago, IL. She is also the director of the Ethics Case Consultation Service and codirector of the Multidisciplinary Ethics Lecture Series at the university.

SALLY SATEL is a psychiatrist and lecturer at the Yale University School of Medicine. She is a resident scholar at the American Enterprise Institute in Washington, DC.

TERESA A. SAVAGE is the associate director, Donnelley Family Disability Ethics Program, Rehabilitation Institute of Chicago, and the assistant professor—research, Department of Maternal-Child Nursing, University of Illinois at Chicago College of Nursing.

JULIAN SAVULESCU is the Uehiro Professor of Practical Ethics, Oxford University, and the director of the Oxford Uehiro Centre for Practical Ethics.

CARL E. SCHNEIDER is the Chauncey Stillman Professor for Ethics, Morality, and the Practice of Law at the University of Michigan Law School, Ann Arbor, Michigan. He is also a professor of internal medicine at the medical school.

SARAH E. SHANNON is an associate professor, biobehavioral nursing and health systems, University of Washington, Seattle.

SUSAN W. TOLLE is a professor of general internal medicine and geriatrics at Oregon Health & Science University and the cofounder and director of the University's Center for Ethics in Health Care, Portland, Oregon.

HOWARD TRACHTMAN is a physician at Schneider Children's Hospital, New Hyde Park, New York.

DAVID WAISEL is an associate professor of anesthesia at Children's Hospital Boston.

ROBERT F. WEIR is the director of the Program in Biomedical Ethics and Medical Humanities in the College of Medicine at the University of Iowa. A professor of pediatrics, he is also on the faculty of the university's School of Religion.

JAY WOLFSON is the distinguished service professor of public health and medicine, associate vice president for health law, policy and safety at the University of South Florida. In October 2003, he was appointed to serve as the special guardian ad litem for Theresa Marie Schiavo, reporting to the Florida governor and the courts.